# A NATION
*to*
# PROTECT

# A NATION
— to —
# PROTECT
## LEADING INDIA THROUGH THE COVID CRISIS

## PRIYAM GANDHI-MODY

Published by
Rupa Publications India Pvt. Ltd 2022
7/16, Ansari Road, Daryaganj
New Delhi 110002

*Sales Centres:*
Allahabad Bengaluru Chennai
Hyderabad Jaipur Kathmandu
Kolkata Mumbai

Copyright © Priyam Gandhi-Mody 2022

Copyright of photographs vests with the respective photographer/organization

While every effort has been made to trace copyright holders and obtain permission, this has not been possible in all cases; any omissions brought to our attention will be remedied in future editions.

The views and opinions expressed in this book are the author's own and the facts are as reported by her which have been verified to the extent possible, and the publishers are not in any way liable for the same.

All rights reserved.
No part of this publication may be reproduced, transmitted, or stored in a retrieval system, in any form or by any means, electronic, mechanical, photocopying, recording or otherwise, without the prior permission of the publisher.

ISBN: 978-93-5520-355-7

Third impression 2022

10 9 8 7 6 5 4 3

The moral right of the author has been asserted.

Printed in India

This book is sold subject to the condition that it shall not, by way of trade or otherwise, be lent, resold, hired out, or otherwise circulated, without the publisher's prior consent, in any form of binding or cover other than that in which it is published.

*To माँ (ma), for without your शक्ति (shakti),
I am powerless, directionless, lifeless*

∾

# CONTENTS

*Introduction* ix

## SECTION 1: FIRST WAVE

1. Advent of COVID-19 — 3
2. India Prepares — 16
3. The Virus Strikes — 22
4. First Responses — 31
5. Junta Curfew — 38
6. Empowered Teams — 52
7. Lockdown — 64
8. Migrants' Distress — 81
9. Plan to Unlock — 90
10. Economic Response — 100
11. Achieving Atmanirbharta — 112
12. Eye of the Storm — 123
13. Vaccine Development — 132
14. Economic Stimulus — 142

## SECTION 2: SECOND WAVE

15. Farmers Protest and the Virus Mutates — 155
16. The World's Largest Vaccination Drive — 165
17. The Second Wave and Kumbha Mela — 179
18. Oxygen Crisis — 195
19. Media Campaign and Role of the Opposition — 222
20. India's Role in Securing the World — 245

*Acknowledgements* 262
*Notes* 263
*Index* 309

# INTRODUCTION

The years 2020 and 2021 have been traumatic for the world as it battled a raging global pandemic brought upon by the novel coronavirus, called the severe acute respiratory syndrome coronavirus (SARS-CoV-2), which causes the disease we now identify as COVID-19. It has been even more agonizing for the bereaved families who lost their loved ones, the brave frontline warriors, healthcare professionals and countries whose health systems collapsed under the sheer numbers and speed at which their citizens were impacted by the unrelenting virus. India, home to 18 per cent of the world's population, had to cope with three particularly strong waves of the virus: the first, from April to November 2020, the second, more ferocious one, between March and June 2021 and the third, which started in January 2022. When the first wave hit us, we braced ourselves having witnessed the devastation already caused by the virus in other countries, despite superior healthcare infrastructure. Doomsday predictions of starvation and mass deaths took over the global media with the inherent assumption that if western nations were unable to rein in the virus, then India, with its weak socio-economic and healthcare infrastructure, didn't even stand a fighting chance.

As the pandemic progressed, Indians united and fought the virus with great tenacity in the face of profound adversity. With timely lockdowns, disciplined mask usage, quick medical infrastructure upgrades, widespread adaptation of digital technologies, science-based regulations and vaccine adoption, we emerged with much lesser damage than many large, developed nations of the world. Hovering at an average of 1.11 per cent through the pandemic, India's fatality has been the lowest in the world, leaving sceptics astounded. Despite totally shutting down our economy for a limited period of time during the initial days of the pandemic, India has managed to get it back on track with sound, strategic regulatory responses. We have also been the quickest country to administer over 1.6 billion vaccine doses in a matter of less than a year flabbergasting critics who predicted that India would take at least a decade to vaccinate its entire population.

However, at such a time when bets were low on India's ability to survive the pandemic and rampant fear spread unchecked in civil society, one man never lost confidence in our capability to fight the virus and overcome the dark times—the prime minister of India, Narendra Modi. As a once-in-a-century pandemic dawned on us, on his shoulders lay the responsibility of protecting the lives of one-sixth of the world's population, and the broader duty of delivering timely, life-saving, affordable drugs and vaccines to the rest of the world. Many sections of the media greatly attempted to divide the country through the pandemic, successfully creating an environment of extreme partisanship and discord. When societal unison and collective response of the people were paramount in defeating the virus, uniting and securing a dichotomous, vulnerable society became an added challenge for the prime minister. A great part of the public discourse was fissured, with his admirers defending the Indian government's response as against those who seemed perpetually dissatisfied with the establishment. However, in this commotion, as I keenly followed the emerging stories, I was shocked to see how superficial this discourse remained. The gatekeepers of information never really got to the bottom of why India managed to positively surprise the world in its pandemic response. I believe, many others, like me, would like to know the story of how India managed to turn the COVID-19 tide into an opportunity for growth. As you will see through this book, the information that I have put out is based on facts, references and hard data presented in a competitive format with the global response situation. As I inched towards completing the book, my takeaway was clear: we are now in the age of a New India, which is stronger, unflinching in its resolve to grow and undeterred by crises. We are no longer discovering our place in the world, but are confident in our contribution towards humanity and the globe.

This vision was truly ushered in by Prime Minister Modi, from the time he took office in 2014. In simple words, it wouldn't be an overture to say that the reason why India's response to COVID-19 was appropriate, adequate and largely effective was because of the culmination of initiatives that the prime minister introduced from the beginning of his first term up until the pandemic. The bureaucracy and the citizens together responded enthusiastically to his every call. Each time he showed vulnerability, seeking help from society and officers, citizens rose to the challenge and outperformed to meet his expectations.

During the journey of the book, I spoke to several senior members of the prime minister's core COVID-19 response team which included his immediate aides as well as senior officials from the Indian government. I was able to also speak with many private folks—ranging from doctors, vaccine manufacturers to researchers and academicians—in order to accurately present the information in the book. As the end of the book drew closer, many unanswered philosophical questions remained with me mainly about what may be going through the prime minister's mind during the difficult days of the pandemic while he made crucial decisions which saved billions of lives. In an effort to understand him, I was able to sit down with him for a short tête-à-tête.

At 7, Lok Kalyan Marg, from the moment I met him, all I could see across the magnificent cobalt-blue-leather-laden, teakwood desk which separated us in his office was a determined, towering human being—replete with human emotions, just like the rest of us. It became all the more important to me to discover the man about whom I had heard so many stories from the media. Some which allude to him being authoritarian, some which say that he takes unilateral decisions and others which paint him as such an intimidating figure who people are afraid to speak in front of. From the many questions I was able to ask him, I will present here those which enabled me to see his vision more clearly than ever. I'd like for you, my readers, to discover him just the way I was able to, vicariously through my words.

At the outset, I asked him, 'Mr Prime Minister, in the darkest days of the pandemic, when there was no hope for India, what kind of pressure did you feel knowing that saving 138 crore lives depended on your decisions?'

'Look,' he said. 'Ever since I took office, it has been my resolve to identify and fix the weaknesses in the way the Indian government functions. Let me give you an example. The biggest weakness of the Indian bureaucracy is that it is an assembled unit, not an organic unit. What this means is that our officers come from various parts of the country, spend years in service in various states, get promoted and finally make it to senior levels of leadership in departments at the Centre. How this plays out is that coordination and camaraderie between officers at senior levels in various departments doesn't come naturally. So, when I took office very early on, I realized that I needed to change the culture of bureaucracy to make it *life-sensitive* versus *file-sensitive*, which had been the case since our Independence. I proactively took several initiatives to form small groups of senior officers, assign them common goals to work on and spent a lot of time with them. Eventually, the officers began to understand what my expectations were from them and began to respond to my calls much more efficiently as a unit. So, when the pandemic struck, I was confident in the ability of my government and the officers to rise to the challenge before us. Now let me give you another example. Look at the way we have adopted digitization. Many nations struggled with getting COVID-19 relief monies to the final beneficiaries either due to political reasons or because their systems weren't equipped to connect the government to the beneficiaries. But thanks to our wholehearted adoption of direct benefit transfers, we were able to promptly and quickly credit funds into the accounts of our most vulnerable folks. To reiterate, I have never been one to feel pressure. However, I do firmly believe in preparation and it is this very preparation that helped us face the crisis.'

I asked further, 'You are the first Indian prime minister to face the Herculean challenge of such a once-in-a-lifetime pandemic. How did you retain your optimism in India and what motivated you during those difficult days?'

He replied naturally, without even thinking about the answer, 'As you may know, only recently I completed two decades of experience in public service. Twenty years ago, my public career began with a crisis in the form of an earthquake in Kutch. So, leading through crises is certainly not new for me. When I was in school, floods in Tapi and Narmada rivers due to overflowing were rather common. There were no dams built on these rivers then. Their flooding used to become big news. I have this image in my mind, perhaps something I may have seen in the media then of Morarji Desai, who was then a Member of Parliament, sitting in a rail engine to go to Surat to visit flood-affected areas. Influenced by actions of a senior leader like him, my friends and I set up a stall in the *shravan mahina mela* organized in our village where we sold some local food products. At the end of the mela, we had collected about ₹25–30 profit as a group which we then donated towards flood-relief measures. Years later, during the unfortunate Morbi Dam burst, where thousands of people had lost their lives, I volunteered to help with rehabilitation. I recollect staying amidst the affected, truly understanding their pain and the ground impact of measures which were undertaken then. One of my big takeaways then was noticing that devastation brought about immense food insecurity amongst grieving folks who had survived. All these experiences remain etched in my memory and looking back, I certainly feel that they do contribute to the decisions I make today—take for instance, the free food grains assistance programme which we started right from the beginning of the pandemic and remains ongoing as we speak.'

'Mr Prime Minister, how do you find strength to deal with the tough days?' I enquired.

'You see, I have a big appetite for risk. I don't believe in religious rituals but find immense strength in spirituality. Having said that, I certainly understand the power of religious rituals and why the path of Bhakti yoga, which is prescribed in the Bhagavad Gita as one of the paths to salvation, is adopted by many. I find great strength in connecting with individuals. In my decades of public life, I have travelled through the nooks and corners of India where I've met with countless people and have managed to stay in touch with them. When the pandemic struck, all my meetings became virtual and I had some time on my hands. To better utilize this time, I would sit by myself and think of the various people I have encountered in my life, especially those who may be senior citizens. I'd imagine how life would have changed for them due to the pandemic and almost make a mental picture of their current circumstances. These people included farmers, grocers, mechanics, businessmen, karyakartas [party workers] and social service workers, amongst others. After a few days, I'd call those folks up and enquire about their well-being. Shocked that the prime minister is calling them at a time of crisis, they'd more often than not tell me they were well and how some initiatives that our government had announced were benefitting them. They'd also encourage me to go on and continue to work harder to ensure that India remained safe and not worry about them. The similarities which I found between the mental pictures I had made of them and their realities in addition to the emotional bond I'd build with them would give me immense strength to bring in more initiatives for easing lives. Similarly, I called up the leaders of the 50 most underdeveloped countries in the world assuring them that India was standing by them in this time of global crisis. Many of them found strength in the fact that an Indian prime minister had reached out to them and I found strength in the fact that many vulnerable nations depended on India in times of adversity.'

'You did face several challenges though, Mr Prime Minister...' I asked.

'Yes. There were certainly many. It remained very important for me that society stayed united. I knew that the pressure of living through a pandemic could only be released by shared experiences. That is how junta curfew and the lighting of the diyas came about. I also realized very early on that doctors were our biggest strength in this war against the virus and it was absolutely critical that people respect them as God. So, I dedicated the junta curfew to the doctors and frontline workers. In addition to that, I asked the Indian Air Force to do sorties and shower flowers from the sky in their honour and also personally held virtual meetings with doctors, nurses, ward staff and ambulance drivers. I was very conscious of what I needed to do to get the Indian people to respond in large numbers to my call to action. In fact, junta curfew was like a rice test—you know how you stick a knife in a vessel of rice to see if it is fully cooked? After the phenomenal response to the junta curfew, I was convinced that the people of the country were willing to put their trust in me. Armed with this knowledge, I kept my communications through the pandemic absolutely clear. I spoke to the people often—I probably did more national addresses in these two years of the pandemic than any other prime minister did through their entire term! Now, take for instance the mask mandate which many countries struggled with and continue to even today. Early on, as soon as our scientists told me that the virus was most likely spreading through aerosol droplets, it was important to mandate masks, but we didn't have as many N95 masks for all our people. If I came on television wearing an N95 mask, people would run to the stores and buy out the available quantities creating a shortage for our doctors, who needed them the most. I had read a scientific paper about the effectiveness of a cloth mask too, so I deliberately wore a shawl around my mouth and nose to demonstrate to the people of the country. I also followed it up and changed my social media profile pictures to an image of me wearing a cloth face-cover and didn't change it till we crossed 1 billion vaccine doses. I wanted to leave no room for doubt that face masks were absolutely essential in our fight against COVID-19.'

My extended conversation with the prime minister features at several places in the book. I have found that his perspective provides meaning behind many of our government's initiatives during the course of the pandemic. I intend for this book to become a definitive account of India's response to the pandemic in comparison to the prevailing situation in the world. For that, I have borrowed heavily from media pieces and books written by various authors around the world. I hope to empower you all with accurate information, because after all, information is strength. And finally, readers, I do sincerely believe that you all will come away feeling the same sense of pride in our country as I have after writing this book.

## SECTION 1
# FIRST WAVE

# 1
## ADVENT OF COVID-19

**15 JANUARY 2020**

INDIA | 0 ACTIVE CASES | 0 DEATHS

WORLD | 42 ACTIVE CASES | 2 DEATHS[1]

The Indian Intelligence, right from December 2019, was privy to hushed chatter coming in from the Hubei province of China. The National Security Advisor (NSA), Ajit Doval, all of 74, was sifting through the messages, calls and reports from a global network of resources he had developed over his 53-year-long career as an Indian Police Services (IPS) officer. All emerging intelligence showed multiple cases of a new, mysterious pneumonia outbreak around a seafood and live animal market in Wuhan, a Chinese city with a population of 8 million.[2] Sources informed him about several cases of hospitalization being kept under wraps. What truly concerned the Indian intelligence was the Wuhan Institute of Virology's location—its proximity to the hospitals where these patients with the mysterious pneumonia were being admitted and to the wet market. Doval's internal radar, trained to perfection, after years of experience in the Intelligence Bureau and over six years as Prime Minister Narendra Modi's NSA, immediately beeped, alerting him that these cases possibly pointed to an emergence of a new virus. It was clear that the origins of this would have to be closely probed to reveal if it was natural or man-made. Also, it would be crucial to probe if it had escaped or was let out.

After working closely with PM Modi for an extended period of time, he knew that the prime minister truly believed that Indians slept peacefully at night trusting that the government was keeping the nation safe. They took solace in the fact that if disaster struck, our defence forces in uniform, following orders from authorities, would step in to save the day. Social psychology theorizes that if fear and panic spread in society with an instinct of self-survival taking over, civilization would quickly collapse. As NSA, part of his job was to keep the prime minister abreast of any potential national security threat, including a biological one, to ensure that all impending disasters could be appropriately dealt with. Trust of the people in the government was paramount to maintaining harmony. Sharing a land border with China, it was important for India to track this minutely.

Ajit Doval is described by most of his colleagues as absolutely reliable and an operational genius. Hand-picked by the prime minister in 2014, only recently, after completion of his first term as NSA, he made history by not only being reappointed for a full second term, but also being elevated to the rank of a Cabinet minister.[3]

Reports of the increasing case count of the mystery virus in Wuhan were disturbing. Our Intelligence knew that the Chinese were not divulging the full extent of the damage. Therefore, to keep an eye on the ball, all hands were needed on deck and other trusted experts including officers in the Prime Minister's Office (PMO) would have to be involved. The PMO is situated in one of the two buildings that flank the Rashtrapati Bhavan, culminating at the centre and top of Raisina Hill. It is lined with large brown stones and a royal dome under which is situated the elegant, circular Waiting Area across from the prime minister's chamber. The security detail of the whole complex is handled by the Special Protection Group, with armed men in camouflage uniforms and sharp suits on duty escorting visitors to their meetings. The PMO's architecture or operation makes no modest assumptions about the power it possesses. Some of India's best Civil Service officers and Officers on Special Duty chosen by the prime minister and who form his core team have offices in the building.

On 31 December 2019, the World Health Organization's (WHO) China country office was informed of cases of pneumonia due to unknown aetiology (unknown cause) detected in Wuhan.[4] By 1 January 2020, 27 people were hospitalized[5] and on 3 January, a total of 44 case patients were reported to the WHO by the Chinese national authorities, of which 11 were reported to be severely ill.[6] The statistics were not good. Although the WHO clearly said there was no evidence of human-to-human transmission and that the spread seems to be contained, the reality was that China had not allowed the WHO team on ground yet.[7] The truth, at that point, was only what the Chinese authorities chose to tell the WHO. China had been a menacing source of some of the most virulent outbreaks: SARS (severe acute respiratory syndrome), H5N1 and H7N9 bird flu. If the new virus was anything like the SARS outbreak of 2002, which started in a bat and transferred to a civet cat sold at the wet market, it would be some solace. SARS wasn't particularly infectious until the fifth or sixth day of the disease onset, by which time the patients would develop severe symptoms. This pattern was considered to have limited human-to-human transmission because people who displayed illness could easily be isolated, thus preventing others from being infected. Having said that, it did claim over 800 lives worldwide. Although India seemed more or less insulated from it, we had put systems in place like temperature screenings at airports, created designated hospitals with isolation wards and ensured effective communication to incoming passengers to watch out for symptoms and report to local health authorities in case of illness. We had also expanded a five-year pilot project undertaken by the National Surveillance Programme for Communicable Diseases (NSPCD) from five to a hundred districts to track, trace and treat. Back then, the former director general of health services in the Ministry of Health and Family Welfare (MoHFW), Dr S.P. Agarwal, noted, 'The SARS coronavirus is neither the first nor the last virus to emerge as a major public health threat. The SARS epidemic should therefore be considered as an opportunity to improve public health systems.' In fact, it was precisely actions from government memory at the time of SARS which greatly contributed to initiate quick strategies when the novel coronavirus (nCov)-19 outbreak hit us. However, if the new virus was anything like the H5N1 in 2006 and H7N9 in 2014 which had claimed the lives of the 60 per cent and 40 per cent of those infected, respectively, it would be extremely worrying.

The PMO and their trusted experts for the job, NITI Aayog[8] member Dr V.K. Paul and Principal Scientific Advisor (PSA) Prof. K. VijayRaghavan got to work. They compiled regular reports on the updated information which was emerging from China. Prof. VijayRaghavan was a distinguished biologist and had served as secretary of the Department of Biotechnology and chairman of the board of Coalition for Epidemic

Preparedness Innovations (CEPI). Over the years, Prof. VijayRaghavan had been deeply involved in the study of various disease-causing agents and had been instrumental in establishing the National Centre for Biological Sciences under the Tata Institute of Fundamental Research. On the other hand, Dr Paul has had a long, distinguished career as a medical expert and a public health expert, serving for over a decade as the head of the Paediatrics department at the All India Institute of Medical Sciences (AIIMS), Delhi. The duo began to study the behavioural patterns of the new virus, which, to them, seemed eerily similar to the coronavirus family. By the first week of January 2020, both had collated more information about the seafood market, which appeared to be the origin point of the infections. As a biologist, Prof. VijayRaghavan knew that the origin of the virus would play a crucial role in determining its core nature. The report he scribbled had details like:

> [T]he Huanan market sold bats (a known super-spreader of diseases which transmit to humans, chicken, cats, dogs, marmots, snakes, seafood and other animals). Currently it seems that the market has been closed for environmental sanitisation and disinfection. Several vendors in the Huanan market are primarily said to have been infected. A river separates the market and the Wuhan Institute of Virology lab. It is not clear if all infections are reported from the market side of the river. Was it a zoonotic spill over or a lab leak, must be investigated![9]

Dr Paul observed, 'The market was located next to a mainstream, busy train station which served as a major transportation hub at the centre of China's domestic train routes.' In his report, he also noted patterns of the clinical symptoms which were observed in the 27 cases reported till 1 January 2020; which were fever and difficulty in breathing, specifically in those who demonstrated bilateral lung infiltrates on chest x-rays. Much to their relief, they were also hearing that there had been no evidence of human-to-human transmission. In fact, no infection of hospital staff had been reported till date. Spread of the disease in hospital staff is generally one of the initial patterns observed in human-to-human transmission. In the first week of January, the Wuhan municipal health commissioner released a statement that laboratory testing was underway to determine respiratory pathogens.[10]

They communicated their findings to senior officials in the PMO who then decided it was time the prime minister was briefed without further delay. Principal Secretary Dr P.K. Mishra and Cabinet Secretary Rajiv Gauba were looped in, so that planning for measures to be taken could begin. Mishra, unassuming and low-key, a 1972-batch Indian Administrative Service (IAS) officer belonging to the Gujarat Cadre, worked closely with Modi in several capacities over the last two decades. In 2001, he was the then chief minister Modi's principal secretary when the devastating earthquake shook the Kutch region of Gujarat and was largely instrumental in shaping relief and rehabilitation policies, which helped the people emerge from helplessness and changed the face of Kutch. He held several positions thereafter mostly focusing on his expertise in disaster management for which he recently received the United Nations Office for Disaster Risk Reduction's (UNDRR) prestigious Sasakawa Award in 2019. He was brought into the PMO as additional principal secretary in 2014 after the prime minister's landslide victory in the general elections. Whereas Gauba, a 1962-batch IAS officer, has held a mixed bag of high-profile appointments in several ministries, namely Home Affairs, Urban Development and Defence.

On 8 January, news arrived that although the Chinese authorities had ruled out MERS (Middle East Respiratory Syndrome), seasonal influenza and some other respiratory pathogens, SARS was still a serious possibility. Information also came in that the case count had now gone up to 50 people.[11] Dr Paul and Prof. VijayRaghavan agreed that the doubling rate —the number of days in which the number of infected would double—did not look comforting at all. As with most information that came his way, Dr Paul played devil's advocate and decided that he wasn't convinced that all these cases were occurances of animal-to-human transmission. The statistics told a different story; human-to-human transmission was a more likely cause of such a rapid doubling rate which would increase the likelihood of a major outbreak. He would divulge his doubt to the prime minister when he would see him, he decided. More importantly, Hong Kong, Taiwan, Singapore and the Amur region in Russia had already begun border screening of passengers arriving from Wuhan. He needed to check with the PMO if India should wait a few more days for the story to fully develop, or begin similar precautionary measures. After all, we do share a land border with China.

By early second week of January, confirmed cases in the Wuhan region had gone up to 59 and information from our Intelligence sources on ground had also come in; there was an increased demand for N95 masks in the Hubei province. Sources added that 'mysterious viral pneumonia in Wuhan' had been a trending topic in Chinese social media and that authorities were actively censoring a particular hashtag—#WuhanReportedMysteriousPneumonia.[12] Reinforcing doubts was intel about a whistle-blower doctor in Wuhan, Dr Li Wenliang, later censored by the authorities, who had warned of a SARS-like virus after examining seven patients and advised doctors treating these patients to wear PPE (personal protective equipment) kits along with N95 masks. In fact, after raising the alarm, this doctor was summoned to the Chinese Public Security Bureau, where he was told to sign a letter which read, 'We solemnly warn you: if you keep being stubborn, with such impertinence, and continue this illegal activity, you will be brought to justice—is that understood?' Underneath the letter, Dr Li had signed in his handwriting, 'Yes I do.'[13] Thailand and Vietnam were the next two countries which seemed to have begun border screening Wuhan returnees.

Chatter had gotten louder about this mysterious pneumonia and had made its way to the prime minister through his personal network of individuals. He had alerted Dr Mishra in early January that he had heard about the pneumonia-like cases in China and that we should keep our guard up and track developments closely. This was not a new phenomenon at the PMO. The prime minister was more often than not ahead of the information going around. Over the years, he had meticulously developed a foolproof network to help him stay on top of things. People close to him say that he relies on four major sources: the first being the official network of government and Intelligence officers working at the PMO, the second, his colleagues and party workers from the Bharatiya Janata Party (BJP), the third, his Communications team and the fourth, his own personal network of relationships he has built with individuals over the years. He makes close to 50 calls per day at the minimum and it is this people-to-people connect which really helps him keep his ear on the ground, making him sensitive and reactive to even the smallest rumblings. In the meeting with Dr Mishra, he had also added that he would like to be briefed on what kinds of proactive measures India would be taking in order to tackle the outbreak, if it made its way to us. He particularly was of the opinion that it would be better to be overly responsive than underprepared and caught off guard in this situation. There was definite concern in the PMO that we were a country which had underdeveloped medical infrastructure; if a large-scale pandemic were to hit, India would have to make several upgrades and stopgap arrangements to save lives. Any and all preventive measures which needed to be taken would have to be taken immediately assuming that this infection would reach our doorstep sooner or later. Dr Mishra has been one of the key players in the drafting of the National Disaster Management Act of 2005, following his and the then chief minister Modi's experiences reviving Gujarat post the earthquake. As fate would have it, he would once again be in a similar position; primarily advising the prime minister as he steers the country through the pandemic and resurrects the economy.

Minister of Health and Family Welfare, Dr Harsh Vardhan and the secretary of the MoHFW were looped in and advised to set up a surveillance and response system. This system would be responsible for keeping a close watch on how other countries were responding, and learn from their disease monitoring and response systems to therefore adopt best practices.

◆

On 8 January 2020, the secretary of Health and Family Welfare convened the first meeting of the Joint Monitoring Group under the chairmanship of the Director General of Health Services with stakeholders from related departments and the WHO. This meeting was the starting point in reviewing the preparedness of the public health systems and core capacities: those which were in existence and those that needed to be built for timely detection and management of nCoV.[14]

Meanwhile, outside of India, things were progressing swiftly. On the same day, *The Wall Street Journal* published a story about the Chinese state media having reported that the results from preliminary studies showed that the unidentified pneumonia making people sick 'is believed to be a new type of coronavirus'.[15] On 10 January, China published online the genome sequence of the new virus, opening the possibility for scientists around the world to begin research and development work on possible treatments and vaccines.[16]

On 13 January, the first COVID-19 case outside of China was detected in Thailand in an infected traveller from Wuhan.[17]

By 17 January, in India, the MoHFW in coordination with the Ministry of Civil Aviation began thermal screening of passengers from Wuhan at major airports. In-flight announcements and travel advisories for passengers travelling to and from China were issued. The National Institute of Virology (NIV) in Pune, under the Indian Council of Medical Research (ICMR), had begun coordinating samples for testing for nCoV. ICMR would also begin preparations immediately to isolate the virus, identify a capable indigenous company and provide the isolated strain to it in order to begin the vaccine-development process. Protocol for infection prevention and control (IPC) was prepared and communicated with the states. The Integrated Disease Surveillance Programme (IDSP) was activated in order to gear up for community surveillance and contact tracing. The status of hospital availability and preparedness was reviewed too. Also compiled was an existing inventory of medical equipment like PPE kits, masks and pharmaceutical products which would be required.[18] Notably, other countries of the world were also similarly responding to the viral threat. Reports were coming in that the United States (US) had joined the list of nations which had begun screening passengers arriving from Wuhan the same day.[19] The US's Vaccine Research Center had also initiated research on making a vaccine.[20]

Scientists have pointed out time and again that airport screenings are only useful in identifying symptomatic infected patients.[21] This works in case of viruses which display symptoms and are infectious after the onset of the symptoms like in the case of SARS or MERS. However, those viruses like SARS-CoV-2, which can become infectious even before the onset of symptoms or can be infectious even in asymptomatic hosts, can easily escape the screening system. For health systems of countries this means that although relying on temperature screenings and health advisories buys time and helps collect contact information, which is useful in surveillance and tracking, it is rarely beneficial in blocking the import of infected passengers. However, most countries brought back first responses from government memory in case of epidemics and pandemics, commencing thermal screenings, in the absence of any known behavioural pattern of the new virus.

◆

## 22 JANUARY 2020

INDIA | 0 ACTIVE CASES | 0 DEATHS

WORLD | 970 ACTIVE CASES | 17 DEATHS

It was only on 20 January 2020 that COVID-19 infection became national news in Chinese media and President Xi Jinping issued his first public comment on the situation revealing the scale of the outbreak. He stated that the outbreak 'must be taken seriously' and that every possible measure must be pursued to control it.[22] On an instinct, on 22 January, Vikram Misri, the Indian ambassador to China, advised his team to start preparing to evacuate Indians from the Hubei province. This would entail establishing exactly how many Indians resided in Hubei and where—the challenge was daunting since Indians were not required to register with the embassy and with popular social media channels like Facebook and Twitter blocked in China, outreach would be difficult. The next day, he attended a reception hosted by the embassy on the occasion of Republic Day, in which the Chinese vice foreign minister Luo Zhaohui was the chief guest, and was attended by several Chinese dignitaries and members of the Beijing-based diplomatic community. It was at this event that Misri heard hushed and off-the-record talk of the true scale of the infection and relayed his concern back to the Ministry of External Affairs in India, solidifying his stance on the need to evacuate Indians in the province.[23] The Indian embassy had planned to host a larger Republic Day ceremony on 26 January but announced on Twitter on 24 January that it stands to be cancelled. 'In view of the evolving situation due to the coronavirus outbreak in China as well as the decision of the Chinese authorities to cancel public gathering and events, @EOIBeijing has also decided to call off the Republic Day reception scheduled to be held @EOIBeijing on January 26th.'[24]

By this time, there were several travel-related cases detected in the US, Thailand, South Korea and Japan. In China, the death toll stood at 25, with confirmed cases at 830, including 26 cases reported in Beijing. China had by then locked down eight cities, including Wuhan, to prevent the virus from transmitting.

On 24 January, the Indian mission in China launched hotlines to track Indians based in Wuhan and provide psychological support by asking about their welfare in terms of supply of essential items.[25]

Meanwhile, Misri was constantly communicating with the secretary of External Affairs, Vijay Keshav Gokhale on the urgency to evacuate Indians. Gokhale was further communicating with the PMO and External Affairs Minister Dr S. Jaishankar to take a final decision on evacuation. On 25 January, Principal Secretary Dr Mishra convened a high-level meeting to discuss and finalize details on evacuation. This meeting was attended by the Cabinet secretary, secretary of Home Affairs, secretary of External Affairs, secretary of Defence, secretary of Health and Family Welfare and secretary of Civil Aviation.[26] By the next day, 26 January, they had confirmed information from WeChat, a WhatsApp-equivalent mobile application used in China, that out of all the Indians who were contacted, about 750 wanted to return to India. The others wanted to either stay put or travel to different parts of the country. Half of those who wanted to return lived in deeper areas of the Hubei province and the other half of them in Wuhan. The decision to evacuate wasn't easy. The prime minister was aware that many countries had decided against taking out their citizens from China, mainly because of the fear that they wouldn't want to provide an opportunity for an unknown virus to spread in their countries. Pakistan, for instance, had already announced that they will not take their citizens back. In fact, their envoy had said, 'Students should stay in Wuhan as Pakistan cannot treat coronavirus.'[27] The prime minister was certain though, if there were Indian citizens who felt unsafe and sought to return home, India should enable their homecoming, no matter how large a risk it was. He gave his go-ahead to evacuate Indians and instructed the officers to begin making all required preparations. The PMO then effectively advised all concerned bureaucrats to work out the logistics and prepare to evacuate on short notice. Simultaneously, negotiations regarding evacuations were ongoing, as natural for any other country; China's stand was that it would keep people safe. At this point, no other country had evacuated its citizens from China; however, Vietnam, which had suspended all flights[28] to and from Wuhan, permitted special flights between 23 and 27 January to bring back stranded citizens. However, many countries were in talks with the Chinese authorities seeking permission to be allowed to extradite their citizens. On 28 January, even as Misri and the deputy chief of mission worked to obtain clearances, the outgoing secretary of External Affairs, Gokhale with his incumbent, Harsh Vardhan Shringla worked closely with the Ministry of Civil Aviation, Air India (our national airline carrier), the Bureau of Immigration and the Indian Army. Air India was asked to put together two aircrafts and an experienced crew on standby, whereas the Indian Army was to set up quarantine facilities for the returnees.

On 28 January, resistance came in from the Chinese when the Chinese ambassador to India Sun Weidong posted on Twitter that the WHO did not recommend evacuation of nationals and persuaded the international community to remain calm and not overreact.[29] Meanwhile, on the same day, Chinese president Xi Jinping met with WHO Director-General Tedros Adhanom Ghebreyesus.[30] While the details of the meeting remain confidential, the next day, on 29 January, Australia, New Zealand, the US and Japan were allowed to run flights to Wuhan in order to evacuate their citizens.[31] [32] [33] [34] Indian diplomats stayed consistently engaged with the Chinese, pressing them for permissions to evacuate our citizens. And on the morning of the 29th, the in-principal approval came in. Each city and each province in China has a Foreign Affairs Office. For matters related to foreigners, embassies must connect with these Foreign Affairs Offices. In addition to connecting with them, the Indian embassy had to then engage with authorities down the chain to the level of provincial authorities so that none of them blocked Indians making their way to the airport. Each point of authority in the chain of command starting from central government authorities, authorities of the Hubei province and Wuhan municipal corporation authorities to even the police had to be looped in and this exercise was aided by the regional Foreign Affairs Office.

On 30 January, WHO Director-General Tedros declared the epidemic a Public Health Emergency of International Concern. The WHO was finally waking up to the tragedy which would soon engulf the world.

The looming task at hand for the Indian diplomats was to get Indians scattered across the city to the airport. Due to the lockdown, free movement was not allowed and people could not be asked to assemble at a certain pickup point or even get to the airport. So, private transport companies were hired who would then be in touch with the staff at the Indian embassy, including Chinese-speaking staff, in order to make logistics and coordination smooth. The Foreign Affairs Office in Wuhan played an important role in this exercise. The formal approval for the airlift came in at 3.30 p.m. on 31 January.[35] Air India, in its preparations, had put one of its Boeing 747 jumbo passenger jets on standby. The 34-member rescue crew that would man the jet included three doctors and four nurses. The visas of all the 34 identified crew members were promptly sent for approval. The Chinese embassy in India was especially helpful in ensuring that all of the crew visas arrived on time. Captain Amitabh Singh, the director of Operations of the AI1348 flight, after returning from the successful evacuation operation recalled that the deathly silence in the aircraft that was devoid of any radio chatter and the eerie quietness of a locked-down Wuhan felt apocalyptic while descending. A second flight brought back 323 Indians on 2 February that year.[36]

The returning passengers were then sent to the two quarantine centres set up by the Indian Armed Forces at Manesar and Chawla Camp near New Delhi. From the returnees, those with any symptoms or comorbidities were sent to Safdarjung Hospital for monitoring.[37] A 30-something-year-old specialist, Dr Nitish Gupta was on the frontline monitoring and preparing the hospital to treat in case of COVID-19-positive cases. He and his team were studying infection-control practices emerging from China and Italy and putting in place standard operating procedures (SOPs) for the hospital which would include use of PPE kits, N95 masks for all healthcare and frontline staff attending to the patients, negative suction doors, isolated rooms for those testing positive and so on. None of the Wuhan returnees tested positive for the virus but Dr Gupta would later say, 'The whole team at the hospital was on its toes. In the absence of clarity on how the virus spreads and how it can be treated, not only were the patients afraid, but even the hospital team was extremely fearful.'

From the Indians in Hubei who wanted to return to their country, there were several Indians who weren't allowed to board the flights on account of their body temperatures being higher than what the Chinese government had allowed as part its travel protocol. On 8 February, Prime Minister Modi wrote to Chinese president Xi, conveying the solidarity of the people and the Government of India (GoI) with the people of China and the readiness of the Indian government to provide assistance.[38] Following that letter, India sent about 15 tonnes worth of medical equipment comprising surgical masks, surgical gloves, infusion pumps, enteral feeding pumps, defibrillators and N95 masks.[39] These supplies were delivered by an Indian Air Force C-17 special flight, which after delivering the equipment to the Hubei Charity Federation, ferried back the remaining Indians who wanted to return but were not allowed to board the two previous flights due to high body temperature.

Eventually, India ended up evacuating not only its own citizens but also helped about 80 other countries bring back theirs. India solidified its footing as a 'first and fast' responder during the crisis, be it during Wuhan or the Yemen crisis or Nepal earthquake, efficiently rescuing not only Indian nationals but people from across the world.

# 2
## INDIA PREPARES

**27 JANUARY 2020**

INDIA | 1 ACTIVE CASE | 0 DEATHS

WORLD | 4,835 ACTIVE CASES | 110 DEATHS

The invisible hitch-hiker made its way to India in the first known case of an infected student who had returned home from Wuhan on 23 January, before the city went into lockdown. Patient Zero, a 20-year-old female, presented herself at the Emergency Department in General Hospital in Thrissur (Kerala) with a one-day history of dry cough and sore throat.[1] In her history, she said that she was asymptomatic between 23 and 26 January. She had most likely been exposed to the virus in the train from Wuhan to Kunming during her journey back home, where she noticed people with respiratory symptoms in the railway station and train. Her sample was sent to the NIV laboratory in Pune and was reported positive for COVID-19 infection to the District Control Cell. Detailed contact tracing was carried out by the Government Medical College along with district health authorities. She was placed in the isolation ward at the hospital and her samples sent for testing every alternate day. By day 17, she had tested negative.[2]

The enemy was at the doorstep. This was no surprise. On 26 January, the mayor of Wuhan had acknowledged that five million people had left the city in the week before the Chinese government locked it down.[3] As Bloomberg News dubs it, the 'world's biggest human migration'—the Chinese New Year celebration—would begin on 24 January, spanning 16 days, with an estimate of about three billion trips taken within China and to other countries for the holiday.[4] Despite the raging march of the virus, the Chinese government did not suspend outgoing international flights until other countries suspended travel from China which was only in the end of January, allowing folks to travel out of the country, potentially carrying the virus. To note here especially is that, they did put stringent curbs on domestic travel in late January 2020 from the virus hotspots.[5]

Given the density and sheer population of India, once the virus had officially arrived, the possibility of coming in contact with a COVID-19-positive person was very real. This was our very first known case, but it was a solid possibility that there were other patients who had simply gone unnoticed because they hadn't presented themselves at hospitals. If a COVID-19-positive person took a train or an Uber, shared a taxi, bus or autorickshaw or lived in close quarters in our socially tight-knit communities, imagine the number of people they were coming in contact with daily!

As early as 27 January, a German doctor, while exploring Germany's first COVID-19 case had concluded that the infection had gotten transmitted to the country's 33-year-old patient zero from a Chinese business partner, who had displayed no symptoms whatsoever, when they met for meetings near Munich on 20th of that month (a week earlier). Later it was noted that the Shanghai resident who returned to her country on 26 January and began to display symptoms only on her flight back home, had also tested positive.[6] Around the same time, we were hearing in the international media about the viral spread of the pathogen in ski-barns[7], churches[8] and soccer stadiums[9] in Europe. One of the first international outbreaks of the virus was on *Diamond Princess*, a luxury cruise ship stuck in quarantine off the coast of Japan, on which 744 people had tested positive and were locked in their cabins. A hundred and thirty-eight Indians were on board. When health workers on the ship were interviewed, the information all pointed to symptomless spread—they vouched that 70 per cent of the positive patients displayed no symptoms at all.[10] The scientific community also learned innumerable lessons which would be extremely useful in prescribing further strategies, i.e. lessons published in *Infectious Disease Modelling* revealed that locking down people in cabins did have a measurable impact on restricting the contagion and that the ship's waste water and ventilation systems did not seem to worsen the spread of the disease.[11] The international health community debated the concept of asymptomatic spread for a long time: The *New England Journal of Medicine* published two papers on the possibility of asymptomatic spread, one of which was the German doctor's who studied the first few cases in Germany and wrote a letter to the editor on 30 January specifying, 'The fact that asymptomatic persons are potential sources of 2019-NCoV infection may warrant a reassessment of transmission dynamics of the current outbreak.'[12] In early February, the WHO noted in a report that patients might transmit the virus before showing symptoms. It also added that patients with symptoms were the main cause of the spread of the epidemic.[13]

◆

On 27 January, in a meeting at the PMO, the Cabinet secretary was informed that India had screened almost 30,000 passengers from 137 flights and that 12 samples had been sent out for further testing to the NIV. India had started distributing health cards on all flights with direct or indirect connectivity to China. Screening began on all international ports with traffic from China and of all visitors travelling across the Nepal border. Health staff were assigned to checkposts and all immigration officers and border security force officers manning these checkposts were sensitized.[14]

On 31 January, foreseeing the increased domestic requirement for PPE kits and N95 masks, the Indian Directorate General of Foreign Trade banned export of all categories of the former.[15]

◆

## 3 FEBRUARY 2020

### INDIA | 4 ACTIVE CASES | 0 DEATHS

### WORLD | 20,061 ACTIVE CASES | 433 DEATHS

Principal Secretary to the PM, Dr Mishra assembled a high-level group comprising senior officials in the PMO, NSA Doval, Chief of Defence Staff General Bipin Rawat and secretaries of several ministries.[16] The message from the prime minister was to immediately constitute a select group of ministers who would take responsibility and provide ground feedback from their respective constituencies regarding several logistical aspects as the pathogen makes its way through the country. He also wanted to enquire about the passengers who had been evacuated from Wuhan and were still housed at Army camps. The prime minister, in his monthly radio programme, would speak to several of them about their experience a few weeks later.[17]

Another big decision taken at the meeting was to suspend e-visa facilities for Chinese citizens. This was a starting point of putting restrictions on international travel. There was no doubt that this would have an impact on the markets; however, considering that very little was known about this virus and the fact that protecting our citizens was priority, this decision was made.

In order to bring them up to speed, the Group of Ministers were briefed by the MoHFW on the status of the (now) three cases in Kerala as well as the preventative measures we had begun taking.[18]

The central government suffers from peculiar strengths and weaknesses. One of its strengths is that officers from almost all parts of the country work together based on their experiences and insights attained from various postings across states. But the same quality often becomes a weakness because there is nothing to bind these officers to one another. Perhaps the only thing common between officers is that either they were in the same batch/year or that they work in the same ministries. In the words of the prime minister, the Indian administration is an 'assembled unit' and not an 'organic unit'. Often what this situation does is that it doesn't provide a common vision or mission for the officers to work on, with the officers working in the narrow silos of their departments.

The prime minister has been working to address this problem over the last seven years. He had made officers work together in various sectoral groups on issues larger than the ambit of respective departments and ministries—be it in sectoral groups or even in policy reforms like PRAGATI meetings and PM GATI SHAKTI. Due to these interventions, the GoI is now witnessing an evolving culture of team-building. With time, officers who have been working closely with the prime minister began to recognize his insistence on bureaucrats being able to work together across ministries in a 'whole of government' approach.

It is in this context that when the pandemic struck, while the 'business as usual' approach would mean that the entire pandemic-related decision-making and subsequent action would be managed by the MoHFW, but in line with the PM's thinking, the GoI decided to take a different approach. Dr P.K. Mishra chaired a meeting with secretaries of various ministries and thought too that if this was going to snowball into a global pandemic, all of the government would need to be actively involved. He was going to have to deal with this problem as soon as possible.

◆

The Ministry of External Affairs was in close contact with the US Secretary of State and the Indian ambassador to the US. Both countries were tracking the development of the spread of the disease very closely. President Donald Trump was scheduled to visit India in the third week of February, but naturally that would change based on the status of the spread of the pathogen in both countries.

As the month of February progressed, the virus spread most prominently in Italy, Asia and the Middle East. Global markets began to take big hits. President Trump did not cancel his state visit. In fact, his meetings with Prime Minister Modi helped reinforce relationship between the two largest democracies of the world. They established an understanding that although there was some friction on both sides regarding the new trade deal, it wouldn't spill over on strategic areas of convergence such as defence and security cooperation.[19] Since India was still pretty much insulated from the virus, a grand event—'Namaste Trump'—was organized in Ahmedabad, with an audience of over 1,10,000 people. The president and the first lady were given a red-carpet welcome at the ceremonial state reception at the Rashtrapati Bhavan. It was only when Trump boarded Air Force One to return was he informed that a senior director of the US's Centers for Disease Control and Prevention had during a media briefing earlier in the day indicated the possibility of closing down schools, remote working and using internet-based teleschooling, if the COVID-19 cases kept going up. She had warned that the situation was 'rapidly evolving and expanding' and that 'it's not so much a question of *if* this will happen anymore but rather more a question of exactly *when* this will happen and how many people in the country will have severe illness.'[20]

When he was in India, both India and the US hardly had any

COVID-19 cases and hence the state visit and the gatherings looked par for the course. However, a few months later, in May 2020, Gujarat Congress claimed that the 'Namaste Trump' event was responsible for the spread of the virus and deaths in Gujarat, notwithstanding the fact that even the initial cases in Gujarat came more than a fortnight after the visit.[21]

♦

Finally, in late February, China released the report[22] prepared by the team of scientists deployed by the WHO to investigate the virus with highly misleading information on the lines that asymptomatic spread of the infection was 'relatively rare and does not appear to be a major driver of transmission'. The report also extensively praised China for its containment efforts adding that the country has undertaken 'perhaps the most ambitious, agile and aggressive disease containment effort in history'. However, it also contained a stark warning: 'Much of the global community is not ready, in mindset and materially, to implement the measures that have been employed to contain COVID-19 in China. These are the only measures that are currently proven to interrupt or minimize' the spread of coronavirus. These were measures which included surveillance, public engagement, cancellation of mass gatherings, traffic controls, rapid diagnosis, immediate case isolation and rigorous tracking and quarantining close contacts.[23] If India had any chance of fighting the virus, all of the aforementioned measures would have to be meticulously put in place.

# 3
# THE VIRUS STRIKES

**4 MARCH 2020**

**INDIA | 26 ACTIVE CASES | 0 DEATHS**

**WORLD | 43,611 ACTIVE CASES | 3,288 DEATHS**

Reality struck India when 15 people from a group of Italian tourists tested positive for COVID-19 in New Delhi. A male tourist from the group after experiencing flu-like symptoms first tested positive in Jaipur. Following which, his wife, 14 others from the group as well as their driver tested positive.[1] The authorities got their first taste of COVID-19 management when all of the groups' contacts—the places they visited, the restaurants they dined at and the hotels they stayed at—needed to be traced, isolated and put under surveillance.

RD, who had returned from Italy via the Middle East with his brother, had hosted a birthday party for his son in New Delhi's Hyatt Hotel. Several kids from two neighbourhood schools attended this party.[2] Only the next day, when he began to show symptoms, he got tested and turned out positive. Both schools had to suspend classes immediately. The kids and their parents had to be closely monitored and the schools had to be sanitized. This gentleman also met with a bunch of people in Agra who had to be traced and tested. After contact tracing, it emerged that none of his primary contacts had tested positive except his brother, who had travelled with him. And by great good fortune, none of the children tested positive either.

Once again, Dr Nitish Gupta and his fearless team were on ground zero at Safdarjung Hospital treating these new cases. They too had children, parents and spouses to go home to. They too worried about carrying the infection home. But as of this moment, the country needed them and they pushed back their fears and stood on the frontline in service of our country.

While in no uncertain way was this perceived as a one-off event, it did raise immediate crucial questions. Did we need to shut down schools nationwide to protect our children? What if kids at the birthday party caught the infection? How would the virus play out on their health? Would it be fatal? Just the thought of these scenarios was shuddering and SOPs needed to be framed to protect our vulnerable populations on priority.

◆

Even as regional authorities were busy putting teams in place to smoothen out tracing, testing and isolating procedures, Dr V.K. Paul and Prof. K. VijayRaghavan were meeting frequently in Delhi in NITI Aayog to closely track the developments and research solutions. They had been closely observing the devastation that the virus was causing in the countries in its grip. Based on fatality and doubling rates, the need of the hour was to do some mathematical modelling in order to provide various estimates of the spread in India. Their thinking was to investigate different mathematical scenarios, pre-empt and prevent the worst outcomes as much as we can. The best analogy that Prof. VijayRaghavan later used to explain why accurate mathematical modelling was important at that point in time for India was one comparing the spread of the virus to a growing tree: 'Modelling would be able to tell us in which direction and how much the virus would grow if it was left unchecked versus if preventative measures were taken. It would give us a very fair idea of where and how much that tree would need to be trimmed.' A range of possibilities would have to be presented to the prime minister and the principal secretary for urgent, important restrictions to be put in place.

There were several expert modelling groups across the globe as well as in India. The agreement between the two gentlemen was to get as many opinions and as much meaningful data as quickly as possible. After about a fortnight of reaching out to about 10 such groups, calling them in for meetings or holding meetings with them virtually, a consensus was reached on which seemed to be the most accurate model. Immediately after, having seen very grim numbers, they requested time from the principal secretary to present their findings.

Just the day before, on 3 March, the prime minister had held extensive briefings with a team of scientists and bureaucrats from the PMO and across ministries.[3] Just like every political leader in the world, he was facing a quandary. What was India's balancing line? Should we protect the vulnerable and minority populations while allowing the contagion to spread through society or lock down the country and the economy to keep the virus at a manageable level? How quickly would the disease overwhelm our healthcare system? Did we have enough doctors, nurses and frontline workers to be able to afford to let the virus run unchecked? What about hospital beds, oxygenated beds, ventilators and other such essential supplies?

Most medical and scientific advice regarding the evolution of COVID-19 was provided first hand to the prime minister by the team comprising primarily Dr V.K. Paul, Prof. VijayRaghavan, Prof. Dr Balram Bhargava of the ICMR, AIIMS Director Dr Randeep Guleria and the in-house bureaucrats in the PMO, some of whom were qualified medical doctors and community medicine experts. This team briefed the prime minister about how social distancing, wearing face masks, handwashing and repeatedly sanitizing seemed to be the only ways to keep the virus at bay. Although evidence on how the virus was spreading was still emerging, and most research around the world was focusing on surface transmission as the main source of spread, our team of scientists seemed to be convinced—based on data from emerging case studies globally and the high doubling rate—that the most likely scenario was of the virus spreading through suspended aerosols in the air when an infected person spoke, coughed or sneezed. This was deeply concerning for us, since not only were we the second most populous country in the world but our population density was almost as high as 460 people per sq. km. It would be a formidable challenge to educate the Indian people on what COVID-19 measures would entail. Clear, firm communication would be paramount.

In the meeting, Dr Paul expressed to the prime minister, 'This is a war that science will win for us, Sir, through ground-breaking drugs and vaccines. We must support and encourage our scientists, industry and scientific organizations to develop this ammunition for our arsenal.'

Following the meeting, the prime minister put out on his Twitter account along with an infographic with a few points to follow for basic protective measures: 'Had an extensive review regarding preparedness on the COVID-19 novel coronavirus. Different ministries & states are working together, from screening people arriving in India to providing prompt medical attention. There is no need to panic. We need to work together, take small yet important measures to ensure self-protection.'[4]

The festival of Holi, which is celebrated all over India by meeting friends and family, was coming up in a couple of days. If it was going to be celebrated as usual, there would be a lot of people-to-people contact, thus providing a fertile ground for the virus to spread. The prime minister knew that he needed to send out a cautionary message. This was the beginning of increasingly ominous warnings about the impending cataclysmic crunch point that the prime minister would have to give. It was his unique way of impressing upon the country on what not to do—the first of many such call-to-action sermons—that would follow over the course of the pandemic. He tweeted on 4 March 2020: 'Experts across the world have advised to reduce mass gatherings to avoid the spread of COVID-19 novel coronavirus. Hence, this year I have decided not to participate in any Holi Milan programme.'[5] Several other political leaders across party lines followed suit.[6]

India was, in no uncertain terms, unprepared for an epidemic and the briefings that the prime minister held would make that crystal clear to him. On the Global Health Security Index published in 2019, India ranked 57th in the world to produce a 'rapid response to and mitigation of the spread of an epidemic.'[7] There was no doubt in the prime minister's mind that in order to stand steadfastly against the virus, the whole country would have to follow the doctors' orders: social distancing, self-quarantining, ramping up testing and scaling up capacities. And he would have to respond as the leader of a nation at war with this hidden enemy.

◆

On 4 March, at noon, Principal Secretary Dr Mishra chaired a review meeting in the PMO which was a prelude to an important briefing meet in which the prime minister would be informed on crucial matters.[8] The list of high-ranking bureaucrats and experts who attended the meeting gave off the seriousness of the agenda. Attendees included Dr Paul,

Cabinet secretary, secretary of the MoHFW, secretary from the Ministry of Shipping, foreign secretary, secretary of Civil Aviation, secretary of Tourism, secretary of Pharmaceuticals, secretary of Information and Communications, secretary of Border Management from the Ministry of Home Affairs, Dr Bhargava, a member from the National Disaster Management Authority, chairman of the Airport Authority and director general of the National Informatics Centre. During the course of the meeting, Dr Mishra asked, 'How many testing laboratories can we expect to increase in two months?'

Someone in the room answered, 'In all probability, Sir, we can have about 70 additional functional labs.' Dr Mishra was not pleased, knowing that the prime minister wanted infrastructure to be ramped up to suit the country's requirements and not merely the government's abilities in 'business as usual' circumstances. *That number is not even close to where we should be*, he thought. (In real time, we were at 151 labs as on 1 April, 254 by 1 May, 676 by 1 June, over 1,056 by 1 July and are over double that number as of August 2021.)

Next, he asked about the availability of masks, PPE kits, ventilators etc.

As a response, a problem of gargantuan proportions emerged; it was the pressing need to augment the availability of masks, PPE kits, sanitizers, test kits and ventilators. From the experience of countries where the virus was spreading rapidly, it was learned that these were essentials which would be needed in large quantities. The grim reality was that India was manufacturing very few N95 masks, the kind which frontline healthcare workers would need. At this point in time, it was estimated that we had only 3.35 lakh N95 masks stockpiled with us. We weren't manufacturing a single PPE kit and had only 2.75 lakh kits in reserve. We were in very short supply of ventilators too—we only had about 20,000 of them and since the virus seemed to have a pneumonia-like debilitating effect on the lungs, ventilators would prove to be life-saving devices.

To the principal secretary, this was not a satisfactory outcome of the meeting at all. He briefed the prime minister of his concerns. The prime minister thought back to his experience in 2015, when he had created small groups of senior bureaucrats and given them common goals to work on which he would discuss with them over personal meetings to instil camaraderie and coordination. The red-tape culture was so disturbing to him that he had spent a lot of time trying to find a way to inspire officers. In one such exercise, as soon as taking office, he had directed some senior-most officers in the Indian government to take time out to visit the place where they first started service. He had insisted that they take their family along if it was possible. He had urged them to ask themselves, 'What is the condition of the place where I first started duty?' Many officers returned disappointed in the growth of that place. The exercise turned out to be an eye-opener. The prime minister had then explained to them, 'You see how little your service has contributed to the overall growth of that place? We must work together as a unit towards common goals for the nation, to bring in maximum progress.'

Just as he did then, even now he needed to find a solution that could cut bureaucratic red tape, thus improving government response time once again. He thought about solutions which may have been explored in the past. In time of such an emergency which was impacting millions of lives worldwide and was poised to hit India like an avalanche, a well-planned and coordinated emergency response strategy was key. The challenges which would confront the government on a daily basis were going to be new and their magnitude and gravity would be severe. In order to confront these, the solutions would also have to be innovative and there would be a desperate need to augment and synchronize efforts by cutting across ministries and departments. We would need to create 'empowered groups' on each major challenge, which would constitute a mix of subject-matter experts and highly ranked government officers. As the name suggests, these groups would be empowered to delineate policy, formulate plans, strategize operations and take all necessary steps for effective and time-bound implementation of these decisions in their respective areas. Details of the breakdown of empowered groups and their constitution was then mulled over with the scientists and other officers in the PMO, after which the home secretary in his capacity as chairperson of the National Executive Committee and the powers vested in him under the Section 10(2)(h) and (i) of the Disaster Management Act, would have to issue the official order to constitute such groups.

In addition to all this, the prime minister was also receiving simultaneous feedback from his own network of individuals he had cultivated over decades of public service. This was his distinct working style—he was adept at gathering information on a certain matter from multiple sources, only after which he would make a decision, thus eliminating overreliance on any one individual or a certain group of individuals.

◆

Meanwhile, only in late February had China admitted that 2,236 people had succumbed to the virus in Wuhan.[9] Even while the accuracy of the number was debated amongst epidemiologists and scientists, nations in Europe including the United Kingdom (UK), were just about upgrading risk levels to 'moderate' from 'low'. These were perhaps Europe's final days of innocence—in Codogno, a small town in Lombardy, north Italy, doctors had just started to treat a man suffering respiratory symptoms, with zero suspicion that there was anything unusual.[10] In less than a month, pictures and videos in the media showed horrifying signs from the streets of Italy displaying a nation in crisis, convulsed by fear, in the tight grip of the new disease. The rise of the cases was so swift that the healthcare system quickly became distressed to a point where doctors had to make the gut-wrenching choice of which patient presenting in the emergency ward had a higher chance of survival over admitting those with a low probability. The sick were either abandoned in their homes or lying on the hospital floors.[11] Soon, Lombardy would be completely locked down, being one of the first cities in the western world to use the 'physical suppression' method to stop the spread of the infection.[12] Being jolted into the reality that the COVID-19 threat was very real, countries like the UK updated their mathematical models and arrived at a new 'reasonable worst-case scenario' where about 80 per cent of Britons would be eventually infected, out of which one per cent would die. With mitigation measures, the team of scientists from the UK's Scientific Advisory Group for Emergencies concurred that the death toll could reach 2,50,000 and the existing intensive care units (ICUs) would be overwhelmed eight times over when the virus spreads in the community. However, the UK government took a more modest view and its National Security Communications Team warned that with 80 per cent of the population infected, 'the current planning assumption is that 2–3 percent of symptomatic cases will result in a fatality.'[13] With this statistic, they said, 'the country planned to create some kind of herd immunity, whereby a large proportion of the population has had the virus and is therefore inoculated [which] is clearly the objective—well, not the objective; rather, it is one of the results of the virus passing through, as flu viruses do regularly. It is expected that it will be a one-off experience, so herd immunity will actually provide resistance to future visits by the virus.'[14] All across, the media headlines splashed that the UK was about to shut down schools and that £100 billion had been wiped off the value of leading shares after the government's warning of potential five lakh deaths.[15] This just about coincided with the US's Centers for Disease Control and Prevention's announcement of school closures, remote working and the Dow market crash.[16][17]

While the global search for information on the virus continued, experts had almost arrived at a consensus about transmission through aerosol droplets in human breath, echoing what our scientists had been indicating since several weeks now. The unresolved problem which remained and was more difficult to solve was to define the rate of asymptomatic infection. Three weeks after Lombardy locked down, all of Italy, following examples of Asian countries, had locked down.[18] An odd observation was the Europe Union's (EU) silence to Italy's request for help and the behaviour of every EU country which acted in its own interest by closing borders.[19] International collaboration was minimal.

Asian countries where the virus had made its presence were handling measures rather differently from the West. Based on its experience with SARS and MERS, South Korea, in one of its first steps, prepared itself to intensify aggressive testing in over 50 laboratories.[20] Seoul's authorities were empowered to compel every infected person to move without their family to a special quarantine accommodation/facility for two weeks. In addition to this, they were using facial recognition on CCTV, personal data from credit card transactions and technology to identify anyone who the infected person would have come in contact with to track, test and quarantine.[21] Due to this measure, and strict COVID-19 behaviour protocols, they were able to avoid a national lockdown and keep casualties at about 10 per day. Singapore and Taiwan had only two deaths at this point; the former had opted to keep schools and restaurants open and was actively discouraging remote working to protect the economy, while the latter had introduced mass temperature screening while keeping shops and restaurants open.[22]

There was much debate across nations whether measures imposed were draconian or not. Could folks be penalized for not following sanitary, lockdown and hygiene rules? Could governments enforce countrymen to wear masks? Could governments track infected people on CCTV for contact tracing without violating their right to privacy? How far could governments go in order to keep their people safe while also protecting human rights and their right to privacy?

Back home, there was no doubt on Lok Kalyan Marg that the prime minister would have to make some tough choices. Unless strict rules and stringent enforcement were the focus in policymaking—looking at our sheer numbers, demographic, the urban–rural divide, rampant illiteracy and compromised hygiene—lakhs of Indian lives would be lost. The only other leader in the history of India who had run historic mobilization campaigns with an emphasis on hygiene and sanitation was Mahatma Gandhi. Although the prime minister initiated and ran a successful Swachh Bharat Abhiyan (Clean India Mission) during his first term, with a goal to increase access to toilets and make the country open-defecation free, the kind of mobilization which would be required to ask people to make urgent behavioural modifications could not be compared to any recent initiatives in the history of modern, independent India.

# 4

## FIRST RESPONSES

**13 MARCH 2020**

**INDIA | 70 ACTIVE CASES | 2 DEATHS**

**WORLD | 1,01,266 ACTIVE CASES | 5,446 DEATHS**

A global religious Muslim organization, the Tablighi Jamaat held a mass congregation of over 9,000 missionaries at New Delhi's Banglewadi Nizamuddin Markaz centre in the first two weeks of March.[1] Thousands of people, including various preachers and attendees who had only the previous month gathered in Malaysia for a four-day global meet which *The New York Times* reported at the time as 'the largest viral vector in Southeast Asia'[2] made their way to the Nizamuddin Markaz. These included 800 preachers from Indonesia, Bangladesh, Malaysia and Thailand who entered the country on 'tourist visas' which categorically do not allow missionary work to be undertaken during the time of stay in India. The event in Malaysia had been such a super-spreader that about 620 people connected to the event had tested positive due to which Malaysia had to quickly seal its borders. Travel restrictions were not initiated then, owing to very low caseload in India, due to which thousands of Indian Muslims belonging to the Tablighi Jamaat from across the country too, made their way to New Delhi for the event.[3]

New information about the virus and its nature of spread was emerging each day. It was learned that during super-spreader events, one infected person had the ability to infect over six people, almost doubling its pervasiveness. However, this number could be volatile and increase dramatically if no COVID-19-appropriate behaviour of masking up or social distancing is followed. Numbers would also significantly increase if people were cramped in an indoor, non-ventilated, humid space.

The Nizamuddin Markaz mosque is a standalone, six-storey building with a capacity to house over 2,000 people, sharing a wall with the local Hazrat Nizamuddin Police Station in West Delhi. On 12 March, following the transmission scare at a children's birthday party and persistently growing daily new cases, the New Delhi government, invoking powers granted by the Epidemic Diseases Act of 1897, announced the shutdown of schools, cinema halls and colleges. Private offices too had begun to operate via remote working.[4] On 13 March, over 3,400 people were reported to be inside the mosque. On 16 March, the Delhi chief minister Arvind Kejriwal announced that no more than 50 people would be allowed at religious, political or social gatherings. While some attendees at the Markaz began to leave and make their way to several parts of the country, others continued to stay put, defying government orders.[5]

♦

Meanwhile, Prof. VijayRaghavan and Dr Paul had a meeting scheduled with the principal secretary and other officials at the PMO to discuss their grim findings after extensive consultations with modellers. Numerous heads of states and their deputies have walked the same wide red-stone hallways through which the two gentlemen made their way to Dr Mishra's first-floor chamber, adjacent to the prime minister's. In the pyramid of India's government, the person empowered to advise and expected to urge caution to a prime minister is the principal secretary. As the bureaucrat-in-chief, he is not only the prime minister's eyes and ears, but is also the official responsible for knowing whether the government machinery is functioning as directed. In this time of crisis, Dr Mishra's job was cut out; one of his main tasks was to understand the developing crisis and assess the advice the prime minister was receiving, especially from scientists.

Although new techniques of modelling have not reached a point where they can make accurate predictions on the rise of an unknown agent beyond two to four weeks[6], a relatively safe bet was to use various different kinds of models using data points from around the world where the contagion was significantly spreading and input them in an instrument which was tailored for Indian demographics and patterns. The challenge was to find, produce and rely on a finely tuned piece of programming which would be able to distinguish between particular people's susceptibility to the virus. For instance, a frontline healthcare worker would be more likely to transmit the virus than an asymptomatic child.[7] Programmes used for other infectious diseases would not work; since SARS, influenza and MERS were mostly symptomatic transmissions, models developed for those outbreaks would not be able to provide precise results. In the case of COVID-19, there were simply too many fundamental unknowns to accurately predict the course of the contagion. Most large countries in the West were making the rookie mistake of using severely flawed models by over-relying on the ones already used for known epidemics like influenza or SARS.[8] Hence, it was prudent for Dr Paul and Prof. VijayRaghavan to also think about the extent to which outputs from models would matter in the context of policy relevance in India's response. Emerging evidence was showing that the 'rate of infection'—passing the virus on to another person—was no longer four to six days but had accelerated to two to three days. This had a direct effect on the doubling rate—the number of days in which the number of infected would double.[9]

The two scientists informed the principal secretary of the various scenarios; the greyest of them being that if immediate sufficient mitigation measures were not undertaken, the peak of the COVID-19 wave was four–six weeks away where we would see a total of 15–25 crore people infected and about 12.5 lakh fatalities. Of these, 18 crore infections would likely occur at the peak in early June and almost 20 per cent of those would have moderate to severe disease and require some kind of medical supervision in a hospital due to lack of proven treatment and about 10 per cent would require oxygen support.

India would have to immediately work on aggressive strategies to what the experts were calling 'flatten the curve'. This would mean taking measures to artificially push the intensity of the infection's growth by taking immediate measures. This would buy us time for capacity building, stocking of essentials, disseminating information to the last mile as well as preparing healthcare infrastructure in order to handle the cases. If we would fail to sufficiently flatten the curve, a tsunami of cases would hit us, out of which lakhs would require hospital beds, ICU beds, ventilators and doctors in numbers which India simply did not have readily available at that point in time. Our entire healthcare infrastructure would quickly crumble. As per the Dr Paul and Prof. VijayRaghavan-led team's estimates, for a surge of 1,50,000 patients on a given day during the peak, about 30,000 people would require hospitalization due to moderate and severe disease. Further, they derived that using the estimate of 15,000 beds which would be required for 1,000 new admissions, approximately 4.5 lakh beds would be needed—out of which 1,50,000 would have to be ICU beds and 3,00,000 would have to be non-ICU beds with provision for oxygen. This number was 40 per cent of all existing bed capacity in India—which meant that 40 per cent of all beds in the country would have to be augmented for COVID-19 patients only.

The first step to be taken was to stop the exchange of travellers from COVID-19-hit countries and airports. India would have to suspend all visas, except a few select categories like diplomatic and employment visas. A recommendation on the lines was made by the Cabinet secretary which further trickled down to the Empowered Group of Ministers, who agreed to green light the decision in their sixth meeting, under the chairmanship of the Union health minister.[10] Starting 13 March, the suspension of visas came into effect. Indian nationals arriving from countries with high caseloads, such as China, Italy, Iran, the Republic of Korea, France, Spain and Germany after 15 February 2020 would be quarantined for a minimum of 14 days. Indians were also strongly advised to avoid non-essential travel.

After the intensity of the projected peak figures, it was clear to everyone present in the meeting with Dr Paul and Dr VijayRaghavan at the PMO that locking down the country for a limited number of weeks in order to break the chain of transmission was the only solution. The chief economic advisor, along with other economic experts would have to put together a report on the impact of complete economic shutdown. In the month of February, the total Goods and Services Tax (GST) collected was ₹1.05 lakh crore, consistent with collections of the past quarter. Based on those numbers, India would need to evaluate the GDP and growth impact and draw up financial measures which would help individuals and businesses sustain.

Only a day before India announced visa suspension, the WHO had announced that COVID-19 was a global pandemic.[11] With states beginning to shut down public spaces, offices and schools and the risk of the contagion levelling up to community spread, the business sentiment was at an all-time low. On 12 March, following the 10 per cent Dow Jones crash in the US, the worst since 1987, the Sensex plummeted 8.03 per cent (2,919 points).[12] More dominoes fell as the Indian Premier League (IPL), which was scheduled to begin soon, made an announcement that considering the coronavirus situation in the country, all scheduled matches would be postponed to 15 April at least, after which the Board of Control for Cricket in India (BCCI) would consult with the government and other stakeholders to decide the schedule of matches.[13] The IPL is the biggest sporting event of the year in India, with thousands of crores of ad revenue and ticket sales at stake.

◆

Panic was quickly spreading countrywide. Indians returning home from oversees were falling sick and many were presenting in emergency wards of hospitals with complaints of shortness of breath. In the absence of guidelines from the state government, private hospitals were admitting these patients, without being equipped to handle COVID-19 cases. They hadn't created isolation wards, or trained the staff on SOPs to follow for appropriate handling of such cases.

Mr MP, a 64-year-old resident of an eastern suburb of Mumbai, had returned to India from the United Arab Emirates (UAE) on 6 March 2020. Following some increasing restlessness and shortness of breath, he presented himself at Hinduja Hospital in Mahim, Mumbai, where he was immediately admitted under the care of leading pulmonologist Dr Zarir Udwadia. Some pneumonia patches had shown up on his chest x-ray and he was being treated for pneumonia. Just to double check, the hospital had collected his nasal and throat swabs and sent them for COVID-19 testing. The authorities were so sure that he just had a bad case of pneumonia that they didn't fast-track testing. By the time the test results came back, it had been about four days and the patient had shown early signs of recovery. In early March, the samples had to be sent to NIV (Pune) and the turnaround time for the results to come back was anywhere between four to five days. He had tested positive for the novel coronavirus. The Maharashtra state government guidelines at that point had disallowed private entities to treat COVID-19 patients. Thus, in a hurry, in the following few hours of MP testing positive, he was shifted to the government-run Kasturba Gandhi Hospital, where he was placed in a separate isolation room. All his primary contacts were traced and placed in an isolation ward at the same hospital, and their samples collected for testing. Havoc followed at Hinduja Hospital as 82 doctors and frontline workers who had come in contact with the patient had to be isolated and quarantined, since the hospital did not follow any COVID-19 protocol, in the absence of SOPs. The out-patient department was temporarily shut down.[14] A day after being shifted, MP's shortness of breath got worse and his oxygen levels suddenly dropped. Unfortunately, Kasturba Gandhi Hospital was not equipped with an ICU or even a ventilator and MP had to be put on a BiPap machine, instead of a ventilator, in order to stabilize his oxygen concentration. His family pleaded to the hospital authorities and even tried to reach out to the state government to make an effort to shift him back to a facility with a ventilator and an ICU. Sadly, due to the prevailing guidelines, they were not allowed to do so.

The subsequent day, on 14 March, patient MP's oxygen levels dropped further and he passed away.[15] From his primary contacts, his wife and son also tested positive. Due to the prevalent stigma, the building complex where they resided refused to let staff or services reach their door. The family who had tested negative and were quarantined at home were not able to order groceries, their garbage remained uncollected and people were banned from entering their floor. Not only was the loss of a family member devastating, but societal isolation made it insufferable for the family to bear.[16] Panic pausing of Hinduja Hospital due to their staff in isolation was attributed to the rumour that the family had not disclosed MP's travel history (which they did as per the hospital's medical history record). Media hounded the gates of their housing complex and the blame game took centre stage, compounding the stigma they were already facing. Eventually, the Municipal Corporation of Greater Mumbai (MCGM) had to send social workers and councillors to sensitize and educate the neighbours. The grieving wife and son in the adjacent isolation ward at Kasturba Gandhi Hospital were not allowed to see the body. It was wrapped in a plastic body bag, transported to the nearby morgue by officials of the MCGM and the local police. Relatives who had tested negative were not allowed to perform the last rites of the Hindu man or go anywhere near him. The only glimpses they got of their beloved family member were from a distance and that too of the body bag tied up with ropes to a wooden stretcher as it was being ferried out of the ambulance for mandatory electric cremation. The whole experience was mortifying—unheard of and unseen.

In MP's case, the Maharashtra state government along with the MCGM should have ensured that he received appropriate oxygen support and medical care instead of announcing a blanket ban on private hospitals treating COVID-19 positive patients prematurely. They should have strengthened their own infrastructure first without shoving patients in facilities which weren't even equipped with ventilators or ICUs. Several lives could have been saved if it wasn't for such instances of policy paralysis in many state governments. However, a crisis like this was going to be beyond the scope of a state government and would turn out to be highly challenging even for a competent central government. Countries simply did not have at their ready disposal the tools to fight an unknown biological enemy. Very few governments are capable of building new hospital structures on an emergency basis. And even fewer have the manufacturing companies to make new medical supplies in quantities which India's projected need was. However, after the initial shock of COVID-19 fatalities, many states set up state-specific COVID-19 task forces and specific teams of experts to help form state response guidelines.

As case studies of such episodes made their way to the ears of the Health Department and the PMO, there was agreement that although health is a state subject, in a pandemic of such sort, the Centre would have to lead with detailed guidelines, policies and orders.

# 5

## JUNTA CURFEW

**14 MARCH 2020**

**INDIA | 88 ACTIVE CASES | 2 DEATHS**

**WORLD | 1,14,719 ACTIVE CASES | 5,869 DEATHS**

A renowned Washington D.C.-based epidemiologist gave select media interviews painting a dire picture of the coronavirus situation in India and the doomsday which lay ahead for the country. He predicted using a mathematical simulation model that India was likely to be the next COVID-19 hotspot, with 40–50 per cent of Indians eventually infected by the month of July 2020, thus amounting to 300–500 million people on the higher end. He also said that about four to eight million patients would require ICU beds which we only had about 70-something thousands of. This prediction was based on his 'IndiaSim model', a generic simulation, mathematical model of the Indian population which his team had been using for other infectious diseases and had adapted to coronavirus specifics. In order to produce India-specific predictions, the model was further adapted to include Indian demographic data such as age and medical facilities data. He stated in his interviews that the UK had recently admitted that they had underestimated the number of cases by a factor of 12 and insisted that India must give itself a similar report card. In his media bytes, he also imparted several suggestions to the GoI and insisted that they immediately consider them in order to allay his predicted apocalyptic situation. His choice of interviewers was controversial and more often than not, he let the interviewer get the better of what should have been a neutral scientific conversation by politically charging the discussion. However, intrigued by his confidence in the predictions, the PMO invited him to make a presentation explaining the model behind arriving at those figures. If there was credibility in the science, the PMO and authorities in the Ministry of Health were most certainly open to taking up his recommendations. When he made the presentation, there certainly was merit in his suggestions to build capacity on a war footing. Just like many other scientists and political leaders, he too opined that the country must go into immediate lockdown, albeit with a caveat that India did not have the luxury to lock down. Other suggestions from him about not mandating mask wearing or not conducting RT-PCR (reverse transcription–polymerase chain reaction) tests on asymptomatic patients didn't seem to be backed by new, emerging, evidence-based practices.

Just like him, several other Indian scientists and doctors were also reaching out to the PMO before speaking extensively to the media. One prominent name was Dr Devi Shetty, cardiac surgeon and founder of Narayana Health, a chain of 21 medical centres in India and a recipient of the Padma Shri and Padma Bhushan awards in 2004 and 2012, respectively, for his contribution to the field of affordable healthcare in India. Dr Shetty was in touch with the PMO right from early March, providing insights and advice on capacity building that India should undertake, right from building temporary facilities, onboarding more doctors and nurses, increasing testing capacities and guiding the GoI on SOPs for patient care.

In mid-March, with the onslaught of new cases within the country on the verge of entering Stage 3 of the disease, which would mean community transmission of the contagion, Dr Shetty reached out to Principal Secretary Dr Mishra, who advised that we could no longer consider a partial lockdown as a mitigation measure since the virus was extremely contagious and transmissible. Only a complete restriction on movement would reduce viral transmission dramatically. In one of his interviews later that week to *The Times of India*, Dr Shetty reiterated what he communicated to Dr Mishra, that if India didn't shut down now, we would be forced to shut down a month later, when cases would have exploded and our healthcare facilities would be totally overburdened. He added that most western countries in the grip of the pandemic were too late in responding with locking down. If Lombardy, a city with the most advanced healthcare system in the world, couldn't ventilate all its elderly population presenting at emergency wards, then India would not stand a chance without significantly upgrading capacities in the weeks of locking down.[1]

Similarly, Dr Shashank R. Joshi, Padma Shri awardee, noted endocrinologist and a member of Maharashtra's COVID-19 Task Force, in an opinion piece in *The Indian Express* titled 'Smart-locking India' expressed that, 'As health is both a central and state subject, there is an urgent need to clamp down on all major cities and towns, in all aspects: From travel to mass gatherings, to schools, colleges and workplaces. Only then can we prevent an Italy- or China-like situation in India. It's time to halt COVID-19 by smartly locking the country at home so that we can have a better tomorrow. This needs a political will which we currently have.'[2]

◆

The prime minister chaired a meeting in the second week of March which was attended by most senior officials of the PMO including the principal secretary, the PM's advisors, Cabinet secretary, officers on special duty, secretaries, joint secretaries and high-ranking officials of various departments. In this meeting, he was briefed in detail on the status of the rising cases, the economic impact of a lockdown, the status of essentials and capacity building efforts along with timelines. Consensus was achieved in the meeting that India, in order to protect its people, would need to go into an immediate and complete lockdown. There would have to be a complete shutdown of movement, nationwide.

It was discussed that we would have to start with a 21-day lockdown, monitor the status of the viral transmission as well as the status of our healthcare infrastructure before deciding on any extensions. A huge concern was of our most vulnerable sections of the society, those who sustain their family on daily wages. It was anticipated that lakhs and crores of people would lose their day jobs and would most likely run out of their meagre savings in a matter of days, if any. The prime minister categorically insisted that minute details of how the government would supply food to these workers and their families be planned. The officials discussed an option of the lockdown to be announced in a phased manner so that their approach could be tweaked as per the evolution of the case trajectory. However, the team agreed that if people were given an advance ultimatum, they would travel back to their villages, crowding in public transport and take the infection to remote parts of the country where the state of health infrastructure was extremely poor. Our rural health infrastructure would certainly at that point in time be unable to handle a new disease and a high caseload, and we would lose lakhs of lives. The migrants would have to stay in the cities. At least until we were able to build some capacities in terms of beds and testing kits, and supply essential medicines and ventilators to the rural and semi-urban hospitals. The last time the Indian government was needed to rise to a challenge of this magnitude was perhaps during the time of Partition in 1947, when it had to mobilize all of its bureaucracy and security forces to rehabilitate people arriving in the country while ensuring that the security situation remained under control.

When the suggestion to announce lockdown within the next couple of days was made, the prime minister put his foot down. He opined that with no notice at all, we cannot ask 1.3+ billion people to stay where they are. Parliament was in session, Members of Parliament would need to return to their home constituencies to assist the people in the difficult times that lay ahead of us. Citizens may have other kinds of emergencies as well like aged parents living alone to be moved, or children in boarding schools to be brought home. Some sort of preview of the upcoming weeks to prepare the citizens must be offered. The prime minister has made it a practice to involve people in every major initiative that he undertakes in the spirit of *jan bhagidari* (people's participation/people partnership). The steps India had to take in the days ahead would not be possible without that spirit. He had been keenly observing the trends in various parts of the country and knew that high-handedness would not work. As a man who has spent at least a night in almost every district of India, he has a tremendous grip on the psyche of the Indian people. With the richness of this experience, he fully understood the challenges associated with the diversity, the geography and complexity of India. As a result, he thought of a day-long, self-imposed curfew—a junta curfew, just a couple of days before completely locking down. Even though the curfew would be self-imposed, it would be crucial for every single Indian to get the prime minister's message. The question arose: how would we get important messages across to every single Indian in such a limited time frame? This question would occupy the prime minister's mind frequently over the course of the next few months. As someone who frequently referred to history pages for reference and inspiration, the prime minister was well aware that for Mahatma Gandhi too, it was challenging to get the entire nation behind the freedom struggle, especially the Northeast. In fact, at the time before Independence, the central leaders of the Congress believed that the independence of India would be delayed due to the stand of the political leadership of Assam (which then included most of today's Northeast—Arunachal Pradesh, Nagaland, Mizoram and Meghalaya).[3] If the usual means of information dissemination were to be activated, it would take at least a couple of weeks for information to pass down to the last mile. A televised address at prime time would be viewed by about 30–40 million people, social media activation would at best be seen by another 20–30 million from his 70 million Twitter and 46 million Facebook followers. That would still leave out over half of the country. The prime minister was also very aware that to effectively communicate with the people, he would have to develop a relationship of trust by stating facts in a language that every Indian could relate to, so that they could accept and follow the plan. He then suggested that they adopt a call to action which would involve asking people to come out to their balconies and doors and clap, play an instrument or even just bang together some vessels at a given time during the junta curfew. This call to action would be dedicated to the frontline and healthcare workers who were risking their lives by being on the call of duty, out of their homes to keep the rest of us safe. This would achieve multiple aims. First of all, hearing the clamour in the neighbourhood and experiencing the positive spirit, even the people who hadn't heard of the self-imposed curfew via messages in the media, would learn of it. This would be the power of 'one to many' exponential communication. Second, this would create an atmosphere of motivation and positivity when the entire country of 130 crore people was going to pass through uncharted territory, not knowing what lies ahead of them. And third, the prime minister knew that with rising cases, there would be a possibility of friction and altercation between people and healthcare workers. By reminding the society right in the beginning of our war against COVID-19 to be grateful to the healthcare workers, he tried to address this problem as well. So, it was settled then, the prime minister would make a televised address to the nation in the next few days asking folks to follow a self-imposed curfew and a day after that, he would announce a total countrywide lockdown.

The officials would use the few days between the meeting and the call to lockdown to streamline the supply of essential items. By this day, India had already expanded its network of labs to test COVID-19 to 52. The Ministry of Home Affairs had also guided the states and Union Territories (UTs) to draw funds from the State Disaster Response Fund (SDRF), in addition to the funds granted by the National Health Mission to expand medical infrastructure and testing capabilities.

◆

## 15 MARCH 2020

### INDIA | 99 ACTIVE CASES | 2 DEATHS
### WORLD | 1,31,723 ACTIVE CASES | 6,581 DEATHS

On 13 March, the prime minister, via his Twitter handle, announced that the South Asian Association for Regional Cooperation (SAARC) nations should get together in their fight against COVID-19: 'I would like to propose that the leadership of SAARC nations chalk out a strong strategy to fight Coronavirus. Together, we can set an example to the world, and contribute to a healthier planet.'[4]

The last SAARC Summit was held in November 2014 in Kathmandu, immediately after the prime minister was sworn in. The next scheduled one was to take place in November 2016, but due to heightened tensions between India and Pakistan over an attack on our military camp in Uri, the Summit was called off.[5] However, the prime minister always maintained his firm belief in his vision to emphasize the centrality of India's neighbourhood in its larger foreign policy agenda—Neighbourhood First Policy. With the COVID-19 pandemic looming and nations such as Sri Lanka, Bangladesh and Nepal strongly advocating for SAARC to take action before the case numbers reached alarming levels, it was time for India, as a regional powerhouse, to extend and even lead strategic efforts which would benefit all the neighbourhood nations in the combined fight. In fact, hours after the prime minister's tweet, several SAARC leaders hailed the prime minister's move.[6]

PM Modi's tweet read, 'I would like to propose that the leadership of SAARC nations chalk out a strong strategy to fight Coronavirus. We could discuss, via video conferencing, ways to keep our citizens healthy. Together, we can set an example to the world, and contribute to a healthier planet.' The Prime Minister of Bhutan Lotay Tshering tweeted in a reply to his Indian counterpart Modi's tweet, 'This is what we call leadership. As members of this region, we must come together in such times. Smaller economies are hit harder, so we must coordinate. With your leadership, I have no doubt we will see immediate and impactful outcome. Looking forward to the video conference.'[7]

Nepali Prime Minister K.P. Sharma Oli replied, 'I welcome the idea advanced by Prime Minister Modiji @narendramodi for chalking out a strong strategy by the leadership of the SAARC nations to fight Coronavirus. My government is ready to work closely with SAARC Member States to protect our citizens from this deadly disease.'[8]

The President of Maldives Ibrahim Mohamed Solih showed his support as well, 'Thank you PM @narendramodi for taking the initiative on this important endeavor. COVID 19 requires collective effort to defeat it. Maldives welcomes this proposal and would fully support such a regional effort.'[9]

Bangladeshi Prime Minister Sheikh Hasina, too, showed her readiness and enthusiasm to engage as per a tweet by Bangladesh's Minister of State for Foreign Affairs. Adding to the list, the Afghan envoy in New Delhi Tahir Qadiry also acknowledged PM Modi's call. Pakistan, too, conveyed via diplomatic channels that its Special Assistant to the Prime Minister would join the video conference.

On 15 March, the video conference of SAARC leaders on combatting COVID-19 was held. In his opening remarks, the prime minister advocated for collaboration over confusion and preparation over panic.[10] He pointed out that SAARC nations face similar challenges in terms of dense population, our interconnected societies and access to healthcare. He informed the leaders on various proactive steps that India has been taking such as upgrading our response mechanism, screenings at airports, gradual increase in travel restrictions, increasing public-awareness campaigns on television, print and social media, efforts to quickly ramp up our healthcare system, including training of healthcare staff, increasing diagnostic capacities (going from one to 66 in two months), developing protocols for managing each stage of the pandemic, contact tracing of suspected cases, management of quarantine and isolation facilities, evacuating over 1,400 Indians and citizens of neighbourhood nations from different countries and building protocol for such evacuations including carrying out testing by deployed mobile teams.[11]

In his remarks on the way forward, the prime minister proposed the creation of a COVID-19 emergency fund based on voluntary contributions. He added that India would begin by offering $10 billion and that any of the member nations could utilize the fund in their fight against the virus.

He also added that India would assemble a rapid response team of doctors and specialists equipped with testing kits and other essential items which will be on standby to be placed at the disposal on any nation's requirement. He further stated that India can provide online training for emergency response teams of member nations based on the model we have used to raise the capacity of our emergency personnel. He further informed that India has set up an integrated disease surveillance portal to better trace possible virus carriers and their contacts which we would be happy to share along with training on how to use it. He insisted that the SAARC Disaster Management Centre must collate the best practices among all of us and set up a common platform for research on controlling epidemics in the South Asian region. He added that the ICMR can help to coordinate this exercise. As a parting note, Modi mentioned that India will ask its experts to brainstorm on longer economic consequences of COVID-19 and how we can insulate our internal trade and local value chains from its impact.[12]

In his concluding remarks, the prime minister expressed his desire to work on strengthening cooperation between the SAARC nations to together fight the pandemic and share knowledge-based practices, capacities and resources wherever possible.[13]

Even before the announcement for a SAARC video conference, the prime minister, on 12 March, had spoken with the British prime minister, Boris Johnson and Israeli prime minister Benjamin Netanyahu on the evolving COVID-19 crisis and the response mechanisms of both countries. In the spirit of collaboration, on 17 March, he had a conversation with the Crown Prince of Saudi Arabia Mohammed bin Salman on what both countries were undertaking in their fight against the virus.

◆

## 18 MARCH 2020

INDIA | 152 ACTIVE CASES | 3 DEATHS

WORLD | 1,92,164 ACTIVE CASES | 9,070 DEATHS

After New Delhi announced a ban on religious gatherings of over 50 people on 16 March and effectively began to gradually shut down, several attendees at the Banglewadi Nizamuddin Masjid Markaz vacated the property, taking buses, trains and planes fanning out to different parts of the country. Two initial incidents raised the alarm that the masjid may have become a COVID-19 hotspot, with thousands of missionaries still housed inside the building. A man, from Karimnagar district in Telangana who was hosting a group of 10 preachers and had arrived by train on 14 March from the Markaz, tested positive for coronavirus after displaying symptoms. On contact tracing, the state authorities tracked down all the 10 preachers, out of which eight tested positive for the virus. As soon as the results came back, the state government announced restrictions in a 3 km radius around their movement area, making it a 'containment zone', the first of many to come over the next couple of months.[14]

Earlier in the week, on 13 March, a frail-looking Thai national who had returned from the Markaz was stopped by the authorities at Coimbatore airport. He was admitted to the hospital but passed away on 17 March due to renal failure. The authorities were able to contact trace members of the group of Jamaat returnees he was travelling with before he passed away and send their samples for testing.[15]

As per information received from these groups, even though the congregation itself was a three-day event, several groups of missionaries were travelling to various parts of the country before and after the congregation to recruit more people. It was more of a rolling affair which was taking place in the first two weeks of March. As per an estimate, 2,100 foreigners visited India for Tablighi activities since 1 January, while approximately 824 of them, as on 21 March, had disseminated to various parts of the country for recruitment and missionary work after being present at the congregation.[16] About 216 foreign missionaries were estimated to still be in the masjid, in addition to over 1,500 Indian Jamaatis.

◆

## 19 MARCH 2020

### INDIA | 170 ACTIVE CASES | 4 DEATHS
### WORLD | 2,20,366 ACTIVE CASES | 10,198 DEATHS

By now, most state governments had announced strict restrictions on movement, closed down restaurants, cinemas, schools and colleges and banned public gatherings. Within the next couple of days, even before the prime minister would announce a national lockdown, Bihar, Chandigarh, Chhattisgarh, Delhi, Haryana, Himachal Pradesh, Karnataka, Kerala, Madhya Pradesh, Maharashtra, Manipur, Odisha, Punjab, Puducherry, Rajasthan (first state to issue complete lockdown), Sikkim, Tamil Nadu, Telangana, Uttar Pradesh, Uttarakhand and West Bengal would issue various curbs and curfews. A noteworthy piece of information is that none of these aforementioned states gave any prior warning before issuing total curfew or lockdown orders. Several large groups had begun to reach out to the prime minister calling for an immediate, total restriction in movement. A group of venture capitalists and leading start-ups appealed to the prime minister, 'While containment efforts should continue, imposing a lockdown and Section 144 now, versus 30 days later, might reduce deaths by 5x (saving nearly 10,000 lives).'[17]

Leaders from opposition parties had also begun to actively advocate locking down instantly. A case in point, former Union home minister during the UPA regime, P. Chidambaram, posted a series of tweets on 19 March tagging the prime minister, PMOIndia, chief minister of Maharashtra Uddhav Thackeray and (now former) chief minister of Tamil Nadu Edappadi Palaniswami:

> After WHO Director General's statement yesterday, there should be no hesitation in ordering an immediate lockdown of all our towns and cities for 2–4 weeks. Even after we have witnessed what is happening in Italy, Iran and Spain, why is the government refusing to take the logical step of a lockdown? Some states that are ahead of the central government should go ahead and lock down their towns and cities. Since ICMR's random sample testing has revealed that there is no community transmission (Stage 3) so far, this is the moment to announce a temporary lockdown and contain the disease at Stage 2.[18]

While some of them, like the aforementioned examples, offered data and scientific facts in their advice, others gave headline-making statements to the press without offering any useful suggestions. For instance, Congress leader Rahul Gandhi spoke to media outside Parliament, 'India should be preparing itself not just for COVID-19 but for the economic devastation that's coming. I am saying it again and again. I am sorry to say this but our people are going to go through unimaginable pain in the next six months.' He added, 'I will tell you a story... In Andaman and Nicobar, before the tsunami came, the water went out. When the water went out, everybody went to get the fish. When they went, the water (levels) came up. I have been warning the government. They are fooling around... they are not clear about what to do. Coronavirus is like a tsunami.'[19]

◆

In perhaps the most difficult speech to give in his tenure, the prime minister was scheduled to be on national television in the later part of the day to prepare the country for the tough days that lay ahead. Effectively communicating key points was absolutely crucial, now more than ever. As he sat down with his speech writers deliberating the important points which should absolutely find mention, one of the challenges was to explain the concept of social distancing to the people. How does one even begin to explain to the people who live in such congested, interconnected societies like ours that staying physically apart from each other would be a lifesaver? Like all of his national addresses, Hindi would be the language of delivery. But in Hindi, social distancing literally translates to *'samaajik doori'*. *Samaajik doori* has negative connotations as it alludes to creating a distance between social classes in our caste-based system, so using that literal translation would certainly not be appropriate. On further thought, he suggested that he use the term *'do gaj ki doori'* instead, which in English translates to a 'two-yard distance'.

To accurately depict the seriousness of the situation, he would have to allude to a human tragedy of this scale and thus he would make a reference to the World Wars I and II, in which even, these many countries were not impacted as were by the novel coronavirus. He would also use the war analogy to remind senior citizens about times of blackout where towns and cities would turn off all lights in the night and restrict movement so as not to be spotted by enemy planes from the skies.

He would have to be a commander-in-chief, a unifier and a consoler-in-chief who India can trust with their lives.

So, when he went on television, the dismal situation reflected on his face. His eyes were grave and his words, measured. He admonished the attitude which had developed in the community—the attitude that India has escaped the wrath of the virus and that life should go on as is. He warned that this attitude would cost Indians many lives.

> Till now, science has not been able to find a definite solution to save us from the Corona pandemic, neither has a vaccine been developed. In such a situation, it is very natural to get worried. Study of the countries most affected by Corona virus has revealed another aspect. In these countries, the spread of the disease has witnessed almost an explosion after the initial few days. The number of people infected by Corona has grown at a rapid pace. The Government is tracking the spread of the disease around the world closely. And we see that there are a few countries which have controlled the situation by taking swift decisions and isolating its people as much as possible. This burgeoning crisis of Corona is not an ordinary occurrence for a nation like India with a population of 130 crore, striving for development. Therefore, as we witness the wide-spread impact of the Corona pandemic even in major, developed countries today, it is wrong to assume that India will not be impacted by it.[20]

He went on to explain that preventing one's self from contracting the disease was the best measure at this point, in the absence of proven treatments or vaccines. And the way to do that would be to follow 'social distancing'.

> During such a pandemic, only one mantra can take us through: *'Hum swasth, toh jag swasth* (If we are healthy, the world will be healthy, too)'. Patience is an essential virtue to avoid this disease, and keep oneself healthy. Practising this patience would mean staying away from crowds and avoiding leaving your homes. This is called 'social distancing' nowadays, and is critical in these times of the global corona pandemic. Our determination and patience will play a crucial role in containing the impact of this global pandemic. It is wrong if you believe that you are okay and nothing can happen to you,

that you can continue roaming around in markets and streets as usual and remain unaffected. By doing this, you will not only be risking yourself but also your family. Keeping this is mind, I appeal to you all that for the next few weeks, step out of your homes only when absolutely necessary. As far as possible, try and do your work, whether related to business or job, from home.

While it is essential that those who are in government services, healthcare services, people's representatives, media personnel remain active, everybody else must however, isolate themselves from the rest of society.[21]

He went on to announce that all Indians, except those involved in essential services, should follow a self-imposed curfew on 22 March, the coming Sunday, from 7.00 a.m. to 9.00 p.m. He added that this people's curfew will be a litmus test for us, as a nation, to assess how prepared we are in spirit to fight off the COVID-19 pandemic.

He insisted that not only on that particular day should people refrain from venturing out of their homes, but even on other days they should avoid stepping out in public places. Backed by the fatality numbers coming from other countries, he added that senior citizens were at an increased risk and must stay put in the safety of their homes.

In the spirit of *'seva parmo dharma* (service to humanity is the supreme duty)', as a tribute to healthcare workers and those in essential services who risk their lives on a daily basis so that others can stay safe at home, he appealed to the people to 'express our gratitude to all such people. On Sunday at exactly 5.00 p.m., we must all stand at the doors, balconies and windows of our homes to give them a five-minute standing ovation by clapping hands, playing instruments, beating utensils or ringing bells to boost their morale and salute their service.'[22]

As a parting note, the prime minister announced that the government was mindful of the disruptions that COVID-19 restrictions would cause to businesses and, consequently, the economy. Therefore, to address these upcoming challenges, he declared the creation of a COVID-19 Economic Response Task Force under the leadership of Union Finance Minister Nirmala Sitharaman. He ended his speech by asking the people of the country, especially businesses and high-income segments of the society to show empathy to the middle class, lower middle class and the economically backward and continue to keep them on their payroll and offer as much financial assistance as possible. With a final piece of advice to not fall prey to unnecessary rumour-mongering and superstition, the prime minister ended his address to the nation.

# 6

## EMPOWERED TEAMS

**20 MARCH 2020**

**INDIA | 221 ACTIVE CASES | 5 DEATHS**

**WORLD | 2,54,394 ACTIVE CASES | 11,623 DEATHS**

As the multilayered COVID-19 Economic Response Task Force assembled, comprising the chief economic advisor and several high-ranking bureaucrats from the Finance Ministry, experts discussed the potential economic hit due to disruptions caused by the pandemic. They were in agreement that the pandemic would vividly expose inequalities in the Indian society. The bottom 10 per cent in the economic spectrum would most likely lose their jobs. The folks who were on day jobs and had migrated to cities would be the first ones to lose their income, making it hard for them to put food on the table. Evidence shows that the bottom half of the income tier is the one who suffers the most in a recession and hence, our schemes and packages would have to be created to alleviate the pain that these folks were about to endure. But what kind of stimulus package would be good enough? The prime minister had made it amply clear that no Indian must starve to death. This would mean putting food on each Indian's table. What kind of arrangements in terms of finances, stockpiling of grains and transportation would need to be made to achieve that goal? What other kinds of stimulus outflows would be required for businesses and the middle class to ensure sustenance?

At this point, it became imperative to take a look at what other countries were providing, and the economic theories supporting those decisions. The US was about to pass a $2.2 trillion Coronavirus Aid, Relief, and Economic Security (CARES) stimulus package, which would include increased unemployment benefits, one-time cash payouts to citizens ($1,400) and forgivable loans to small businesses. Chair of the Small Business Committee in the US Senate, Marco Rubio, observed, 'I would never vote to support the payroll of small business in normal times. I believe in free enterprise, it's the best way to generate growth. But the purpose of the economy is to serve people, not people to serve the economy.'[1] Japan gave out $900 cash in hand to all citizens as well. In a number of European countries, the governments had resorted to extensive loan guarantees to help keep businesses afloat. But ultimately, this was money which would have to be paid back. It is imperative to note that a number of European countries already have strong social programmes in place. European countries decided to pay companies so that they could continue to keep people on their payroll piggybacking on the theory that the employer–employee relationship must not suffer. The US, on the contrary, was offering increased unemployment benefits to those laid off.

The cornerstone of framing economic policies for governments world over still remains an amalgamation of theories propagated by two magnetic and influential economists of the twentieth century—John Maynard Keynes and Friedrich von Hayek. Keynes's work *The General Theory of Employment, Interest and Money* (published in 1936) defines the role of the government in capitalist societies leading to increased regulation and the creation of global institutions such as the World Bank and the International Monetary Fund. His theory hugely propagates that in times of crisis, substantial government spending would kick-start consumption and cause businesses to expand, thereby reducing unemployment.

In contrast, Hayek's work *The Road to Serfdom* (published in 1944) and, subsequently, his paper titled 'The Use of Knowledge in Society' (published in the September 1945 issue of *The American Economic Review*) theorizes that government control of the economy inevitably crushes individual freedom, leading to tyranny. He argued that central planning can never replace market forces.

If we were to apply these theories to the economic impact due to the COVID-19 crisis in India, Hayek would have argued that trying to return to the status quo, by extreme handholding by the government would block the opportunity to create the economy of the future, leading to long-term stagnation which the fastest-growing, large economy like India's couldn't afford. Keynes, on the other hand, would have proposed vigorous government intervention and spending like cash handouts and putting large amounts of money in people's and business' pockets, thus awakening demand and lifting spirits of the businesses to hire more people. He would have advocated that in a major recession, only the government has the resources to prod society back on its feet. For India, this would be a major challenge, since we were still not a 'rich economy' and several billion pockets would need to be filled, causing extreme strain on the exchequer. The solution, as the members of the COVID-19 Economic Response Task Force concurred, lay somewhere in the middle of the two theories. It was certainly clear to them though that this could possibly be the greatest economic crisis India would see since Independence.

And hence, the immediate relief package that India would give out would include some cash handouts by way of direct benefit transfers to limited, vulnerable groups. Money would be transferred to Women Jan-Dhan account holders, 8.69 crore farmers, widows and handicapped persons under the poverty line. Wages of those employed in the government's rural employment guarantee scheme and pensioners would be increased. Families below the poverty line would also be given free gas cylinders for the next three months. A majority of the immediate stimulus would go towards supply of free food grains—5 kg of rice/wheat and 1 kg pulses to 80 crore people, in addition to what they were already receiving. Insurance cover for frontline workers would be increased and some initiatives for workers of the organized and construction sectors would also be carved out.

◆

Meanwhile, the frequent meetings that Dr Paul and PSA Prof. VijayRaghavan were having, right from January 2020, were now expanded to include 18 more members comprising scientists, doctors, modellers, academicians and bureaucrats. Constituted by the PMO, it was called the R&D Task Force for COVID-19 Research and was primarily responsible for providing sound scientific advice on aspects such as spread of the virus, the role of science, the direction that the country should take to shape its response and so on. They were also responsible for closely studying emerging evidence and responses by other nations hit by the virus.

At around the same time, ICMR constituted a National Task Force (NTF) too, chaired by Dr Paul and co-chaired by secretary (Department of Health) and Dr Bhargava to focus on epidemiological matters related to the pandemic. Members in the NTF ranged from celebrated clinicians such as Dr Guleria and epidemiologists such as Dr Raman Gangakhedkar to top-ranking leadership from the National Institute of Allergy and Infectious Diseases, the Public Health Foundation of India, the WHO, the National Institute of Epidemiology, the National Centre for Disease Control and the Enterovirus Research Centre, alongside several scientists from the ICMR system. The NTF looked at downstream research, seeking solutions to COVID-19-related clinical epidemiology issues such as how the disease was spreading and establishing a clinical registry on COVID-19. The NTF also deliberated upon and issued guidelines on testing criteria which would include advice on who would need to be tested and when it would be appropriate to use RT-PCR versus antigen and antibody tests. The group also considered emerging treatments by looking at all the available evidence from global scientific papers—peer reviewed as well as unpublished, after which it would make a decision on whether that particular treatment protocol should be used and under what caveats, i.e., the considerations to be made for people with comorbidities, dosages to be used for varying levels of the infection and such. It is in the NTF that the need to lock down the country was first discussed. The prime minister stayed on top of the information relayed by the scientists in the NTF and it was on their recommendation that he decided to lock down the country.

Closing the chain of hassle-free communication, the empowered groups which were to be created after the prime minister's instructions following the 4 March meeting in the PMO were now in place. Eleven empowered groups would be formed to begin with. Each group would consist of experts in the subject area of the group, senior bureaucrats from ministries which would be needed in order to achieve the objectives set forth by that particular group as well as one senior official from the PMO. The groups would not have a chairperson or a leader, but a convener instead, so as to allow senior forces across spectrums to put forth their ideas equivocally, without a clash of egos. Although the official order from the Ministry of Home Affairs was yet to come, the groups had not only been constituted but had also begun to conduct meetings on a daily basis.

The R&D Task Force for COVID-19 Research and NTF would outline policy, evidence-based practices and administrative requirement for capacity building. These decisions would then trickle down to the specific empowered group which would then find a way to implement the Task Force's recommendations, streamline procurement and troubleshoot problems which cropped up in real-time basis. In the event the groups were unable to find a solution or there was a hold-up, the matter would be immediately raised for the attention of the two advisors to the prime minister. If solution of the matter was not found even then, it would be further put to the attention of Dr Mishra, who would then either find a solution or, depending on the scale of the matter, bring it to the prime minister's notice for guidance.

The broader areas of the 11 empowered groups were:

1. Setting up a medical emergency management plan;
2. Ensuring the availability of hospitals, isolation and quarantine facilities, disease surveillance measures and testing and critical-care training;
3. Ensuring the availability of essential medical equipment such as PPE kits, masks, gloves and ventilators as well as looking into their production, procurement, import and distribution;
4. Augmenting human resources and capacity building;
5. Facilitating supply chain and logistics management for the availability of necessary items such as food and medicines;
6. Coordinating with the private sector, NGOs and international organizations for response-related activities;
7. Taking up economic and welfare measures;
8. Introducing information, communication and public awareness measures;
9. Augmenting technology and data management;
10. Responding to public grievances and suggestions;
11. Considering strategic issues relating to lockdown.

As more travel restrictions were imposed across the world, several Indians living in various countries expressed their desire to return to India. Similarly, several foreigners in India also wanted to return to their home countries. This task would require coordination between governments and embassies of each country from which we would either need to bring back our citizens or send the foreigners to. Even within our government infrastructure, inter-ministerial coordination would be required to arrange for flights, visas, health status checks and so on. For this purpose, the Ministry of External Affairs set up a COVID-19 Cell, which would oversee all of the above. Over the next few months, India initiated and executed the largest evacuation exercise in the world called 'Vande Bharat Mission', which would go on to bring home 3.9 million stranded Indians between May and December 2020.

◆

The prime minister, as people who work closely with him point out, frequently draws on his experiences from his role as the chief minister of Gujarat for over 12 years. This experience, almost always urges him to think of policy decisions from the perspective of states. He truly believes that states require autonomy in decision-making as well as financial independence to excel at governance. In his view, large-scale and major policy changes or actions don't reach their potential without strong participation from the state governments. Also, deriving from his over four-term-long experience as the chief minister and one complete term as the prime minister, he had formed a strong opinion that *jan bhagidari* was crucial in ensuring success of our COVID-19 measures and for controlling the spread of the contagion. And without the state governments' wholehearted participation, *jan bhagidari* could not be achieved. It would have to be local governments and regional authorities through whom information, schemes and containment measures would need to percolate. Therefore, as an attempt to take the state leadership on board, the prime minister, flanked by the Union health minister, the secretary of the MoHFW and Dr Bhargava of the ICMR, held the first of over 15 video conferences with chief ministers of all 28 states and eight UTs, apprising them of the efforts that the central government had been taking to respond to the COVID-19 crisis. He categorically asked the chief ministers to remain vigilant and strictly follow containment measures as the next three to four weeks were going to be absolutely vital in India's fight against the virus.

◆

The global and Indian media were constantly reporting coronavirus-related stories. In Italy, the grim situation of patients being denied treatment, convoys of trucks carrying coffins through Madrid's empty streets and overflowing crematoria, and even visuals from New York of hotels being converted to quarantine centres were spine-chilling. Fear amongst the Indian masses compounded when news broke out about a celebrity singer Kanika Kapoor testing positive for coronavirus after returning from the UK and attending a party in Lucknow. When efforts to contact trace began, one after the other news of politicians and celebrities in attendance at the party isolating and testing themselves took over social media home pages. Former Chief Minister of Rajasthan Vasundhara Raje and her son, Member of Parliament (MP), Dushyant Singh were at the party and had come in contact with the singer. Raje announced that the duo would get tested and go into isolation. But before that, Dushyant had attended a breakfast meeting with the President of India, Ram Nath Kovind along with several other MPs and marked his attendance in the Lok Sabha. All those who came in contact with him including Defence Minister Rajnath Singh, Union Minister of Jal Shakti Gajendra Singh Shekhawat, actress Hema Malini, BJP MP Rajyavardhan Singh Rathore, Trinamool Congress MP Derek O'Brien and several others made announcements that they would get tested and isolate themselves as well. The same day, one of the Italian tourists who had tested positive for the virus, passed away in the hospital where he was being treated. Alarm was rapidly spreading.

The MoHFW, in an effort to ensure clear communication, disseminate any panic arising amongst the people as well as to ward off rumours and superstition began to hold daily video briefings outlining the status of the COVID-19 situation in India. They announced that there would be no issues in the supply of essential commodities at any point in time during the lockdown. They also started a COVID-19 helpline number, which would be useful in getting any kind of facts about the virus. They repeatedly assured the people that the measures taken by the government at this point were preventative, so there wouldn't come a time when the virus would get the better of us.

◆

## 22 MARCH 2020

**INDIA | 364 ACTIVE CASES | 8 DEATHS**

**WORLD | 314,668 ACTIVE CASES | 14,992 DEATHS**

As per the prime minister's orders, the country, in all its essence, followed the junta curfew. People stayed indoors, in the safe haven of their homes. All businesses, establishments, restaurants, malls and public places remained shut. Only essential and frontline workers stepped out of their homes. The usually buzzing streets went silent, with not a man in sight. At 5.00 in the evening, people came to their balconies and doorsteps to applaud and show their gratitude for the services of the doctors, nurses and essential workers who were risking their lives, akin to soldiers fighting a war at the border. Social media was abuzz with images and videos from the length and breadth of the country. From celebrities, politicians and sportspersons to the last man standing outside a small, remote hutment with a broken roof—each Indian showed this collective spirit of unity. It was a reminder for us of our grit, determination and fighting spirit; that we were all in this together. India's spirit to fight and its spirit to conquer were in full display at 5.00 p.m. for five minutes, on 22 March 2020. The prime minister's plan for his message to reach out to every single Indian was a success.

◆

During a briefing with his communications team, the prime minister expressed that he would like to receive two media reports a day going forward for his briefings, versus a single daily report. He specifically instructed them that the reports should be segmented as per the broader subjects of the empowered groups. The team henceforth would submit their media reports to him at 1.30 p.m. every afternoon and then again at 8.00 p.m. The briefing would include global news reports (from media and social media) of best practices and problems that various governments were encountering and overcoming, adversities that people within the country would face on account of the new curbs as well as remarks from the ground situation. He further instructed that he would like to keep communication channels to him and the PMO as open as possible in order to receive and respond to public grievances. If he came across any complaints in his briefings, his team would further send it to the empowered groups, who would then need to act on it immediately and submit to the PMO an action-taken report within 24 hours. Not only did he indicate that he would be personally very involved with this, but he also made it the PMO's mandate to solve these issues on-ground very quickly on a real-time basis.

In the last 10 days of March, the prime minister interacted with people from all walks of life through video-conferencing, taking their inputs, motivating them and, most importantly, involving various sections of society in the collective fight. An aide recollected how he insisted on interacting with people from diverse backgrounds because he wanted their direct suggestions and also wanted to instill a sense of confidence in them as India braced to face its biggest crisis since Independence.

On 20 March, the prime minister interacted with all the chief ministers of the country through a video conference wherein he called for tackling the challenge together. He directed them to maintain constant vigilance and monitor the spread of the virus. He insisted that the Centre and states must work closely together to combat the pandemic.

In an interaction with members of the industry, he requested them to encourage employees to work from home as well as to not cut down on workforce.

He also scheduled a video conference with leaders from the pharmaceutical industry and prodded them to expedite the manufacturing of Ribonucleic acid (RNA) testing kits which we would require in millions in order to quickly scale up testing. He assured them that the government is committed to maintaining supply of active pharmaceutical ingredients (APIs) and encouraged their manufacturing within the country. He also directed them to maintain supply of essential medicines and prevent black marketing and hoarding. By now, India had expanded its testing capacity to conduct over 50,000 to 70,000 tests per week in government laboratories. But the natural next step would be to expand the network of laboratories to include the private ones as well, in order to increase testing coverage. For reference, at this point, France was conducting 10,000 tests per week, the UK about 16,000, the US about 26,000, Germany approximately 42,000, Italy about 52,000 and South Korea approximately 80,000.

On a separate call with representatives from the media, he asked them to help spread awareness about how coronavirus spreads. He asked them to inform people about the locations of testing centres, who should get tested, whom to contact to get tested and follow home isolation protocols. He also urged the media to act as a link between the government and the people and provide continuous feedback, at both national and regional level.

Additionally, he spoke with radio jockeys (RJs) from across the country where he explained to them views of experts and steps taken by the government. PM Modi also requested the RJs to provide feedback about the difficulties and challenges faced by the people so that the government can proactively resolve them. He also exhorted the RJs to disseminate positive stories and case studies, particularly of those patients who have fully recovered from coronavirus infection, and also interplay such stories in different parts of the country, thus bringing the entire country together. He appealed to them to showcase and celebrate the contributions of the local heroes like police officers, doctors, nurses, ward boys and other frontline workers at the national level.

He also connected with AYUSH practitioners across the country who spoke about the advantages of using traditional practices in immunity boosting and yoga.

He then interacted with social welfare and spiritual organizations and suggested that they play an important role in arranging for basic necessities for the poor. He appealed to them to dedicate their medical facilities and volunteers to serving patients and the needy in this time of crisis. The prime minister also pressed that they play an active role in countering superstitions, misbeliefs and misinformation. He observed that in the name of beliefs, people have been gathering in various places flouting social-distancing norms. He added that the social welfare and spiritual organizations should actively spread the importance of maintaining social distancing to check the spread of the virus.

The pandemic was a global one and so the problems and solutions would also have to be such. Thus, perhaps in a first-of-its-kind interaction, the prime minister spoke with heads of Indian missions across the world. He directed them to attend to Indians who remain in various foreign countries, given the uncertainty of continuing international travel restrictions. He advised them to help boost the morale of compatriots abroad, and help them address issues arising from their unplanned stay, with their host governments. He also asked them to be compassionate to other problems which Indians might face abroad, including arranging shelter. He added that they stay vigilant and identify in their host countries best practices, innovations, scientific breakthroughs and sources to procure medical equipment to strengthen India's fight against COVID-19. He also advised them to focus on ensuring seamless coordination with foreign partners so that trade in essential supplies, logistic chains, remittances and such remain unaffected.

◆

India was preparing to go under a prolonged lockdown. All train services were suspended at least until 31 March, including suburban rail services and metro services. Goods trains were exempted from this. All interstate passenger transport was also suspended. Domestic flights were to be suspended with effect from the midnight of 24 March.

Meanwhile, it was no joke for the NTF to decipher between what would and would not work in India's context from constantly changing emerging experiences from other countries. Due to the very limited information that the world and the scientific community at large had about the new virus, the questions that they needed to find answers to were how would due processes and SOPs be decided? For instance, as of last week, the UK had withdrawn items of critical advice which had previously stated that asymptomatic patients could not spread the infection. A few days later, their National Health Service instructed hospital trusts to urgently discharge all medically fit patients as soon as it was clinically safe, ideally within three hours. The directive essentially was to get people out of the hospitals to their homes as soon as possible with the right support. They were calling this model 'discharge to assess (D2A)'. This model did not require testing patients for COVID-19 and waiting for them to test negative in order to discharge them. How could we be sure that we are not releasing asymptomatic carriers of the infection back into the community? The challenge was for how long could we afford to let patients occupy hospital beds if they appeared clinically healthy even though they were not testing negative on the COVID-19 test versus freeing up hospital beds faster? In such a scenario, would we be risking releasing potential spreaders into the community?

Since the ICMR constituted the NTF, it was important for them to take a comprehensive look at how most countries were competing for the same products—PPE, masks, sanitizers and ventilators—essentially coming out of Asia. The US, in fact, announced that all states must make their own arrangements to stockpile these products, essentially pitting one state against the other. While India was manufacturing some of these, we didn't have nearly enough of the essentials. To compete with other wealthier economies, the NTF and subsequently the Empowered Group No. 6 mandated to ensure availability of medical supplies, would have to figure out how many orders would need to be placed and within what time frame to ensure steady supplies to India. In order to streamline supplies could we locally manufacture products that we weren't currently?

# 7

## LOCKDOWN

**24 MARCH 2020**

**INDIA | 485 ACTIVE CASES | 11 DEATHS**

**WORLD | 3,90,352 ACTIVE CASES | 19,584 DEATHS**

The prime minister was scheduled to deliver yet another difficult address to the nation. However, the overwhelming response to his call to stay home for a day-long junta curfew bolstered his spirit—especially the *bhagidari* from the Northeast. So positively overpowering was the response, that *The Telegraph*, which most often takes an anti-establishment stand, published a piece titled, 'Junta Curfew unites Northeast' with heartening quotes that reporters on ground had collected from people. One individual who was playing a guitar outside his home had said to the reporters, 'Thanking people who are working tirelessly for [the] welfare of humanity is a good gesture. Now we cannot thank them in person by shaking hands, but I am sure this resounding thanksgiving will do wonders for them.' Another woman seen beating a steel plate had said, 'This is a unique call by the PM. I am happy to be a part of it. We should not forget the sacrifice of the emergency workers and all those who are working tirelessly to prevent the spread of the disease and also for those who have lost their battle while fighting.'[1] The prime minister now had the confidence that although the stringent restrictions he was about to announce may come across as draconian to a few, his mantra would be *'jaan hai toh jahaan hai* (if you are alive, you can have the world)'. With a resolve to save as many Indian lives as possible, he was going to ask 1.3 billion people to stay put for the next 21 days, at the very least.

Strategically, he scheduled his address to the nation for 8.00 p.m., when shops and activity for the day would have died down. Had it been earlier in the day, people would have crowded at shops and markets to stock up on items, leading to panic buying and risking rampant community spread of the contagion.

The prime minister started his address by acknowledging the efforts of the people who followed junta curfew and for making it a success. He then went ahead to talk about how experiences of other countries within the grip of the virus have taught us that social distancing is the only way to break the chain of the infection. He explained further,

> You are also witnessing how this pandemic has rendered even the most developed countries of the world helpless. It is not that these countries are not putting in adequate efforts, or that they lack resources. The fact is that the Coronavirus is spreading so rapidly that despite all preparations and efforts, countries are finding it hard to cope with the situation.[2]

He clarified that social distancing wouldn't just mean staying away from sick people, it would mean staying away from each other. He further added that:

> Keeping in mind health sector experts and experiences of other countries, the nation is about to take a very important decision today. From 12 midnight today the entire country, please listen carefully, the entire country shall go under complete lockdown. In order to protect the country, and each of its citizens, from midnight tonight, a complete ban is being imposed on people from stepping out of their homes. Every state of the country, every Union Territory, every district, every municipality, every village, every street, every locality is being put under lockdown. This is in effect a type of curfew only. A few levels more than Janata-Curfew, it is more stringent. This is a critical step in the decisive fight against the Corona Pandemic. There is no doubt the nation will have to pay an economic cost for this lockdown. However, at this moment, my utmost priority, and that of the Government of India, state and local governments is to protect the life of every Indian. Hence, it is my plea and prayer to you to continue to remain wherever you are right now in the country.

He explained how the best experts in the country were recommending 21 days to break the chain of the infection. He further advised that according to WHO's experts, it may take days for symptoms to manifest after being infected with the virus and that a person infected with this virus can transmit it to hundreds of people within the span of seven to 10 days. However, this asymptomatic person may unknowingly spread the virus to several others who come in contact with him.

The prime minister added another statistic to drive the point home,

> Another estimate given by the World Health Organization is very important. It took 67 days for the count of people infected with Corona to reach the 1st one lakh all over the world. After this, it took only 11 days for another one lakh people to get infected. It took the world 67 days for the number of Coronavirus infected persons to reach the first one lakh, but only 11 days to reach two lakh thereafter. What is even more alarming is that it took only 4 days for this number to go from 2 lakh to 3 lakh infections. You can imagine how rapidly Coronavirus spreads. And once it begins to spread, it is very difficult to contain.

He added that there would be no shortage of essential supplies at any point in time. He particularly urged people to come forth and help the poor. He also assured the people that the government was constantly working to better equip healthcare facilities and also making decisions as per advice from the WHO, our country's top medical and research organizations and experts.

He concluded his address by warning people against taking medication without consulting doctors and falling prey to rumours and fake news. As a parting note, as always he expressed confidence that India will emerge victorious in this challenge.[3]

◆

Union Finance Minister Nirmala Sitharaman announced a slew of relief measures as part of a ₹1.70 lakh crore relief package. The highlight of this ongoing package was the Pradhan Mantri Garib Kalyan Anna Yojana (PMGKAY), which would put 5 kg of wheat or rice and 1 kg of pulses per month on the table for all poor families, which amounted to about 80 crore people. This would be in addition to the 5 kg of wheat and rice and 1 kg of pulses that they were already entitled to get. She highlighted that this package would focus primarily on migrant workers and daily wage labourers and was essentially designed to help the nation's poor tackle the financial difficulties arising out of the outbreak. She said, 'A package is ready for the poor who need immediate help like migrant workers and urban and rural poor. No one will go hungry.'[4] In addition, she announced, 'Safai karamcharis [cleaners], ward-boys, nurses, paramedics, technicians, doctors and specialists and other healthcare workers would be covered by a special insurance scheme. Any health professional who while treating COVID-19 patients meets with some accident, then he/she would be compensated with an amount of 50 lakh rupees under the scheme.'[5] Several direct cash transfers were announced for some of our most vulnerable groups. Nearly 8.9 crore farmers would immediately receive the first instalment of ₹2,000 as part of the PM-Kisan Samman Nidhi. Wages under the Mahatma Gandhi National Rural Employment Guarantee Act (MNREGA) would also increase by ₹2,000 per worker as additional income for daily wage workers. Three crore senior citizens, persons with disabilities and widows would also be entitled to receive a one-time additional amount of ₹1,000 in two instalments. Twenty crore Jan-Dhan women account holders would receive a direct transfer of ₹5,000 per month and that families below the poverty line would receive free gas cylinders for the next three months. In addition, collateral-free loans would be doubled to help seven crore women working in self-help groups. The government would bear the cost of the employee provident fund contribution on part of both the employer and the employee over the next three months. She also permitted workers to draw up to 75 per cent advance from the existing credit in the employee provident fund or three months' salary. More funds were announced to benefit construction workers as well.[6]

◆

The lockdown itself and subsequent infection-control measures that the government would put in place would have to stand in the court of law. For this, the National Disaster Management Authority, of which the prime minister is the chairman, exercised its powers under the National Disaster Management Act, 2005 and issued an order directing the ministries and departments of the GoI, the state and UT governments to take effective measures to prevent the spread of COVID-19 in the country.

During a briefing at the prime minister's residence where the Minister of State for Chemicals and Fertilizers Mansukh Mandaviya (now Union health minister), senior bureaucrats from the Department of Chemicals and Fertilizers and our scientific experts were present, it was discussed that India would need to not only scale up the manufacturing of all artificial respiratory apparatus, oxygen therapy apparatus and any other breathing appliances or devices, but we would also have to ban exporting these for the time being. It was also decided on the same day that India would ban the export of sanitizers as well.

Over the past few days, the use of anti-malarial drug hydroxychloroquine (HCQ) as a potential prophylactic drug was being heavily discussed in the international media. President Donald Trump's endorsement of it in mid-March especially fuelled the scientific community to seriously look at the capability of this drug in fighting the novel coronavirus.[7] Fox News also interviewed Gregory Rigano, the co-author of a new study showing the benefits of two drugs widely used to treat malaria. The Fox News anchor asked Rigano, 'How big a game-changer would chloroquine and its sister drug hydrochloroquine be if say, we began using it fairly promptly to treat Americans who are highly at risk?' The author replied, 'The drugs were effective in treating COVID-19 and could be used as a prophylactic to prevent contracting the disease.' He pointed out to another study of 30 patients, half of whom had received HCQ and the other half a placebo and said, 'Within a matter of six days, the patients taking HCQ tested negative for coronavirus... the patients that took the control tested positive.' Several other studies from around the world published in reputed journals and outlets highlighted the effectiveness of the early use of HCQ in inhibiting SARS-CoV-2 infection.[8]

Assessing the potential of this drug and the huge demand it would create worldwide, the attendees of the meeting at the prime minister's residence recommended that India ban supply of the drug in order to first meet needs of its own population. However, the prime minister looked uncomfortable with that suggestion. He wasn't one for this kind of hyper-nationalism during a humanitarian crisis. He said, 'In the interest of humanity, it would be wrong to ban a potentially lifesaving drug. This is a moment when India can save lives and we can't let it go. We should look at increasing manufacturing capabilities in order to meet demand.' Although he allowed a ban for a limited period of time,[9] he asked Mandaviya and other officials to get in touch with manufacturers of the drug in India, map out our requirement in the worst-case scenario, find a way to bring all stakeholders together, scale up manufacturing and look at the timelines of such an exercise. He instructed the officials to ensure that no bureaucratic hold-up came in the way of increasing production to meet demands not just of India's but of other countries as well. Once again, deriving from his experience in Gujarat, which is also a manufacturing hub of the pharmaceutical industry, the prime minister had a rough idea of the processes which would be needed to significantly scale up production and he was aware that this would not be an impossible task to accomplish. After the meeting at his residence, he reached out to Pankaj Patel, Cadila Healthcare's CEO, to urge him to increase manufacturing as soon as possible. Just in a fortnight, Patel would say to the media, 'PM Modi motivated the industry by saying this is the chance for India to make a mark globally and the results are for all to see. This month our industry produced twenty crore tablets. My company alone will produce active pharmaceutical ingredients (APIs) worth fifteen crore tablets next month.'[10]

It took about a week for the officials to report back to the prime minister that India would be able to quickly scale up production to suffice not only internal requirements but also be able to meet new demands arising from other countries. With that information, the ban on HCQ was lifted[11] and India began to supply it to several countries initiating its crucial role during the COVID-19 years as the 'pharmacy of the world'. Several world leaders also appreciated India's timely help in HCQ supply. President Trump, on a phone call with the prime minister, said, 'We'd appreciate you allowing our HCQ supply to come out.'[12] A few days later, the President of Brazil Jair Bolsonaro tweeted a thank you note for the prime minister with an image of Lord Hanuman carrying Sanjeevani.[13]

◆

## 26 MARCH 2020

**INDIA | 727 ACTIVE CASES | 21 DEATHS**

**WORLD | 4,80,180 ACTIVE CASES | 25,367 DEATHS**

To mask or not to mask was becoming a rather sticky subject around the world. Since the beginning of March, our scientists, specifically Dr Guleria, were adamant that the contagion was spreading through aerosols and the best way to stop transmission would be to have face masks.

Taiwan was heavily relying on mask mandates. A country with a population of 23 million was manufacturing 13 million masks per day.[14] Similarly, Hong Kong too, one of the most densely populous cities in the world, was strictly enforcing mask mandates and seeing a great amount of success in controlling the pandemic. To understand how stringent the masking mandate was for them, a scientist advising the Hong Kong government commented in the media, 'Not wearing masks in Hong Kong is like not wearing pants.'[15]

However, larger nations were struggling to enforce these mandates. In February, Dr Anthony Fauci, the director of the National Institute of Allergy and Infectious Diseases in the US, almost condemned healthy people wearing masks. The US's Centers for Disease Control and Prevention (CDC) and its then director Robert Redfield echoed a similar tune. However, as more behavioural patterns of the virus came to be known, some high-ranking Americans began to advocate their strict usage. There was a popular story of the former deputy NSA to President Trump, Matthew 'Matt' Pottinger, doing the rounds at the time. He was on a call, while driving to the White House, with a doctor in China in the first week of March, trying to figure out all the things that had helped China contain the contagion. He made notes on the back of an envelope, while using the other hand to navigate traffic. The doctor on the line was giving out very useful information which included something about the prudence of an antiviral drug remdesivir. But then he specifically talked about masks and the fact that they were even more effective in combatting COVID-19 than influenza. He stressed, 'It's great to carry around your own hand sanitizer, but masks are going to win the day.' However, in the US, masks had become a political litmus test where many conservatives condemned mask mandates as infringements on liberty.

So much was the resistance that even the president chose not to wear a mask, in private meetings or in public.[16]

The scientific advisory group in the UK too was advising against mask usage in the early days, leaving Prime Minister Johnson in an uncertain situation.[17]

China had undertaken several case studies which were only now coming out in public portals. One such anecdotal study was where the researchers were studying a typical case of cluster outbreak caused by public transportation exposure. In the study, a male passenger took two bus rides. He had begun coughing on the first ride, unaware that he may have been infected with COVID-19. After the first ride, he purchased a face mask and put it on before getting on to the second ride in a minibus. The results were so telling. Five passengers out of the 39 in the first bus ride came to be infected, whereas none of the 14 passengers in the minibus were found to have contracted the infection.[18]

Another study where viral shedding was observed in a group of over 3,000 individuals noted that mask intervention significantly stratified it. Both, respiratory droplets as well as aerosols were compared between participants wearing masks and those not wearing masks. Both the above studies demonstrated a dramatic reduction in transmission when masks were worn.[19]

The prime minister, convinced by the studies and best practices put forth during a meeting on 26 March, advised the PSA to draw up guidance on how to make and use home-made face masks. Subsequently, the prime minister's close aides together with the joint secretary for health in the PMO were putting together experiences of other countries for him to look at. The prime minister requested to read some peer-reviewed papers before making a final decision on masks. After all, it was about mandating individuals to use a piece of clothing. And he wanted to be absolutely certain about its effectiveness. As his advisors frequently note, it is no easy job for a leader to accurately sift through fast-changing information and developing science and conclusively make decisions which had the potential to upset political stability. Several world leaders were facing the flack. Chinese president Xi Jinping was being criticized for his opacity, Prime Minister Boris Johnson for overreliance on scientists' advice which was not accurately presented to him and President Trump for disregarding scientific advice.

Prime Minister Modi was certain: we would have to leave aside political consequences and make difficult decisions, as long as they were backed by strong evidence-based studies. The team presented to him several aforementioned studies in addition to another one worked upon by a spectrum of respectable researchers from the University of San Francisco, Brown University, Center for Quantitative Biology (Beijing), Institute of Chemical Process Fundamentals (Czech Republic), University of Oxford, University of Cape Town, Stanford University, Massachusetts Institute of Technology, Hong Kong University of Science and Technology, University of California Los Angeles, University of Pennsylvania and Vrije Universiteit Brussel which came out in the early days of March, conclusively studying how mask wearing could be used as an effective mitigation measure in the management and spread of COVID-19. The study presented simple cloth masks as a pragmatic solution for use by the public. It also synthesized literature across various relevant topics such as population impact, transmission characteristics, source control, wearer protection, and sociological and implementation considerations. In addition, it went on to clearly recommend that given the shortages of medical masks, the adoption of public cloth mask wearing was an effective form of source control.[20] In the meeting which followed after the prime minister had browsed through the literature, he directed the officials present that since mask wearing was more effective at reducing the spread of the virus when compliance was high, he would discuss it in his address to the nation scheduled soon. All departments of the GoI would push awareness of mask wearing and perhaps the states could even look at mandating it. He was much relieved that cloth masks were also quite effective making it possible for millions to make their own masks versus having to purchase them. For a country like ours, where a majority was still trapped in the cycle of poverty, a directive from the government to purchase a mask from the open market would just not work. Thus, just a few days after the PSA published guidance on how to use cloth face masks, the Department of Health recommended wearing home-made masks. Incidentally, it was around the same time that the US CDC also put out masking guidelines.[21] To offer a comparison to attest to the timeliness of this decision, there were over two lakh cases in the US as compared to less than a thousand in India at the time of publishing mask mandates.

On one hand, while the global media as well as subject matter experts were hailing the Indian leadership's efforts to act quickly and decisively in an effort to rein in the spread of the contagion, several critics were attributing the low caseload to inadequate testing. By the last week of March, India was testing about 31 people for every COVID-19-positive case. As a matter of comparison, the US was testing about nine, South Korea about 38, Taiwan about 111 and Russia about 200. In total, we were testing about one person in every one million people, but our test positivity rate was 2.10 per cent.[22] According to WHO guidelines at the time, 'a general benchmark of 10% or even better, lower than 3% could be considered a sign of adequate testing'. However, all experts at the time opined that higher the testing, better the possibility of successfully tracing contacts and thus, higher the chance of curbing the spread of the infection. India had to depend on importing testing kits mostly from China to fulfil its requirements. Due to every country in the world scrambling to source COVID-19-fighting essentials from China and the other limited Asian countries where they were available, demand was huge and largely unmet. Often, products of compromised quality would be provided, leaving the countries in a lurch at an extremely sensitive time. India too, early on, received about five lakh faulty testing kits from China.[23] While the two countries tried to discuss the issue through diplomatic channels, the damage on ground was that several false negatives were marked. Those individuals were let out into the community, assuming they didn't carry the infection, when in fact they could have been potentially spreading the infection to tens and hundreds of people.

Over the past six weeks, a group of nine women, many of them mothers and one gentleman led by an eight-month pregnant virologist Minal Dakhave Bhosle worked tirelessly in the laboratories at Mylab Discovery Solutions in Pune trying to find a cheaper, Indian alternative to the imported testing kits which India was relying upon.[24] This group had been actively involved in making PCR kits for several other diseases for several years. However, the usual timeline of four to six months to come up with a test kit was just not acceptable to them anymore. Since mid-February, the team was determined to dive into their experience of developing Deoxyribonucleic acid (DNA) and RNA tests for applications in clinical, veterinary and food safety settings and connecting with researchers who had worked on the SARS family of viruses in India. The WHO guidelines for COVID-19 tests came in handy as the team put together the reagents they would need to extract nucleic acids from patient's saliva samples in order to carry out real-time PCR. They even gathered material they would require to use as controls for positive and negative tests. All of this in a matter of weeks! On 18 March, they consolidated their data and submitted their test kit to the ICMR for approval. The next day, Minal was in labour. However, at the end of her difficult pregnancy, which was laced with complications, she delivered a healthy baby girl. Six days later, on 26 March, ICMR approved the testing kit that Mylab submitted after which the company went on to manufacture millions of kits in a matter of weeks. Not only did the kit yield results with commendable accuracy, it was also half the price of the imported test kits and delivered PCR results in half the time. In a matter of weeks, the company began to manufacture over 2 million test kits per week, catering to the rising demand of India's testing needs at a critical juncture in the COVID-19 crisis.

When media broke the news, inspiring many young girls and several citizens to turn to problem-solving, igniting a ray of hope in dejected citizens, Minal in her interviews would say, 'It's like I've just had two babies! Despite complications in my pregnancy, it was my national duty to do this!'[25]

◆

## 28 MARCH 2020

### INDIA | 878 ACTIVE CASES | 25 DEATHS

### WORLD | 5,87,695 ACTIVE CASES | 332,799 DEATHS

Earlier in the week, the Ministry of Home Affairs, after confirming that Tablighi missionaries who had spread out to different parts of the country were testing positive, sent out an intimation of the developments to all state governments. The order issued specifically asked the state governments to track down and test the returnees from the Markaz as well as people they have come in contact with in the community.

Ever since the ban on religious gatherings announced by CM Arvind Kejriwal on 16 March, the Delhi Police and more specifically the officers of the Hazrat Nizamuddin Police Station, had been engaged in the exercise of persuading those still within the Markaz Masjid to evacuate the premises. Though the Markaz officials said that over 1,500 people had left the building, over 1,000 missionaries were still housed within. Various states in the country were reporting increased cases in the community, linking them back to the Tablighi returnees. Due to the panic and fear of the unknown disease and a perception being built up in the media, folks began to blame the Tablighi Jamaat as the group responsible for spreading the virus in the country. A war of words between the Kejriwal government in New Delhi and police officials, where the former blamed the cops for not being able to get the building vacated and the latter releasing videos proving the actions they had taken was putting even more focus on the role of the group in the speed of transmission of the virus in the early days.[26]

The Markaz officials were of the opinion that after the prime minister announced complete lockdown of the country, the missionaries did not know how to return to their home towns.[27] While the massive manhunt to track down the Tablighi attendees, who had by now spread out to over 19 states, was being undertaken countrywide, the videos of sermons posted by the leaders in the Nizamuddin markaz were outright anti-science and in violation of government orders. In one such released tape (later taken down) but showcased on prime-time news, the chief leader of the Tablighi cult, Ameer Maulana Saad, is heard saying, 'Don't pay heed if they (the government) ask us to lock down mosques. They want us to stop praying in mosques. Allah is punishing us for abandoning mosques. We shouldn't pay heed even if doctors advice not to pray in mosques.'[28] For a society in anger, living in total lockdown akin to blackouts during war, a group of people (regardless of religion) in such abhorrent disobeyance of the law, led to heightened communal tensions. This disharmony was in full display around the Nizamuddin neighbourhood in Delhi. The city had only a couple months ago witnessed ugly communal riots.[29]

Reports from the police indicated that despite repeated urges to vacate, the jamaatis were not yielding; they weren't letting police personnel inside the premises either. However, the jamaatis defended themselves saying that they didn't have the required travel passes and permissions.[30] The situation was very tense. At the PMO, Intelligence had begun to come in that stone pelting and violence was on the verge of breaking out. To avert the violence, the government decided that it would be best to peacefully solve the problem versus using any kind of force through the army or the police to evacuate the masjid. Although the prime minister carries a reputation of being a tough administrator from his Gujarat days, he is also known to have a way with words to on-board all communities in times of crisis. For this, he and his team have over decades developed close relationships with leaders of religious and caste-based organizations—some of these relationships are on display often, whereas some come to light in times like these. National Security Advisor Ajit Doval was deputed to mediate and convince the Tablighi leader to allow the missionaries in the mosque to be evacuated, tested and quarantined. To avoid a scene which would further elevate tensions and garner unnecessary media attention, he made a visit with his team at 2.00 a.m. on the intervening night of 28 March.[31] Although it wouldn't be wise to put out the exact conversation between Doval and Maulana Saad, the actions that followed his visit are very telling. Saad went out of the limelight for the next few weeks, the tapes were taken down and the missionaries lodged in the mosque were allowed to be taken to quarantine centres where they were tested for coronavirus.[32] The future tapes which emerged from the now 'underground' Maulana Saad were significantly more responsible ones, appealing to his followers to follow government directives and laws in an effort to fight the virus in the country.[33] For several months thereafter, Saad remained confined in his home only to resurface in public in June 2020 to offer prayers at a mosque in the national capital.[34]

◆

Needless to say, for a lockdown of this scale, in the second most populous country in the world, several issues cropped up which required committed firefighting on a daily basis. The PMO along with the empowered groups essentially became a war room. The prime minister's directive to everyone was clear: no issue was too small to warrant our attention. To further describe how accessible he wanted to be, there was an episode around the last week of March when Sakal Media Group's managing director, Abhijit Pawar reached out to the prime minister to offer suggestions on curbing the contagion. As evidenced by the audio leak of their conversation, the prime minister not only took note of his suggestions but also assured him that he'd minutely look into the proposals, adding, '*Mujhe koi jadu ki chari mil jaye toh desh bach jayega mera* (If I can get some kind of a magic wand of this sort, then my country can be saved.)'[35]

In the truest sense, following the prime minister's push, many influential personalities walked the extra mile in contributing to the national fight against the virus. For instance, in sync with national priorities, leading names in the film fraternity such as Amitabh Bachchan, Akshay Kumar, Madhuri Dixit, Alia Bhatt, Ayushmann Khurrana, Ajay Devgn, Varun Dhawan, Ranveer Singh, Arjun Kapoor, Shilpa Shetty and many others came together by creating a video to spread awareness on the disease. The industry also came together and released a lovely, emotional song produced by Jackky Bhagnani and Akshay Kumar, composed by Vishal Mishra called 'Muskurayega India' (India Smiles) to uplift spirits of citizens. The video featured several young stars such as Sidharth Malhotra, Rajkummar Rao, Kriti Sanon, Tiger Shroff, Kartik Aaryan, Vicky Kaushal, Bhumi Pednekar, Kiara Advani, Taapsee Pannu, Rakul Preet Singh, Ananya Pandey, RJ Malishka and cricketer Shikhar Dhawan.[36] Leading singers came together for a virtual concert 'Sangeet Setu', hosted by Akshay Kumar, the proceedings of which were donated to Prime Minister's Citizen Assistance and Relief in Emergency Situations Fund (PM CARES).[37]

In the spirit of last-mile outreach, the prime minister instructed his entire Union Cabinet of ministers to provide a daily report of the situation on ground in their respective states and constituencies. A similar directive was issued to his close team as well. The report should not just highlight issues but also add solutions and actions taken to alleviate the troubles that those highlighted issues were causing.

To cite an example, news came in from Belagondapalli near Hosur, Tamil Nadu, that about three tonnes of capsicum that a farmer named Raju had harvested was about to go bad due to transport issues. He hadn't been able to get the capsicum to the market in order to sell it. And, if there was no intervention, due to the short shelf life of the perishable capsicums the entire produce would begin to rot causing great financial damage to the farmer. This news appeared in various regional media outlets and a couple of English news dailies carried it as well.[38] The prime minister's communications team flagged it, included it as part of their twice-a-day media reports to be turned in as well as alerted the PMO official in the concerned empowered group. The empowered group on 'Facilitating Supply Chain and Logistics Management for Availability of Necessary Items such as Food and Medicines' immediately got into action and called the Horticulture Department of the government of Tamil Nadu. They reached out to the farmer and ensured that he faced no issue in transporting his produce. They also made sure that enough labour was arranged for the farmer to load and offload the capsicums along with market access where his produce was eventually sold. The next day, the empowered group filed the aforementioned actions in the action-taken report which was then included in the prime minister's media report the subsequent day.

Another example was of news reports arising from Noida that despite assurances from the chief minister, doorstep delivery of essentials was not being permitted. Once again, the same empowered group was alerted who then reached out to the district collector. The collector confirmed facts on the ground and immediately reported back to the empowered group that the issue was arising not because the vendors were not willing to deliver but because some residential colonies were not permitting access to delivery boys beyond the main gate.[39] The happenings of this episode were filed in the prime minister's media report for his review, as per protocol.

Another problem which came up was that although there were no curbs on transportation of essential products, the truck drivers and the trucks themselves didn't have the required e-passes and there was confusion about how they could access them. Several times, these vehicles would be detained at state borders since interstate transport was also not allowed (barring essential commodities). Due to this, the plying of commercial vehicles carrying essentials had drastically reduced which was an indication that if no action was taken quickly, the supply of essentials and medicines would soon be impacted. Normally, pre-lockdown about 18–24 lakh commercial vehicles would use the Indian roads every day in which 0.8 lakh metric tonnes of food grains would be transported in rakes by the Food Corporation of India (FCI). In the first few days of the lockdown, that number had drastically reduced to merely three to four lakh trucks on an average plying on the roads. Once again the empowered group had to step in and ensure that no local authorities would stop the plying of trucks and other commercial vehicles carrying essential items. They started to maintain a daily tracker to keep an eye on what percentage of the baseline number had the operation of commercial vehicles carrying essentials reached. They also kept a daily tracker of food arrival in major mandis and what percentage of baseline it was on each day of the lockdown. Markers such as traffic of trucks carrying specific items such as packaged food, pharmaceutical products and fertilizers, traffic of rakes and port traffic was also monitored on a daily basis by the empowered group. The efforts yielded results when later it was observed that by the first week of April, FCI was moving about 1.93 metric tonnes of food grains, a significant increase from even pre-lockdown levels.

On further observation, it was noted that most of the outgoing movement was occurring in Punjab, Haryana, Telangana, Chhattisgarh, Odisha and Andhra Pradesh. Induction markers showed that maximum consumption movement was in Uttar Pradesh followed by Bihar, West Bengal and Karnataka. These were also strong indicators that there was a definite increase in the delivery of food grains as promised under the PMGKAY scheme, from the early days of the lockdown. Adding an anecdote, a close aide of the prime minister noted that, 'The PM drew several inferences from studying previous pandemics which led him to believe that food security and an unhindered agricultural sector were what would see the country through the pandemic years. That is when he decided to formulate the PMGKAY. Even after the countrywide lockdown he directed us to ensure that the agricultural sector functioned smoothly and that all their roadblocks were solved on priority as the aforementioned example.'

In the Indian bureaucratic system, typically, procurement and specifically procurement of high-value items is a very tedious and slow process, encompassing several levels of officers across varying levels of authority. This kind of tendering is usually done to keep a check on corruption and leave out favouritism amongst vendors. Owing to this system, officers often hesitate to make quick decisions on procurement, fearing that they would come under the line of fire for impulsive purchases. However, in the COVID-19 crisis, it was imperative that the officers felt comfortable enough to purchase necessary items in high quantities quickly. To enable this, on 27 March, the Finance Ministry released an order providing necessary relaxations and issuing suitable guidelines for specific ministries namely Department of Pharmaceuticals, MoHFW, Ministry of Textiles, Department of Consumer Affairs and Ministry of Civil Aviation.[40] The order further read,

> The prevailing health emergency requires immediate procurement of certain items in quantities which may not be available with a single supplier and/or within the time frame in which they are needed. There is also a possibility that some items may not be available in the country in sufficient quantity within the time frame in which they are needed. Certain items and equipment are currently in global short supply and are effectively in the 'seller's market'. There are also variations in specifications within the same category of item and hence, price differences which may sometimes reflect differences in specifications or quality. With the shutting down of international flights and surface transport routes, international procurement may have to be done through Indian missions. Being a national health emergency of unprecedented and historic scale, delays in procurement will result in loss of lives of citizens. Hence, there is a paramount public interest in ensuring that the necessary supplies are procured in the fastest possible manner and financial procedures have to adapt accordingly.

Owing to this GoI notification, the empowered group on 'Ensuring Availability of Essential Medical Equipment such as PPE, masks, gloves and ventilators; production, procurement, import and distribution' was able to confidently procure ₹30,000 crore worth of lifesaving essentials like medicines, masks, PPEs, testing kits and so on in a matter of weeks.

# 8
## MIGRANTS' DISTRESS

**30 MARCH 2020**

INDIA | 1,116 ACTIVE CASES | 33 DEATHS
WORLD | 6,80,870 CASES | 40,639 DEATHS

When the country locked down, the expectation was that all people, from all strata of society would be compelled to bend over backwards and stay put where they were for the next three weeks in national interest, or in the prime minister's words, *'Joh jahaan hai, wahi rahein* (Wherever you are, stay put).' Unfortunately, for daily wage workers and migrants, the idea of spending three weeks without a wage was scarier than the fear of coronavirus. Possibly because they knew how debilitating hunger could be versus not having enough information on the morbidity of the new disease. Compounding this was the fear of the unknown disease and if infected they wouldn't know where and if they would be treated. In a situation of so many unknowns, several of them craved for the comfort of their villages and their families. Something as basic as being able to stay put with a full stomach was now being viewed as an unaffordable luxury.

Migrants are the backbone of India's workforce. Over the years, over a hundred million people have migrated to the urban areas in search of work. They work largely in informal sectors as helpers in urban homes and shops, cleaners, construction workers, masons, factory workers and such. Although, looking deeper into this demography it is revealed that there are two kinds of migrants who set out to the cities to look for work: long-term migrants and short-term migrants. Long-term migrants are those who have a considerably stable employment in a certain field of work and have been in that particular city for over 10 years. On the other hand, short-term migrants are those who move to cities only for about four to six months but keep returning to their home base after every 'project'. While the exact breakdown of the demographic split between long-term and short-term migrants is not known, it is estimated that smaller and poorer states send out anywhere between 30–40 per cent folks as short-term migrants from all the people who leave. Long-term migrants are more likely to be educated, come from upper income groups, are forward caste and have procured ration cards in the cities of work. In contrast, short-term migrants are less educated and tend to come from poorer sections of the society. A World Bank working paper in 2018, authored by Gaurav Nayyar and Kyoung Yang Kim, demonstrated that short-term migrants are far more likely to migrate interstate and are at the mercy of their 'contractors', whereas long-term migrants tend to stay within the state and engage in more 'permanent' jobs such as domestic help. The study also showed that a third of short-term migrants are most likely engaged in the construction sector and usually the logistics of moving them to the 'city of duty' is arranged by the contractor.[1] Due to the temporariness of the arrangement, it is not possible for short-term migrants to build social capital, which often comes in handy in times of distress as you can rely on communities and their systems to fulfil your needs. For instance, if one was to become infected with the virus, in the presence of abundant social capital one would be able to rehabilitate the rest of their family or room-mates in homes of neighbours or relatives living nearby. The person infected would also be able to access the social ecosystem where someone would supply them food for exchange of a pending favour. They would also likely have better access to government schemes due to a network of folks who are party or government workers in the community. In short, social capital builds the identity of an individual in the community and that identity can then be capitalized to make the best use of the social ecosystem, i.e., social capital. Equipped with the aforementioned information, it would be safe to assume that during a time of crisis like the announcement of a national lockdown and due to the absence of social capital, a large proportion of short-term migrants would have felt extremely financially insecure. They would have been laid off, displaced or left in the lurch by their contractors, not even knowing how to return to their home towns.

Almost immediately after the announcement of the nationwide lockdown, flocks of migrants began to crowd at interstate bus stations and major railway stations in an effort to find a means of public transport to on board.[2] From several accounts, covered extensively in the media, most migrants were of the opinion that with very meagre savings, they wouldn't be able to pay rent and put food on the table. So, instead, they'd use their savings to find a way to get home, to the village. However, due to the curbs on passenger transport since the lockdown, several of them decided to make the journey of hundreds of kilometres by foot. This put the government in a tough spot. They could not, under any circumstance, allow such a mass exodus at this point in time. Health infrastructure in the rural parts of the country was very weak, there was no awareness of the disease and allowing the virus to spread unchecked to the villages would be catastrophic. So, up until the communication about the virus had percolated to rural India and the infrastructure had been strengthened enough to be able to handle positive COVID-19 cases, the government would have to stop the migration. And hence, keeping in mind the safety of the millions of unexposed rural Indians, the Indian government ordered the states to close borders. However, to allay some fears, the empowered group responsible for overseeing logistics ensured that food grains were in ample supply and that every single Indian with a ration card, regardless of domicile, would get free access to their promised quota. Furthering that intent, on 27 March, four days after the announcement of national lockdown, the Ministry of Home Affairs sent out an advisory to state governments and UTs to provide adequate support including food and shelter to the migrants. The same advisory further stated that states and UTs should explore measures, with the support of non-profit organizations, to provide food, shelter and basic amenities, such as clean drinking water and sanitation facilities to informally employed workers, in particular to stranded migrant workers. They were also advised to make these vulnerable groups aware of the measures taken by the government, including provision of free food grains and other essential items through the Public Distribution System (PDS) and streamline the distribution of such items.[3]

However, a huge glitch in the system was the absence of ration card portability which would compel the states to officially provide benefits of the free food grains scheme through the PDS. What this meant was that since migrants, especially short-term migrants, did not have a ration card in their destination city which at this point it was still defined by domicile requirements, they would be left out of the free food grains welfare scheme unless state governments went out of their way, developed special mechanisms and ensured security.

The ball was in the courts of the states and UTs to ensure that temporary accommodation facilities were provided and that access to food, water, toilets and drinking water was granted to those from our most marginalized sections. A disturbing outcome of a study published by the Tata Institute of Social Sciences in Hyderabad showed that out of a sample size of 10,672 migrant workers surveyed between 16 April and 4 May, nearly 97 per cent did not have ration cards in the destination city and thus, would not be guaranteed availability of food and ration benefits announced by the Centre.[4] However, later in June, the prime minister announced the 'One Nation One Ration Card' scheme with interstate portability of the cards and thus opened up access to free food grains from any food provision service store of choice all over the country.[5]

In a disconcerting study conducted by India Migration Now and Dvara Research, between 5 and 11 April 2020, it was found that 47 per cent of the migrant responders were not aware of the relief schemes announced by the government.[6] This translated to chaos amongst this vulnerable population and a feeling of helplessness. In distress, where society at large was relying on the government for their safety and welfare, it was natural for the short-term migrant community to feel orphaned owing to the unawareness of welfare schemes.

While this was in the truest sense a large-scale humanitarian crisis and was initially driven by behavioural psychology, it began to become an issue which the opposition parties could exploit in order to launch an attack at the government. While making reverse migration a subject in their anti-government campaign was malicious enough, it was their indulgence in rumour-mongering and misinformation campaign which egged more migrants to come out on the roads. For over a week when this crisis engulfed the country, the leading opposition party and its top leaders reposted viral videos from Delhi's and Mumbai's transport hubs, forcing those migrants who had made the choice to stay put to reconsider their decision on account of so many deciding to mobilize.

On 28 March, Rahul Gandhi tweeted a viral video showcasing a large crowd gathered at a bus stop in New Delhi with a by-line, 'Out of work & facing an uncertain future, millions of our brothers & sisters across India are struggling to find their way back home. It's shameful that we've allowed any Indian citizen to be treated this way & that the Govt had no contingency plans in place for this exodus.'[7]

Whereas some leaders, despite being from the opposition parties, understood the magnitude of charging up more people to come out on the streets and appealed to them not to do so in the interest of the nation. For instance, on 29 March, the chief minister of New Delhi, Arvind Kejriwal, tweeted in Hindi:

> Some people are urging to go back to their village. The Prime Minister has appealed to us to stay where we are. I also appeal to you that you not return to your villages and stay put where you are. Such large gatherings can make you vulnerable to catching the virus. And through you, the virus can further spread to your villages and your families. It will spread to various parts of the country and if that happens, it will be very difficult for the country to emerge out of the grip of the virus. I assure you that [the] Delhi government has made arrangements for all your food and shelter requirements. It is in the interest of the country at this point that you don't return to your villages.[8]

Chief ministers began to coordinate with each other to ensure that as a united force they provide all possible assistance to the migrants. The chief ministers of states from which most migrants hail which includes states from the Indian heartland comprising Bihar, Uttar Pradesh, Madhya Pradesh and others like Telangana and Andhra Pradesh began outreach measures to the chief ministers of destination states such as Maharashtra, New Delhi and Karnataka to ensure that folks hailing from their states were provided welfare and taken care of.

On 28 March, responding to concerned calls from these chief ministers, Uddhav Thackeray, chief minister of Maharashtra, responded in a televised address, 'If human beings from other states have to survive, then humanity must be shown to them. It is in our culture and is our responsibility to look after them.'[9]

However, this spirit of camaraderie eroded quickly in the upcoming weeks as reports of migrants not being adequately provided for by state governments surfaced. Catalyzing that was the realization by the opposition parties that this could become a major point to politically dent the popularity of the ruling establishment. Therefore, hand in hand with their trusted media outlets, they began to fuel the fire, encouraging more migrants to take to the streets. An expert on Migration Studies later noted,

> The mainstream political opposition failed to make any worthwhile intervention not because it was ignorant of the existence of migrant workers, but because they could not think beyond conventional trade unionism and institutionalised routine politics. Failing to notice the impending crisis, the opposition forgot that the migrant question was a 'social' question.[10]

The Supreme Court intervened on 1 April. A Bench comprising Chief Justice S.A. Bobde and L. Nageswara Rao noted in a report on a petition concerning relief for stranded migrant workers that:

> The migration of large number of labourers working in the cities was triggered by panic created by fake news that the lockdown would continue for more than three months. Such panic driven migration has caused untold suffering to those who believed and acted on such news. In fact, some have lost their lives in the process. It is therefore not possible for us to overlook this menace of fake news either by electronic, print or social media. We do not want to interfere with the free discussion about the pandemic, but direct the media to refer to and publish the official version about coronavirus-related developments.

Invoking the 2005 Disaster Management Act, the court noted that it provides for punishment of up to one year or a fine for a person, 'who makes or circulates a false alarm warning regarding a disaster or its severity or magnitude, leading to panic.'[11]

◆

## 2 APRIL 2020

INDIA | 2,279 ACTIVE CASES | 73 DEATHS

WORLD | 8,44,303 ACTIVE CASES | 57,332 DEATHS

Since the beginning of last month, NITI Aayog members and experts from the technology industry, led by the National Informatics Centre (NIC), had been meeting extensively to perfect a contact tracing app. With the limited number of daily new cases and the fact that community transmission was not yet taking place, it was possible for our health authorities to carry out contact tracing. But if the caseload was to significantly increase, efficient contact tracing would have to be done with the help of technology. Human contact tracing also had limitations of scalability due to limited human resources as well as overreliance on individual memory of the infected. Other limitations would also be the efficient marshalling of contact tracers, distrust from patients as well as exposure to the risk of violence from communities in which they are perceived as unwelcome invaders. Several countries had begun to rely on sophisticated technology for contact tracing which included South Korea, Japan, Taiwan and Vietnam. Eventually, 46 countries had begun to rely on contact tracing apps, despite uptakes remaining low, due to privacy concerns on data breaches as well as low awareness of the existence of the applications. However, the world over, there seemed to be a consensus that despite low usage, having a contact tracing app is a natural adjunct to the manual contact tracing efforts because small effects would accumulate over time.[12]

Not far behind, India had not only developed a sophisticated app but also a secure one: Aarogya Setu, which would use Bluetooth and in the absence of Bluetooth, global positioning system (GPS) to track the phones that a particular device would come in close contact with. Although, the developers maintain that Bluetooth is far more accurate than GPS. The app would alert not just the health authorities but also individuals who could have possibly come in contact with an infected individual, so that they can look out for COVID-19 symptoms or self-isolate. As long as the data accumulated by the app remained on the NIC server, it would be anonymous and secure, as per the design. The security audit was conducted by the Indian Institute of Technology (IIT) Madras.

Once the interface was ready, the team made a presentation to the PMO for consent. As the team put it, 'The effectiveness of the app would be directly proportional to the number of users using it'. India had about 700 million smartphone users and it would be imperative to get as many of them to download and use the app. The question arising thus would be: could the use of this app be mandated? What kind of encroachment on privacy would mandating an app like Aarogya Setu entail? As per a seminal judgement in the Supreme Court, Justice D.Y. Chandrachud had stated, 'If the state preserves the anonymity of the individual, it could legitimately assert a valid state interest in the preservation of public health to design appropriate policy interventions on the basis of the data available to it.' The court had gone ahead to set out three conditions: first, there must be a governing law. Second, this governing law must have a legitimate aim. And third, the law adopted must be proportionate to the objective sought to be achieved. However, until March 2020, India had not passed a data protection law successfully. In the absence of such a law, during a time of national crisis, it would be only natural for the government to use public data for the cause of national safety, as long as they kept the information anonymous.[13] Hence, Aarogya Setu was designed in line with the privacy policy: 'The information on the app would be uploaded to a server every fifteen minutes. This information would then be used in anonymised, aggregated datasets for the purpose of generating reports, heat maps and other statistical visualisations for the purpose of the management of COVID-19 in the country...'[14]

In the first week of April, all of these facts were presented by the NIC and NITI Aayog team to a high-level group chaired by the prime minister, comprising Union ministers Amit Shah, Ravi Shankar Prasad, Piyush Goyal and secretaries of the Ministry of Home Affairs, the Ministry of Electronics and Information Technology, the Ministry of Health, the Ministry of Railways and Ministry of Human Resource Development. Approvals came in fairly quickly and it was decided that awareness campaigns of the app be run at the highest levels, in order to ensure high uptake. The prime minister would also, in his forthcoming address to the nation, appeal to the people to download and use the app in the interest of the nation.

Although, not as high as envisioned, the app has had over 190 million downloads with over 140 million downloads within the first year. It is, as it stands today, the world's most downloaded COVID-19 tracking app.[15] And in the larger scheme of things, it became an important piece of ammunition in India's arsenal of tools to fight the contagion effectively.

# 9

## PLAN TO UNLOCK

**3 APRIL 2020**

**INDIA | 2,780 ACTIVE CASES | 87 DEATHS**

**WORLD | 9,02,387 ACTIVE CASES | 63,600 DEATHS**

Times were grim. Tens of thousands of people had taken to the streets in an effort to return to their home towns. Every arm of the GoI was working in overdrive to provide comfort and necessities to these groups, in an effort to make them settle where they were, and halt their march. The prime minister had spoken over video call with the chief ministers just a day before, on 2 April, specifically asking them to ensure that the poor got food, shelter and clean drinking water. The machinery was overladen with fear and anxiety, what if these folks took the disease to the villages and hinterland? We could potentially witness mass annihilation like never seen before. The invisible enemy would consume our small towns and villages with a vengeance and in the absence of available treatment, there wouldn't be much we would be able to do. Businesses and companies were working from home and several had begun to experience cash crunch. The sentiment was at an all-time low. People were caged in their own homes, fearing that even the air they breathe could possibly be fatal. At this stage, the prime minister, donning his role as the consoler-in-chief, needed to come forth to offer strength and courage. In another effort to increase outreach regarding the virus and COVID-19-appropriate behaviour, especially among the rural folks, he appealed to the people, 'I want nine minutes from you all on 5 April, Sunday. Switch off all the lights in your homes, come to the door or the balcony and light a candle, diya or switch on the torchlight on your phones.'

He added, 'The collective power of unity of 1.3 billion of us will be felt through and this unity will give us the strength to pass these very difficult times.'[1]

Two days later, on 5 April, the country once again came together to adhere to the prime minister's call for unity. The visuals which came in via media outlets were particularly moving. Entire streets were lit up with diyas and torchlights. People even came out to their balconies to play conch shells, ghantis and thaalis and clapped too. Neighbours looked at each other appreciatively, knowing very well that although at the moment they were separated physically by the walls of their respective homes, they were in this fight together. Cities and villages alike reverberated with the positive, hopeful energy—world over it has left observers boggled even after two years of the pandemic as to how a country like India stayed the official line and stood firmly behind our prime minister to together fight the virus. A feat difficult for many large nations to achieve. Out of the many images which cropped up, a certain one with an old, raggedy woman standing outside her hut with a diya in her hand and hope in her eyes particularly touched many hearts, conveying the true spirit of the prime minister's intended exercise.

The PM also joined in and visuals of him lighting a diya at his official residence went viral, gathering around six million likes on his Instagram account, one of the highest ever. Across the country, similar visuals of various chief ministers, Union ministers, film personalities, cricketers and business leaders were also being flashed in the media.

Some people observed that the atmosphere across the country was as if Diwali had arrived early in the year. It appeared as if, for those brief moments, there was no fear or trepidation among the people. As if there was no uncertainty and anxiety relating to the deadly virus. In that moment, the entire nation was united in feeling hopeful and optimistic. Perhaps this was what the prime minister had in mind when he planned it: to instill positivity among the people despite the despair all around. The upbeat energy also encouraged patience in society.

In contrast, some sections worked overtime to peddle fear in an already anxious population. Shashi Tharoor[2], India Today's news anchor Rajdeep Sardesai[3], a state minister for Energy in the Maharashtra Vikas Aghadi (MVA) government from the Congress party and several other ill-informed media influencers touted rumours that India may face a severe grid crisis owing to the lights-out call given by the prime minister. The Union Power Ministry had to eventually clarify that no such grid failure was likely and that all systems had been put in place to avoid any chance of such a failure.[4]

States like Maharashtra were particularly active in spreading discord at a sensitive time and in retrospect it is now clear that Sardesai, who has amassed a huge following on social media owing to prime-time news anchoring, played an active role in perpetrating misleading information. Over the years, it has become clear that once considered a doyen of journalism, he routinely peddles fake news and amplifies propaganda,[5] which has the potential to harm the Modi government. Immediately after 9.00 p.m., when vigil had just about started, several media persons including Sardesai tweeted images of a fire breaking out in a building in Solapur.[6] In fact, instead of quashing such fake news, the guardian minister of Solapur from the Nationalist Congress Party (NCP) tweeted, 'There is nothing to worry about the fire near solapur airport in solapur. As guardian minister I just spoke to collector solapur and all is under control #StayHomeStaySafe.'[7] The truth however was that these images of the fire were two months old. No fire had broken out at Solapur or anywhere else due to the people's response to the prime minister's clarion call.[8]

Sardesai didn't stop here. All through the pandemic, he continued his aggressive misinformation campaign. The next day, on 6 April, he tweeted a letter from the Resident Doctor's Association at Safdarjung Hospital about them seeking donations for PPE kits, N95 masks, triple-layer masks and hand sanitizers with a note, 'What can be more appalling: resident doctors at a leading Delhi hospital seek to raise funds for protective equipment. Can't expect doctors to be soldiers at the frontline in this battle without equipment, can we?'[9] As always in his case, the truth was altered. Safdarjung Hospital, only on 4 April, two days before, had tweeted tagging the Union Health Ministry and the then Union health minister, 'There is no shortage of PPE kits, N95 masks and any other logistics in Safdarjung Hospital to fight with CORONA Pandemic. The Doctors, Nurses and all staff of Safdarjung Hospital are trying their best to beat this virus @MoHFW_INDIA, @drharshvardhan #FightAgainstCoronavirus.'[10] They were merely trying to convey to NGOs that they were accepting donations of the aforementioned medical equipment.

Sardesai's role in spreading fake news and fear-mongering eventually became a menace for India Today when he put out similar factually incorrect tweets in January 2021 and they eventually took him off-air, only to bring him back two weeks later.[11] The India Today group surely understands that people don't watch prime-time news on their channels because Sardesai is on the screen but that they watch Sardesai because the channel puts him on at prime time.

On 5 April, the prime minister spoke to several leaders, including his predecessor Manmohan Singh, Congress chief Sonia Gandhi and former president Pranab Mukherjee, on the situation arising out of the novel coronavirus pandemic. He also called up various leaders, including Mulayam Singh Yadav and Akhilesh Yadav of the Samajwadi Party, West Bengal Chief Minister Mamata Banerjee, Odisha CM Naveen Patnaik, Dravida Munnetra Kazhagam's M.K. Stalin and Shiromani Akali Dal leader Parkash Singh Badal, former president Pratibha Patil and former prime minister H.D. Deve Gowda.

◆

At this point, about 400-odd cases or 30 per cent of all cases in India were linked to the jamaatis who attended the event at the Nizamuddin Markaz in March.[12] Although after NSA Doval's intervention, the Markaz itself had been vacated and the residents escorted to a quarantine centre for testing, several attendees who had gotten out before the lockdown announcement had spread all over the country. In an advisory issued by the Ministry of Home Affairs, the state governments were asked to intensify their efforts to trace these attendees as well as their contacts in an effort to contain the spread.[13] It had also come to light that most foreigners who attended the congregation had violated visa rules and they'd be blacklisted from entering the country again.[14] Unfortunately, in a scenario where most in the country were blaming the jamaat to be a super-spreader event, instances of the jamaatis misbehaving with nurses and doctors at quarantine centres were appearing in the news.[15] Natural social psychology would attribute the mounting anger in the minds of Indians to the anxiety, helplessness and fear arising out of the lockdown. However, such instances of violence on caregivers coupled with irresponsible media coverage would drive a deeper communal wedge, leaving the jamaatis ostracized. In a saddening incident widely reported in the media, at the MMG District Hospital in Ghaziabad, Uttar Pradesh, six quarantined jamaatis misbehaved with the doctors and nurses, using foul language, making vulgar gestures, spitting at them and even roaming around naked. They had to be later shifted to a temporary isolation ward at a private educational institute.[16] In Hyderabad too, at Gandhi Hospital, family members of a jamaat attendee who had tested positive for the virus and were quarantined, attacked doctors who were on call and damaged hospital property.[17] In Madhubani (Bihar), bullets were fired and stones were pelted at policemen on duty who had gone to a community to trace the jamaat returnees. The local police had received intelligence that a crowd of a hundred-odd people had gathered at a mosque. When they reached the mosque, the locals not only attacked them but chased them for a kilometre, eventually leading to the police car being overturned into a pond.[18] Several doctors were also being discriminated against by being disallowed to continue living in their societies.[19] Many such incidents came to be reported concerning the authorities. Several state governments responded swiftly by booking and detaining the attackers under the National Security Act. Others brought in special laws to offer protection to doctors and other medical personnel.[20] However, the existing state laws did not have the wide sweep and the ambit required to ensure complete protection, especially since they did not cover harassment at home or workplace and were focused on physical violence. In addition, the penal provisions contained in these laws were not stringent enough to deter mischief.

The prime minister, in his daily media reports, had been receiving stories of violence against the police, doctors and health workers from all around the country. Not only was it worrying that the frontline workers who were trying to save lives by putting their own at risk were being attacked, but it was also of grave concern to him that the acts of violence were most often communal in nature—pitting Muslims against Hindus and vice versa. Such a situation would also hamper the medical community from performing their duties to their optimum best, killing their morale. The safety of our doctors and healthcare workers was a critical need in the hour of national health crisis. Our healthcare workers were our frontline soldiers in the battle against COVID-19. They deserved our highest respect and encouragement at this moment rather than being harassed or being subjected to violence. We would have to have a zero-tolerance policy against such disgraceful acts, he concurred. Growing increasingly concerned, he immediately directed senior officials in the PMO to find a solution which would stop these attacks and also added that the violators should be subject to the strictest punishment.

This is how, the Ordinance to amend the Epidemic Diseases Act, 1897 which would provide for making such acts of violence cognizable and non-bailable offences was introduced. It would also provide compensation for injury to healthcare service personnel or for damage or loss to property in which these personnel had direct interest in. In the Union Cabinet meeting held on 22 April, promulgation of this Ordinance would be approved, immediately after which the president would give his assent.[21]

◆

In an attempt to make the states more financially secure, during his video call with the chief ministers on 2 April, the prime minister assured the quick release of the Centre's share of the first instalment of the State Disaster Risk Management Fund. After his directions, the Union home minister Amit Shah approved the release of ₹11,092 crore and immediately disbursed them to the states, providing the much-needed financial relief to the states.[22] Unfortunately, many states failed to use these funds to relieve the plight of the migrants.

To specifically cater to the urgent requirements of a pandemic, the prime minister proposed to set up a separate public charitable relief trust fund which would accept voluntary donations from Indian citizens called the Prime Minister's Citizen Assistance and Relief in Emergency Situations Fund (PM CARES). The trust would be chaired by the prime minister and include three ministers from the Union Cabinet who hold the three most important portfolios: Home, Defence and Finance, and would be audited by an independent auditor. As soon as the fund was announced, donations started pouring in from citizens who wanted to show their solidarity with the prime minister's efforts.[23]

Donations to the tune of ₹3,000 crore would be collected in 2020 and several essentials in critical times during the pandemic years would be provided for by this fund.[24] However, it became mired in controversy after sections of the Opposition criticized the opacity of it. The fund was not covered under the Right to Information (RTI) Act since it did not qualify as a government or public authority and received donations which were voluntary and from private sources. On a closer look, this would mean that anyone making donations to this fund, made them in good spirit. In an effort to attract funds which corporations set aside for mandated corporate social responsibility (CSR), the fund was included in the eligibility list in the Companies Act to make CSR donations.[25] Conventionally, CSR contributions to private funds have not been allowed under the Companies Act, since many could use this as a loophole to divert monies in order to make them tax-free and indulge in tax evasion. However, based on this ambiguity, the Opposition used its might to attack the prime minister on charges of possible misspending, in other words, corruption.[26] Interestingly, Congress President Sonia Gandhi wrote in a letter dated 7 April, suggesting five ways in which the government could cut down expenditure and allocate more money towards pandemic management. One of those suggestions included transferring donations from the PM CARES fund to the Prime Minister's National Relief Fund (PMNRF) to ensure 'efficiency, transparency and accountability'.[27] To grasp the absurdity of this suggestion it is important to understand that contrary to popular media stories, the PMNRF is also outside the ambit of the RTI, as it is not a 'public authority' within the meaning of Section 2(h) of the RTI Act, 2005.[28] Even more interestingly, up until 2018, PMNRF's managing committee from the time of its constitution by former prime minister Jawaharlal Nehru included the Congress president, their chosen representatives from the private sector selected by FICCI and a representative from Tata Trustees along with the prime minister and finance minister. Even more strangely, the PMNRF, which was deemed to be a trust, has since functioned without a trust deed making its operations totally ambiguous.[29] More importantly, PMNRF is also audited by a private independent auditor. Interestingly, until very recently, the firm which was auditing PMNRF was owned by a Congress leader who rose to the ranks of a Union minister during the United Progressive Alliance (UPA) regime. In a Great Indian Mystery, funds from PMNRF were used to donate to the Rajiv Gandhi Foundation, thrice (2005, 2007 and 2008), as disclosed in the annual report.[30] What kind of relief measures was the Rajiv Gandhi Foundation engaging in to be considered an eligible beneficiary of the PMNRF, as per the wisdom of UPA leaders?

Changing up this archaic structure to one where realpolitik would take precedence by ensuring that the prime minister's discretion on disbursement of monies would be final at a time of a once-in-a-century crisis was perhaps the driving force behind establishing PM CARES. Moreover, PM CARES was designed to live up to the test of time as it would pass on to the incumbent governments over years to come versus continuing to being managed by one particular political party and its chosen few as in the case of PMNRF.

However, the media noise was so dichotomous that the real intent behind the formation of PM CARES barely came through. However, despite the unnecessary ruckus, contributions to the fund continued to be made generously by Indians—a sign in the truest sense that India placed immense faith in the prime minister's integrity. Moreover, a public interest petition filed in the Supreme Court to transfer the funds collected in PM CARES to the National Disaster Response Fund was dismissed by a three-judge Bench which also noted that 'financial planning was the government's prerogative' and 'no one could question it'.[31]

◆

Several relaxations in the usual tendering processes for building of standalone COVID-19-treatment centres and procurement of medical and necessary equipment to maintain and run these centres were made at the state and city corporation levels. Due to these relaxations, several instances of corruption surfaced where large sums were given out to preferred vendors and builders. For instance, in Mumbai, the MCGM, the richest corporation in Asia, spent over ₹1,200 crore to erect and manage 'Jumbo COVID-19 Centres' from March to December 2020. Due to the time sensitivity, several relaxations in due processes were made and allegations have since surfaced over favours given out by the ruling party, Shiv Sena, to private builders without inviting tenders.[32] Adding fuel to the fire, the MCGM chief was unceremoniously transferred in the middle of a nationwide lockdown.[33] After demands from the opposition party to audit the funds, the MCGM set up a standing committee for the purpose of investigating corruption charges. It remains to be seen if such a body can evaluate itself fairly! If the audit was intended to be fair, an external committee with members of all parties and ex-bureaucrats should have been set up.

On similar lines, several allegations of corruption accounting for over ₹2,000 crore were made against the West Bengal government. Some agencies were favoured for procuring medical items. The agencies failed to meet the standard quality of the supplied items and after multiple complaints and reports in the media, West Bengal Chief Minister Mamata Banerjee formed a three-member panel under the supervision of the chief secretary to investigate the irregularities.[34] Once again, it remains to be seen how fairly the committee will evaluate its own government's wrongdoings, particularly since the chief secretary's political affiliations came to light when he failed to attend a meeting chaired by the prime minister in the visit to the state, thus breaking protocol during early 2021.[35]

Even in BJP-ruled states like Himachal Pradesh, purchase of PPE gear of about ₹1 crore was made without keeping due processes in mind, favouring two organizations pitched for by a certain middleman. When the allegations surfaced, a top health official was arrested and five days later, the then state BJP party president who had links to the middleman resigned.[36]

◆

## 14 APRIL 2020

INDIA | 9,734 ACTIVE CASES | 394 DEATHS

WORLD | 1,413,911 ACTIVE CASES | 137,794 DEATHS

The 21-day lockdown which the prime minister had put in place was to end today. The prime minister, after speaking with the chief ministers to get an update on the status of upgradation of health infrastructure and the spread of the contagion on ground, was urged by them to extend the lockdown. However, after careful deliberation with the health authorities, he was of the opinion that those districts which were not impacted by the contagion must be allowed to operate essential economic activities. He felt that a 'one-size-fits-all' approach shouldn't be used. This district-by-district analysis would be done in the upcoming week and districts would be carefully categorized as red, orange or green based on their caseload. The categories naturally would be dynamic as caseloads would go up or down/fluctuate. Not only did this announcement boost the spirits of people who were low on morale because of losing work but also of local governments who would now strive to achieve low positivity rates in their respective districts in the hope of restarting activity.

This time around, when the prime minister appeared on television for his scheduled national address, he was seen repurposing his scarf as a face mask. Before beginning to speak, he lowered it and wrapped it around his neck. This was a predecided move by him. The emerging science that he had read was strongly recommending mask usage which had the potential of reducing travel of viral load in aerosol droplets up to a factor of two.[37] Although the MoHFW had already published mask guidelines on 3 April, the usage was still low and to penetrate to more people the prime minister decided to demonstrate it. He decided to repurpose his scarf to display that a home-made mask too can be very effective. This would also increase the sales of cloth masks, offering the much-needed employment generation opportunities to self-help groups. Later, he would also use a picture of his in a cloth mask as his Twitter display picture, leaving it unchanged until India administered one billion vaccine doses.

In the address, he sympathized with the pain of the people and presented India's positive report card as compared to other wealthier nations, only because of the bold, drastic steps we had taken very early on. He went on and presented seven mantras, appealing to the people to continue to maintain lockdown discipline until 3 May. His seven mantras were: taking care of the elderly since they were most vulnerable to the infection, following social distancing, staying at home and wearing masks, following instructions from AYUSH ministry to enhance immunity like consuming warm water and kadha (Ayurvedic home remedy), downloading the Aarogya Setu app, taking care of the poor around us and offering as much help as possible, being compassionate to employees and not cutting them off the payroll and last, following lockdown rules until 3 May, by staying put.[38]

# 10

## ECONOMIC RESPONSE

**16 APRIL 2020**

INDIA | 11,213 ACTIVE CASES | 449 DEATHS

WORLD | 14,83,234 ACTIVE CASES | 1,53,514 DEATHS

While India was preparing to exit lockdown in the upcoming weeks, the challenges staring us in the face were unprecedented. China had suffered a huge loss in credibility due to its failure to alert the world early on about the virus and its origins and its refusal to quarantine itself so that the world could be insulated. However, in an effort to build back some reputational positivity, it had begun to supply all kinds of medical equipment necessary to fight the virus to countries across the world. India too, like most other countries, relied on the Chinese to source PPE kits, rapid antigen testing kits, raw materials for medicines and several other necessary products.

However, reality hit us hard when we received lakhs of faulty testing kits and PPE kits. We were at a crucial intersection in our fight against COVID-19, we needed to scale up testing significantly and rapid testing kits would enable us to do just that. These kits were meant to produce results within 30 minutes and could be used by local governments to get an accurate idea of the scale of infection in a particular territory by deploying mass testing, i.e., sero-surveys. Sero surveillance would enable us to further break down the impact of the virus on specific demographics. At a time when India's unlocking strategy was based on classifying districts as red, yellow and green zones and further creating micro-containment zones in areas of high prevalence, rapid testing kits would be a boon. Various Indian states had been pushing the ICMR to allow testing with these kits amidst criticism that we were simply not testing enough. The ICMR was initially reluctant, since the result accuracy of rapid testing kits was much lower than that of RT-PCR tests. However, considering the benefits of sero surveillance, the ICMR cleared the way and imported rapid testing kits from two Chinese companies. India was one of the early recognizers of the usefulness of rapid antigen tests as a community health measure as early April as opposed to countries like the US, who came around to approving their use only in the month of May.[1] Even after these were approved, they weren't really used for mass surveillance. In fact, a popular American cardiologist, scientist and author Dr Eric Topol had been pushing for community surveillance as an effective measure to restrict the spread of the virus since the final weeks of March, however the US government didn't quite see merit in it like India did.[2]

Soon after, several local governments raised concerns over the accuracy of these kits. They complained that the accuracy of the received kits was only about 5 per cent, down from about 78 per cent. This meant that in a normal scenario, if rapid antigen kits were used on a hundred patients who were already tested COVID-19 positive on RT-PCR, 78 of them would turn up positive even on the rapid antigen testing kits. In the case of the five lakh, overpriced tests received from the two Chinese companies, not only did they fail ICMR's quality tests but also only five out of a hundred positive patients were testing positive. In other words, the tests failed to detect 95 per cent of positive cases, raising an alarm amongst the authorities. This wasn't the first time we had received faulty equipment from China and were certainly not the first or only country to encounter this problem. We had recently also received a faulty batch of 50,000 PPE gear from them. Spain, Czech Republic, Slovakia, Turkey and the UK had also received faulty test kits after paying millions of dollars to procure them. Due to these experiences, Georgia cancelled its agreement to procure the kits. The Netherlands also had a salty experience after being delivered about six hundred thousand N95 masks in which neither did the fillers work nor did they fit like they were supposed to. However, when the Dutch officials requested a recall, instead of apologizing, Beijing blamed the Netherlands asking the Dutch government to read the instructions on the box.[3]

The ICMR, needless to say, halted the use of these kits and cancelled the remaining order from the Chinese companies.[4] Not putting all our eggs in one basket, we began to source from South Korea, Germany, Canada and Japan. Taking forward the 'Make in India' initiative, SD Biosensor, a South Korean company manufacturing tests with a facility in Manesar, began manufacturing about five lakh kits per week starting April 2020.[5] The Indian mission in South Korea played an important role in ensuring that the company's unit in Manesar got all the necessary clearances required in South Korea and India. The licences were facilitated without delay by the ICMR and the Drugs Controller General of India (DCGI) in a matter of days. However, the episode of receiving faulty medical equipment from China ended up leaving a rather sour taste in the mouths of countries which were grappling with the virus, and banking on aggressive testing and treating to 'flatten the curve'.

◆

A strong supply chain for essential products had to be established, especially for the equipment which we had scarce stockpiles of and didn't manufacture domestically in large quantities. When the review meeting to forecast the requirement for essentials took place with PMO officials in March, the direction to the empowered groups was clear: become self-sufficient in the production of essentials as soon as possible. The Ministry of External Affairs was instructed to maintain cordial bilateral relations with the countries from whom we would be sourcing essentials in the weeks or months to come, till we became fully self-reliant. This was to be done through the respective Indian missions in these countries. During a meeting in the last days of January 2020, it had become clear that we didn't manufacture a single PPE kit; in fact, we didn't even have SOPs in place to manufacture PPE kits. We only had about 2.75 lakh imported kits stockpiled with us. In the meeting at the PMO in early March, NITI Aayog officials, led by Dr Paul and Amitabh Kant, forecasted that India would need about 20 million of them by July 2020. This meant that India would need to make 20,000 PPE kits with a classification of Class-3 protection level under ISO 16603 standards per day to meet this upcoming target. Even before the meeting in March, looking at the abysmal numbers stockpiled with us, the MoHFW and the Ministry of Textiles had deployed teams to understand the gaps in the existing infrastructure and resources and in the overall end-to-end production, testing and packaging of the kits as per WHO-approved quality standards. On 18 March, the Ministry of Textiles decided to prohibit the export of domestically manufactured PPEs and raw materials for the same, the notification for which was issued the next day. The team, led by Dr Harsh Vardhan and Smriti Irani, involved industry experts and large private players who then put together an SOP document in 24 hours. A pilot was run which involved local manufacturers as well and the South India Textile Research Association was looped in to test samples. However, on 22 March, it emerged that only four manufacturers passed the quality test. Thus, Operation PPE Coverall was launched by the Ministry of Textiles on 24 March under which a working business ecosystem where local manufacturers could be guided by bigger companies in the market or industry associations was enabled. In order to bridge the information gap, the Defence Research and Development Organisation (DRDO), the Alternative Energy Promotion Centre, the Bureau of Indian Standards (BIS) and the Confederation of Indian Industry were involved.[6] The efforts yielded great results, as in a matter of four–six weeks not only had India become self-sufficient in producing PPE kits, but we were beginning to export them. In another two and a half months, by July 2020, not only was our stockpile in surplus, but we had already exported about 23 lakh PPE kits to the US, Senegal, Slovenia, the UAE and the UK.

Similarly, as opposed to the dismal 3.35 lakh imported N95 masks which we had in reserve in March 2020, we strengthened our end-to-end manufacturing chain which led to us being able to produce 40 million N95 masks by July.[7]

While stories of achieving sufficiency in manufacturing of N95 masks and PPE kits are noteworthy, it is India's ventilator manufacturing story which establishes the true spirit of the Indian public–private entrepreneurial state model. In January 2020, India only had about 16,000 ventilators in public health facilities and another 29,000 in private care hospitals in circulation.[8] Most of these were imported from Europe and China at an average cost of about ₹15 lakh per unit. Domestic manufacturing of ventilators or its components was insignificant; as a matter of fact, neither there existed domestic standards for manufacturing of these units nor were they regulated medical devices with a BIS certification. Even the very few which were made in India were heavily dependent on importing components from various countries. In the forecast meeting at the PMO in mid-March, the team had projected India's requirement at about 60,000 pieces. In order to meet immediate demand, the Ministry of External Affairs approached China to supply about 10,000 ventilators at the earliest; however, China expressed its inability to supply since it was facing an acute shortage of components which it was importing too.[9] With a ban on flights there had been disruptions in the supply of vital components across product categories around the world of which China and India were no exceptions. Media reports were emerging from various countries like the UK, EU, US and Brazil about acute ventilator shortage and an inability to procure them.[10][11] After China's rejection, India immediately placed orders with international companies like Hamilton, Mindray and Draeger for urgent sourcing of units.[12] However, relying on these for our bulk, long-term requirement was not feasible. The empowered group for ensuring availability and production of essential medical equipment began to work towards creating solutions for mass supply, which could be completely manufactured in India. Keeping in mind that COVID-19 primarily affects pulmonary functions, the DRDO programme, Society for Biomedical Technology, began efforts to find innovative solutions to create a 'multi-patient' ventilator. After achieving a working prototype with collective effort by the public–private effort of the DRDO and M/s Skanray and Bharat Electronics Limited (BEL), nine companies were identified for design transfer so that manufacturing could be scaled up. The DRDO zeroed down on Skanray to produce critical care ventilators. At the same time, the DRDO began to make efforts towards indigenizing components which would be required to produce these prototyped devices. Eventually, they were able to achieve 70–80 per cent domestic production of components which went into these devices. Two public-sector companies—BEL enabled by Skanray and the Andhra Pradesh MedTech Zone—committed to the GoI that they would make 30,000 and 13,000 devices, respectively, within two months.

Businessman Anand Mahindra, the head of Mahindra and Mahindra group, had indicated early on in March about how the Mahindra Group would immediately begin brainstorming on how their automobile manufacturing facilities could make ventilators.[13] Skanray had the capacity of building only 5,000 ventilators in three months. In order to augment its scale to produce 30,000 units in two months, it needed to tie up with larger players such as Mahindra and Mahindra. To reduce import and development time, automotive components used in Mahindra vehicles were selected to produce a simpler version of the full-fledged mechanical ventilator used in ICUs.

Similarly, Maruti Suzuki rose to the challenge and partnered with AgVa Healthcare to produce 10,000 ventilators in a month.[14] AgVa provided the technical knowledge, whereas Maruti Suzuki used its network of suppliers in addition to its experience in scaling up production. Bharat Heavy Electricals Limited provided the electronic chips which would go into these ventilators and HP Inc partnered with Redington 3D in India to produce 1,20,000 ventilator parts which would go into these 10,000 ventilators. These were parts with complex design and a certain level of tolerance. Typically, it would have taken five months to manufacture them. But HP used its 3D printing technology to produce the same parts in less than a month.[15]

With rigorous efforts from the DRDO and the private manufacturers, the cost of the Indian manufactured ventilators went down to about ₹2–5 lakh for simple ventilators and about ₹5–8 lakh for complex ones. These were paid for by the PM CARES fund, expensing about ₹2,000 crore to make about 50,000 units which would be distributed to government-run COVID-19 centres and hospitals across states and UTs.[16] These were also fitted with geotags so that their location for transport, delivery and usage could be accurately tagged.[17] The MoHFW also created WhatsApp groups with officials from states, doctors from hospitals where they were supplied and suppliers so that issues regarding the use and maintenance of these could be raised and resolved efficiently in real time.[18]

By December 2020, in six months, from being a country which had absolutely no ventilator manufacturing and only about 16,000 units in public health facilities, 36,000 Made-in-India ventilators had been supplied to public health facilities and by May 2021, that number rose to 49,960.[19]

◆

Emboldened by these experiences, the prime minister made up his mind that across industries ecosystems could be created which could spurt manufacturing immensely. The possibilities of the kind of push these new ecosystems would give to the economy and the jobs which would be created were magnanimous. He saw vast opportunity in times of crisis, which could shoot up over the decades to come and decided that it was time for India to become atmanirbhar (self-reliant) across sectors and industries.

World over, leaders and economists were growingly increasingly concerned over the looming economic depression. The emerging trends from the scientific community which showed that the virus would possibly stay with us for a long time were significantly concerning. The mentality in the beginning when the virus started spreading was: 'let's freeze in place, the virus will pass, then we will unfreeze and go back to normal'.[20] However, with no vaccine in sight and no significant proven miracle treatment, there was no chance of returning to 'normalcy' in the near future. The Bank of England had predicted UK's biggest recession in 300 years and the US wasn't far behind.[21] When the pandemic hit, the whole world suffered a supply shock: trade was disrupted, factories closed down, stores and restaurants shut and people lost their jobs. In a world so interdependent, this had brutal consequences. Several economists had begun to worry about the doom loop—a cycle of negative feedback. The cause of worry was that if people didn't start earning again soon, the supply shock would turn into a demand shock which, in turn, would weaken supply, further increasing unemployment and diminishing demand. The doom loop. In order to break this circuit, several countries took difficult policy decisions and offered tailored stimulus packages. Normally, swings of business cycles have a direct effect on people's ability to spend on consumer goods, their income and large personal investments. This situation was a bit different. It wasn't that people didn't have money to buy things or go to restaurants; many had the funds, but they couldn't go to restaurants or malls. Businesses had shut shop to follow lockdown protocol. Airlines and shipping companies had halted operations. Circulation of containers had ceased causing a sharp crunch in their availability. Factories had closed down because of which production ceased. Entire sectors had shut, albeit temporarily, contracting the global economy.[22] As the world leaders and economists assessed the longevity of the crisis, there were hard realizations that thousands of businesses would not be able to sustain the stress of the pandemic, creating permanent paralysing gaps in production and supply chains. Governments would have to intervene with extraordinary relief measures and incentives. The pandemic would come to be a historic disrupter, and only those businesses and companies which were sustainable would be able to endure. In a Darwinian world, it really would come to 'the survival of the fittest', with changed rules of the game.

India for one, foresaw the longevity early. Partly because we were pretty much insulated from the virus for about three weeks after it began to spread in other countries. The three weeks gave us a close insight into its dangerous multiplying ability. We also were very aware that considering the length and breadth of India, breaking the chain of the infection by making hosts unavailable was not possible. So, until there was strong evidenced treatment or a vaccine, right from the get-go, India had to be prepared to live with the virus.

Ever since we had only a handful of cases, the prime minister's economic team had been closely debating the strategy that would work best for our country. Emboldened by the prime minister's insistence on *jaan hai toh jahaan hai*, the goal was to save every Indian life possible, while being acutely aware of what world-renowned economists such as Joseph Stiglitz were preaching: 'The flatter we make the pandemic curve, the steeper the economic cost would be: that's the trade-off'.[23] Indian economists were also closely studying the failures of a moderate distancing approach, where social and economic activity would be allowed to continue only till the rate of infection doesn't explode, followed by disorderly de facto lockdowns.[24] At the time, many world-renowned economists including Nobel Laureates took the view that India's economic response should be one grand re-inflation package which would spend a lot of money trying to re-inflate the economy right upfront as early as April and May 2020.[25]

However, our prime minister, on the sound advice of his economic advisors, took the view, contrary to those opinions, that we were not in for a sprint, but rather a marathon which was going to take us through a great deal of uncertain terrain. So instead of using up all our ammunition right up front, India opted to adopt an adjusted approach: a modified version of the barbell strategy in modern economics.

Now what really is the modified barbell strategy? Let me explain. Imagine a barbell. It has two heavy components on either side, joined together by a small connecting line. Now, let's put it in context of the Indian economic scenario of the time. A modified barbell strategy would mean that the most risky outcomes would be insured against and feedback from restarting economic activity would determine each upcoming response. When the prime minister decided to lock down everything, it was an out-of-normal, once-in-a-century event. It was an extreme step, taken during a time of crisis when there were simply too many unknowns. Had we chosen to have a fairly lenient lockdown, like many other countries, it would not have been as bold a decision. However, we didn't know how long the virus would circulate amongst us, we didn't have proven treatments available, we didn't have enough equipment to safeguard even our healthcare professionals, we didn't have a vaccine in sight and didn't even have the required infrastructure should the virus spread unchecked in our very dense society. In this situation, the prime minister made a strategic decision to impose a stringent lockdown, later rated as the most stringent lockdown in the world by an Oxford University survey.[26] Had we opted for a more moderate strategy, we would have had to be prepared for very negative outcomes. In India's case, the worst outcomes were widely believed to be mass starvation and deaths following the disruption of supply chains and mass bankruptcy.

Let's consider this extreme event of national lockdown as one side of the barbell. In order to balance the barbell on the other side of the connecting line, i.e., when we emerged out of our lockdown, aggressive pumping in of resources would have to be undertaken by the government depending on feedback on how our businesses responded. Speaking on India's economic recovery strategy, Sanjeev Sanyal, principal economic advisor to the GoI, noted,

> This (barbell) approach is often seen as one lacking a grand plan, and this is positively true. However, when dealing in uncertainty—it is impossible to have a grand, prescribed plan. It is only viable to have a broad mission and a broad vision and moving forward based on the feedback loop. It is reactive, yes. But what it does allow you to do, is to feel your way across the river by feeling the strokes. Incidentally, China itself used this approach to build itself up to becoming the world's second largest economy in just three decades.[27]

In a way, fears of mass food shortages were allayed as the government managed to provide substantial rations, free LPG cylinders and cash transfers. While relief measures totalled to only about 1.1 per cent of our

GDP, states were allowed to increase their borrowing limit to 3 per cent of their gross state domestic product (GSDP), out of which 0.5 per cent would be unconditional. The remaining amount would be conditional to the implementation of Centre-recommended policy reforms. However, these measures were only a cushion to soften the blow. Now that the government was evaluating opening up districts in the green zone with almost very little presence of the virus, measures which would have to be put in place to reinvigorate businesses which had gone under due to the nationwide shutdown were being worked out.

Countries with colossal resources offered measures like the furlough scheme in the UK, where the government would cover 80 per cent of the employee wages on behalf of employers[28] or America's CARES package, which offered an extended unemployment insurance programme and a paycheck protection programme where small employers or self-employed individuals would be offered direct cash flow assistance and federally guaranteed loans.[29] Germany, the largest economy in the EU, not only offered a furlough wage cushion in March, but also topped it up with an aggressive surplus package comprising tax cuts and huge loan support programmes.[30]

A ginormous challenge for India was that we had to work with limited resources in our ex-chequer as compared to some of these big economies. Compounding this challenge was that recipients of our programmes were manifold in number as compared to some of these countries. This meant that we didn't have money to throw away. All our money had to be used in a way where we would see multiplying trickle-down effects. Simply reflating of the economy through increased government expenditure could possibly lead to high inflation, and combined with low growth, stagnation. Early on, to prevent a worst-case scenario of business going under, we provided government guaranteed loans to the Micro, Small and Medium Enterprises (MSME) sector and expanded the definition of MSMEs to accommodate more businesses. The Reserve Bank of India (RBI) had stepped in with substantial liquidity support and a cut in the repo rate to 4 per cent. With the fiscal deficit of the government at less than 5 per cent of GDP and more than $490 billion in foreign exchange reserves, there was ample room to begin an infrastructure-led stimulus without causing the currency to depreciate unusually if the current measures proved insufficient. Designing well thought-out, bold structural reforms which would catalyse growth was going to be our key to economic recovery, thus, balancing off the other side of the barbell.

◆

Interestingly, all sorts of theories were being floated in western nations about how COVID-19 infections could be treated—many of them far from scientific. For instance, President Trump was touting the use of disinfectant inside the human body as a COVID-19 cure. An eyewitness reported at the time,

> Let me set the scene, the President had brought along an official for whom this was his first outing in the Briefing Room. At the Department of Homeland Security in their research labs they have been conducting a study on the impact of UV light, temperature and humidity on the coronavirus. And the findings were really interesting—and encouraging. The warmer it gets, the brighter it is, the more humid it is, the less long the virus lives on the surfaces or in the air. The DHS boffin then took us through the impact that [the] disinfectant had on the virus—how it killed it stone dead within a very short time. This clearly flicks a switch in the President's head—and very quickly it is open mic night at Trump University medical school, junior common room. He is riffing on what the potential of this might be. The President starts speculating on putting UV lamps inside the human body. My head is spinning. But then he muses on whether you could inject disinfectant into the human body, just like you spray it onto a kitchen surface: 'I see the disinfectant that knocks it out in a minute, one minute. And is there a way we can do something like that by injection inside, or almost a cleaning? Because you see it gets inside the lungs and it does a tremendous number on the lungs, so it would be interesting to check that.'[31]

Meanwhile, India was focused on strengthening its team of scientists advising the prime minister and the government so that our responses were absolutely, positively evidence-based. In furtherance to that resolve, an important development by mid-April was the constitution of the 'Task Force for Focused Research on Corona Vaccine and other Science & Technology issues' (Vaccine Task Force or VTF, as members would refer to it) with Dr Paul and Prof. VijayRaghavan as co-chairs.[32]

This body subsumed the R&D Task Force on COVID-19 research which was formed a month ago and expanded its membership to now include secretaries of Health Research, Biotechnology, Science and Technology, Scientific and Industrial Research, Telecom, Electronics and Information Technology, Defence R&D, AYUSH, Science and Engineering Research Board, DCGI and the Directorate General of Health Services. VTF looked at mostly upstream research and essentially became a think tank of all national COVID-related issues and responses. Just like how moving towards a source of a river is considered upstream, VTF was vastly the body contemplating the origins of the virus, how it was spreading in other countries and what proved to be effective strategies to curtail it. VTF also began to keep track of all vaccine candidates—national and global—very early on, and essentially became the interface to initiate talks with all organizations engaged in vaccine research. The first outreach to all potential vaccine makers was made by these folks. VTF used the Department of Biotechnology (DBT) as a central coordinating authority for vaccine development. All related assistance, financial and in kind, would be routed to the vaccine manufacturers via them. The first meeting of this task force was held on 16 April and they went on to hold about 23 meetings until July 2021.[33] VTF was constantly briefing the top office of its recommendations which then trickled down to other arms of the government for speedy resolution.

# 11

## ACHIEVING ATMANIRBHARTA

**12 MAY 2020**

INDIA | 47,451 ACTIVE CASES | 2,421 DEATHS

WORLD | 23,06,351 ACTIVE CASES | 3,18,011 DEATHS

All arms of the government, including our Armed Forces had put in night and day to ensure that supply chains of essential items were maintained and healthcare infrastructure significantly updated. Over 588 flights were operated under the Lifeline Udan mission to make sure that even remote corners of the country were not left out of the supply of essentials.[1] We had become self-sufficient in the production of essential medicines, N95 masks, PPE gear as well as ventilators. We had successfully evacuated all Indian citizens who wanted to return home. Time had now come for the country to reopen. Economic measures were put in place and structural changes planned.

The prime minister, after months of cautionary messages, addressed the nation with a message of hope and renewal.[2] Ever since he was voted in as prime minister with a large majority in 2014 and an even larger one in 2019, he has commanded authority from all sides of the political spectrum as a man who could bring drastic changes to catalyse India's growth story. The fact that he presents himself devoid of worldly attachments and as the foremost patriot and a full-time prime minister adds to his credibility. Millions of Indians invest their emotions in his dreams of taking India's growth story to new heights. In his speech on 12 May, he delivered precisely that—his dream for a new, post-COVID, stronger India with a solid plan to achieve it, invoking a rejuvenated spirit of patriotism.

He noted in his speech,

It has been over four months that the global community had been fighting against the Coronavirus. Forty-two lakh people across the world have been infected and tragically over 2.75 lakh have lost their lives. In India too, people have lost near and dear ones. And I express my heartfelt condolences to all. The virus has destroyed the world with crores of people facing the crisis. Across the world, countries are engaged in a battle to save precious lives. We have never seen or even heard of a crisis of such proportion. It a crisis which is unthinkable and unprecedented for all mankind.

*Lekin, thaknaa, harna, tootna, bikharna manav ko manzoor nahi hai. Satark rehte hue, aisi jung ke sabhi niyamo ka palan karte hue, ab hume bachna bhi hai aur aage badhna bhi hai.* (But, getting tired, losing, and breaking down is not acceptable to mankind. By being vigilant and following the new rules of the battle, we not only have to protect ourselves but also move forward.) Today, as the world is in crisis, we have to strengthen our resolve. It is this collective resolve which will be even more powerful than the crisis.

*Hum pichli shataabdi se hi lagaatar sunte aaye hai ki eekisvi sadi Hindustan ki hai.* (We have been hearing since the last century that the twenty-first century will belong to India.) We have had the opportunity to study and analyse in great detail, pre-corona world order and the global arrangements. Even after the Corona crisis has struck, we have been closely and constantly observing the changing global situation. If we look at both of these, from India's perspective, it becomes clear that our dream of the twenty-first century belonging to India doesn't just have to be a dream but also our collective responsibility. But how do we get there? Looking at the prevailing situation in the world today, it is clear that there is only one road to our dream: *Atmanirbhar Bharat* (self-reliant India).

We stand today, as a nation at a very important crossroads. A huge crisis like this has brought to us a warning, a message and an opportunity. Today, the definition of self-reliance has been revisited. The whole world is now looking at human-centric globalization versus the prevalent economy-centric globalization of the recent past. It is here that India's fundamental value of *Vasudhaiva*

*Kutumbakam* (the world is our family) comes in as a ray of hope to the world.³

He proceeded to give out five pillars on which Bharat can achieve self-reliance: first, an economy that brings a quantum jump rather than incremental change. Second, infrastructure which is the identity of modern India. Third, a system which is based on superior technology-driven solutions. Fourth, our vibrant demography which can become the source of energy and lastly, demand. The strength of our demand can drive the cycle of demand and supply chains within our economy, harnessing its full potential. In order to increase demand in the country and to meet this demand, every stakeholder in our supply chain needs to be empowered and our supply chains strengthened by our labour force.

◆

In line with the prime minister's speech, the Union finance minister announced a new liquidity-driven, atmanirbhar relief package worth ₹20 lakh crore—amounting to 10 per cent of India's GDP—to be released over five tranches in the next consecutive days. Keeping in mind the reverse migration which had already started to take place, enterprises which would soon start functioning at normal levels were bound to face a human resource crunch. The fallout of this would pan out as a breakdown of domestic supply chains. In order to attain high growth with moderate inflation, it became imperative to get the supply chain right. With a push in agriculture, coupled with good rainfall, ensured that the workers migrating to villages would most likely occupy themselves in jobs within the agricultural sector. Allotments to the National Rural Employment Guarantee programme were sharply increased so that rural infrastructure could be augmented quickly to support this growing workforce and economic activity. Several measures were announced as part of the package to provide relief to MSMEs, like collateral-free automatic loans as against 100 per cent government guarantee, equity infusion through funds and relaxations in employee provident fund contributions. The package included a special liquidity scheme for Non-banking Financial Institutions (NBFCs), Housing Finance Companies and Mutual Fund Investments, wherein securities issued by them would be fully guaranteed by the government. This also included a partial credit guarantee scheme for NBFCs wherein 20 per cent loss would be borne by the government. In tranche two of the packages, announced on 14 May, the focus was mostly on the farmers and middle-income families. Middle-income families would be provided credit-linked subsidies of up to ₹6–18 lakh a year. It also provided tax breaks of up to 25 per cent in tax collected at source (TCS) and tax deducted at source (TDS) rates. Fifty lakh street vendors were included in the list of beneficiaries as the package provided for up to ₹10, 000 working capital along with a micro-credit facility (PM SVANidhi). The free food grain scheme for migrants was extended for two more months amounting to ₹3,500 crore. Emergency working capital would be provided to farmers and concessional credit to two and a half crore farmers would be provided through Kisan Credit Cards. In tranche three, which the finance minister announced on 15 May, funds were to be provided for agri infrastructure projects, formalization of micro food enterprises, animal husbandry infrastructure development fund, funds for fishermen and funds for promotion of herbal cultivation and beekeeping initiatives. The policy push announced was that the Essential Commodities Act would be amended to free up agriculture marketing.

The borrowing limit of the states had been increased to more than 2 per cent of their GSDP. Interestingly, they were incentivized to adopt certain Centre-led policy initiatives in order to be able to borrow the full 2 per cent. In other words, while the Centre increased the borrowing limit of the states by an extra 2 per cent from what was earlier sanctioned, 1 per cent was made conditional on implementation of certain economic reforms. The Centre hoped that his kind of incentivization would nudge the states to adopt progressive policies to avail additional funds in the spirit of Centre–state *bhagidari*. There was a push for four policy reforms, which came with an attachment to borrowing an additional 0.25 per cent GSDP each. The first reform under the One Nation One Ration card policy required states to ensure that all ration cards in the state under the National Food Security Act were seeded with Aadhaar numbers of all family members. It also required states to ensure that all fair price shops were equipped with electronic points-of-sale devices. The second reform required states to ensure that the renewal of business-related licences under 7 Acts was made automatic, online and non-discretionary on payment of fees. The third reform required states to notify floor rates of property tax and of water and sewerage charges in consonance with stamp duty guideline values for property transactions and current costs respectively, in urban areas. The fourth reform would require the states to introduce direct benefit transfers in lieu of free electricity supply to farmers. The states would have to formulate a state-wide scheme accordingly and pilot it in one district by the end of the year. Kerala, Chhattisgarh and Goa implemented all four reforms availing maximum benefits for their people, whereas Maharashtra, Delhi and West Bengal failed to implement even one.

Several more measures across public and private sectors were announced in the next two tranches, providing a much-needed fiscal boost to reignite the economy.[4]

◆

## 19 MAY 2020

INDIA | 60,855 ACTIVE CASES | 3,311 DEATHS

WORLD | 25,11,431 ACTIVE CASES | 3,55,250 DEATHS

Meena Mukhiya (name changed) heard panicked noises as her husband Ravi Kumar Mukhiya rushed into their 100 sq. feet room in the Nehru Nagar chawl in Juhu. She shared the room with her husband Ravi, his two brothers and her two-year-old daughter. The brothers worked in temporary jobs as house help and cooks in upper middle-class homes in the posh JVPD suburb of Mumbai. After the lockdown was announced, all three brothers were asked to discontinue coming to work. For two months, they were paid their salaries; however, they had been forewarned by their respective employers that they should not expect to be receiving any more. Cash crunch had begun to hit even affluent households and coupled with the uncertainty of when businesses would function at pre-COVID-19 levels, they simply could not afford to keep their staff on payroll.

Lockdown had been hard. The five of them had to be cooped up inside the teeny room. The enforcement on movement restriction by the next-door Juhu Police Station had been very harsh, with folks unable to leave even the narrow lanes which housed their rooms. Entry and exit points to the Nehru Nagar Chawl were blocked by policemen carrying lathis, who didn't hesitate to use them. The family was paying ₹6,000 as room rent and with no income in sight, they had begun to grow increasingly frustrated and desperate to return to their village in Bihar, where the boys' parents had a big farm with a large self-built house. Over the years, the brothers had sent the savings to the parents in the village to build the family home. Her two-year-old had not had a cup of milk in over a month and the family was exclusively relying on the free rice, wheat and pulses provided by the government as their meals in the absence of any money available to buy other groceries. Sometimes, the middlemen distributing the rice and pulses would cut corners and the grains would come in mixed with pebbles or sand even, and at other times, the middlemen would not come through with the grains at all. Desperation was at a peak. If at home, in the village, they would have no shortage of good food, farm-grown vegetables and meat and they would also be able to work in the fields and generate income out of farming.

Every day, there was a new rumour in the drain-lined lane housing their room about many people falling severely ill with the virus and being taken away by the government to quarantine centres. Sometimes those rumours would get serious when news would arrive that the person taken away had not been able to make it alive. Meena was worried about the baby's health and was willing to take any risk to be able to go back home.

Emotions were running high as this was the case in most rooms in the Nehru Nagar Chawl. In a tense situation like this, news came in via some boys in the chawl that the local police station had called and confirmed that the government had arranged for a train scheduled to depart for Bihar late in the afternoon to send folks like them back home.[5] Her husband rushed in and asked her to immediately pack the essentials and the baby and leave as soon as possible so as to make the long 45-minute walk to the Bandra Terminus Railway Station. They didn't have any further details of how many trains were arranged or the timings or the scheduled trains; and in the case with so many unknowns, they decided to follow the flock. Most migrants living in the chawl had also set off towards the Bandra Terminus Station. Hundreds of them rushed out of the chawl, outnumbering the lathi-yielding policemen who were stationed there and began to brisk walk. Most were not even carrying bags with them, which Meena found a little odd, even in the heat of the moment. She had managed to tie the baby's essentials and some water in a cloth which she carried over her shoulder. They made their way to the station by foot in the absence of any available public transport.

As they arrived at the station, they found that no such train was scheduled to depart for their home state and they had just fallen for a false rumour. Like Meena Mukhiya and her family, thousands of other people from chawls in various parts of the city had also fallen for similar fake news, and walked to the same station. Dejected, she sat with her daughter on the side of the platform while Ravi and his two brothers, Basant and Shyam, dived into the angry crowd demanding the police, who had arrived at the scene to disperse them, for answers.

The media, considered essential services, began to aggressively track the story and by mid-afternoon, chaotic images of hordes of angry mobs collected at the station began to appear on various news platforms. Bandra East, Mumbai's western suburb, where the crowds collected, was already classified as a red zone, with high positivity rate. Dispelling all COVID-19-appropriate behaviour of masks and social distancing was a step back for the city in its fight against the virus.

Not only did it throw light on the unfortunate plight of this vulnerable community, but it also exposed the incapability of the state government to act quickly in the interest of the city. Several things could have been done to avoid this: the migrants should have been better provided for by the state government, which was headed by Uddhav Thackeray of the Shiv Sena in an alliance with the Congress and the NCP. On the day itself, it was rather odd to see that none of the crowds making their way to the station were stopped by the Mumbai Police. It was only after the mob got out of control at the station, did the police arrive at the location and lathi-charged. Naturally, it leads one to ask: if the media was able to follow the story since morning, why wasn't the police? Even if we work on the assumption that the cops did not receive the intelligence of such an event taking place, police were stationed all over the city in order to enforce lockdown. Why didn't they act? There were reports in the media that the rumours were spread by local police stations.[6] Were folks instigated to come out on the roads for an underlying political agenda?

From 1 May, the GoI had arranged for Shramik Special trains, which would be operated gradually, in a phased manner, to take the migrants back to their villages. Eighty-five per cent of the cost of these trains would be borne by the Centre, whereas the other 15 per cent would be undertaken by the states. This exercise was taking place in close coordination with the states, where the states would have to raise demands and furnish a list of returnees, on the basis of which the number of trains, their destinations and routes would be planned by the Union Railway Ministry. To get on to the list, migrants would need to pre-register. Extensive safety arrangements to test and quarantine the returnees were made in recipient states so as to avoid the spread of the virus to remote parts of the country. In Maharashtra, political spats turned ugly when Thackeray announced in a televised message that they had been asking the Centre for 80 trains to operate daily, but the Centre was only sending 30-odd ones. Responding to this criticism, the Centre planned 125 trains to be operated in a couple of days, provided the state gave the list of migrants who would be boarding these trains in the next hour. However, several hours passed, but the Maharashtra state government was unable to send over the list.[7] Union Railway Minster, Piyush Goyal, tweeted,

> More than 2.5 hours have passed but still passenger details for 125 planned trains in Maharashtra not received by GM Central Railway from Government of Maharashtra. I hope that these trains will not have to leave empty after arriving at the station like it has happened earlier. I would like to assure you that the trains you need will be available.[8]

The Central Railway issued a press release noting that it had to cancel 65 scheduled trains due to the incapability of the state government to deliver a list of passengers. They added, 'For the last two hours, rail authorities have been waiting for the list of passengers with details of their destination to plan the trains. Planning special trains is an elaborate process, which requires time and unless lists are given in time, Maharashtra government will make it impossible for Railways to run trains.'[9] Eventually, at 2:00 a.m., Goyal tweeted once again: 'Where is the list for 125 trains from Maharashtra? As of 2am, received list of only 46 trains of which 5 are to West Bengal and Odisha which cannot operate due to cyclone Amphan. We are notifying only 41 trains for today despite being prepared for 125 !!!'[10]

Early in the month, when the GoI had just begun the Shramik trains, the official guidelines to cover costs were, 'Sending state may decide to bear this cost or take it from passengers or take it from receiving state after mutual consultation or may charge it to any fund. It is purely their prerogative. Without a ticket, passengers cannot go, so we are issuing tickets to each passenger.'[11] However, coming down heavily on the decision of the Centre to charge the states for migrant travel or possibly take ticket costs from migrants, Congress interim president Sonia Gandhi issued a letter stating that state Congress units would cover the cost of migrants on-boarding the trains.[12] The letter was clearly intended for Ms Gandhi to come away as the premier saviour of migrants, fighting tooth and nail for their justice. The Central Railways had to come out clean on their cost break-up and specify that it was the states which had to cover the costs. With that being said, the fact remains that no money has been borne to date by any of the state Congress units for this purpose. Zilch.

There was one particular nail-biting episode where the Congress committed to arrange for a thousand busses to send migrants from Rajasthan to UP. Priyanka Gandhi Vadra, the Congress general secretary, urged the Yogi Adityanath government to make use of them. What is rather interesting about Mrs Gandhi Vadra is that she surfaces only when elections are around the corner or to create a controversy. In a way, it may be fair to even say that the party mostly uses her only to elevate matters in the national media narrative, possibly to gather more attention. In the quickly unfolding drama, politicizing the matter in a recorded video which she uploaded on social media, Mrs Gandhi Vadra urged the UP chief minister to use the buses, even if they had 'to put BJP stickers on them'. The permission for the buses to enter UP was denied by the Yogi government because many of them were junk vehicles registered as vehicles such as autorickshaws, cars and trucks; many were unsafe and the rest were uninsured. Allowing uninsured, unregistered vehicles into the state could possibly create a law-and-order problem and thus, in retaliation, the UP police filed an FIR against Mrs Gandhi Vadra's personal secretary for cheating and forging documents. Eventually, the Congress party yielded and recalled the deployed buses from the Rajasthan-UP border.[13]

The media developments which had occurred over the past two months since the migrants began to walk home, shortly after the announcement of the nationwide lockdown had been rather interesting. The unfortunate mass exodus was tracked and covered extensively in sections of the media. When it started to appear that the Congress and other opposition parties in the country were able to use this to attack the government over its failure to rehabilitate the migrants before the announcement of the lockdown, the international media too began to extensively cover the story. Pictures were published on a daily basis of tired, hungry, desperate migrants trying to walk back home. Stories of people dying on the roads due to dehydration or hunger were also extensively published with gut-wrenching videos. An interesting pattern came to be observed, Left-leaning international media became hyperactive in covering these stories; most often with anti-establishment freelancing journalists based in India.[14] Several Indian journalists like Barkha Dutt even revived their careers tracking 'on-the-road' micro stories of the journey home on their YouTube channels.[15] To give you a better idea of why I cautiously use the word 'revive', her YouTube channel Mojo Story attracted fewer than 7,000 views in October 2019. After the grotesque coverage of selling miseries and Hindu pyres, the channel began to attract over 2 lakh views per video. Several folks in the film industry made documentaries and several authors wrote books detailing the miseries the migrants faced.[16] [17] Due to this increased coverage, it began to take up lot of prime-time space in news channels, print media as well as social media. As a consequence, success stories of how India was saving most lives per capita as compared to the rest of the world became buried, putting the government on the back foot in terms of media perception. However, despite going all out, these loaded tactics failed to dent the approval ratings of the prime minister.

Let us take for instance, the Bihar Assembly polls, which took place in November 2020—the first state-level elections to follow after the COVID-19 crisis. Prof. Shamika Ravi of Brookings Institution authored a paper with an in-depth post-poll analysis of the results, which were in favour of the prime minister-led National Democratic Alliance (NDA) government. The paper revealingly concluded that the poorest districts of Bihar, from where most migrants come from, voted for the BJP. The paper also made the scientific assumption that the post-COVID schemes announced by the prime minister were truly reaching the last Indian on the ground, a significant chunk of who were migrant returnees in Bihar, as intended. This analysis also discredits the jingoism fed into the media by the political opposition about the migrants being angry, ignored and unhappy with the Modi government.[18]

Now, coming back to the Mumbai episode with an understanding of the prevalent media narrative of the time, there were several pertinent questions to be asked. Could one draw a conclusion that the Shiv Sena-led government wanted to instigate and create an episode displaying migrant desperation which would continue to push the anti-government media narrative? Were the cops asked to deliberately ignore the crowds walking to the railway station? Was any investigation conducted to find out if the rumours of a planned migrants' train were ignited by the police as many media sections reported?

While several migrants died on the journey home, the truth remains that lakhs of lives and mass deaths in rural India were averted due to the decision of not sending them home in the early days of the pandemic. In national interest, the government took on the attacks and didn't budge on their decision to start migrant movement from the cities until they were fully prepared.

# 12

## EYE OF THE STORM

**1 JUNE 2020**

**INDIA | 96,990 ACTIVE CASES | 5,626 DEATHS**

**WORLD | 27,50,337 ACTIVE CASES | 4,19,796 DEATHS**

While the country was unlocking itself and economic activity picking up, our scientists were making immense progress as well. The COVID-19 NTF had been working in close contact with various agencies to fill the gaps in production of indigenous medical supplies.

As countries were beginning to cope with the new normal, heartening news was coming in from the global scientific community regarding progress being made in vaccine development. The US, under President Trump's $10-billion fund under Operation Warp Speed, invested about $2.5 billion to help research and develop Moderna's vaccines and buy doses. Pfizer had partnered with BioNTech and produced a working messenger ribonucleic acid (mRNA) vaccine in a record 63 days and had already begun Phase I trials. The UK, on the other hand, in January 2020 had announced the allocation of £40 million in search for a vaccine.

Early last month in May, the prime minister had chaired a meeting with top bureaucrats from concerned ministries, Dr V.K. Paul, Dr VijayRaghavan and officials from the ICMR in which the agenda was to discuss India's vaccination strategy. Dr Bhargava had informed him that the ICMR along with the Department of Biotechnology had successfully isolated a strain of the virus at its Pune-based facility, the NIV. This is one of the foremost critical steps in the road to vaccine development. The prime minister had insisted that India push the model of an 'Entrepreneurial State' even in crafting its vaccine strategy. He had added that the government should look at credible private players as partners in the common goal of making vaccines available to all Indians in the fastest possible time. He particularly had insisted that the government mustn't distinguish between public and private players, and keep the eye on the target of achieving the collective goal. Following the PM's approval, the ICMR tied up with a Hyderabad-based private company called Bharat Biotech International Limited (BBIL) to develop a fully indigenous COVID-19 vaccine. Globally, eight candidates had already entered the human trial stage and India was in no mood to be left out of that race. After the official tie-up, the isolated strain was transferred by the NIV to Bharat Biotech. Other Indian private companies were not far behind either. The Serum Institute of India (SII) had already partnered with University of Oxford's vaccine project, becoming one of the seven institutions globally capable of mass manufacturing the vaccine. Zydus Cadila, too, was attempting to develop a DNA-based vaccine.

In view of these developments, Dr Paul and Prof. VijayRaghavan led VTF-initiated conversations with all potential vaccine manufacturers in India as well as abroad. The main foreign players in the advanced stages targeting mass production and availability by the third quarter of 2020 seemed to be Pfizer, Moderna, Johnson & Johnson and Sputnik. Initial conversations mostly indicated the kind of logistics required to be able to import, distribute and administer these vaccines successfully without wastage.

Meanwhile, Bharat Biotech had successfully developed its vaccine based on an inactivated virus which would trigger an immune response in the body to draw up a defence system against the infection. During the rest of the month, they would undergo toxicity studies in rats, mice and rabbits and submit their data to the DCGI in order to be cleared for Phase I human trials. Likewise, Zydus Cadila, too, would successfully develop the worlds' only DNA-based vaccine a few weeks into June, which would be capable of generating an immune response and pass the test for safety.

◆

## 15 JUNE 2020

INDIA | 1,52,761 ACTIVE CASES | 9,945 DEATHS

WORLD | 30,52,471 ACTIVE CASES | 4,92,092 DEATHS

While the National COVID-19 task force, the empowered groups and all arms of the government were fighting on a war footing against an invisible, unknown and unpredictable enemy, our soldiers stationed in the Galwan Valley along the 3,488-km-long Sino–Indian border engaged in a violent face-off with the People's Liberation Army's (PLA) forces: a first since the 1962 India–China War. This stand-off would have long-term consequences on India's bilateral relationship with China as well on the Indian political psyche to focus on reducing dependability on China in trade. Eventually, India's atmanirbharta would enable us to significantly improve our position in the global supply chains which were reforming due to the pandemic. In fact, in the first state visit to India post-pandemic, when the Prime Minister of Denmark Mette Frederiksen gave her remarks to the press, she noted, 'Can't rely solely on China, India needs to become part of global supply chain,' echoing sentiments of several other world leaders.[1]

The Galwan River Valley, with its harsh climate and high-altitude terrain, has more or less been peaceful despite being in the disputed Himalayan border region. The clash occurred during the night time hours along the Galwan River, which originates from Aksai Chin, a disputed area claimed by India, but controlled by China, reaching the Shyok River.[2] At a certain point along the route, at a height of 14,000 ft on a steep terrain, the river takes a sharp left turn before merging with Shyok. Patrol Point 14 (PP14) is just a little bit ahead of this confluence and has traditionally been a point up until where Indian and Chinese troops regularly and jointly patrolled. However, a structure has never been built at this level due to bipartisan understanding. Since over a month, tension had been building up around this point: the Chinese first built up a tent along this point in an area considered to be part of the Indian territory and attempted to trek down the Shyok River. After confrontation by the Indian troops, they dismantled the tent and retreated. However, after this one-off event, both sides built up troops at their camps near PP14, raising tension in the area. Early in

June, a meeting was held between the Indian Corps Commander and his Chinese counterpart where it was decided that both sides would retreat by two kilometres from their current positions in order to maintain peace in the area. Both troops retreated accordingly. But in a few days, the Indians discovered that the Chinese had once again built two structures on a slope leading down to the river, one of which seemed to be an observation point. The Commanding Officer held talks with his counterpart and agreed that both sides would strictly honour the talks which were held between the Corps Commanders, which would involve the Chinese having to dismantle those structures. Later in the day, when the Indian troops visited PP14 to check if the structures had been dismantled, they observed that, in fact they hadn't. The Indian Commanding Officer ordered the Indian troops to dismantle the structure which was met with a small group of Chinese soldiers who engaged in a verbal spat. However in less than an hour, while this brawl went on, a larger group of Chinese soldiers arrived with iron rods, stones and sticks, outnumbering the Indian troops. The Indian Commanding Officer was hurt and fell into the freezing river, charging up our troops who wrangled the weapons from the Chinese. This fight seemed to be happening over a ledge, leading to several soldiers falling over into the icy-cold river. After learning about the brawl breaking, the Indian contingent too sent more soldiers armed with sticks. Both sides engaged in hand-to-hand combat, in which several Chinese soldiers were gravely injured. The main area of the fight was narrow and at one point the Indian troops had outnumbered the Chinese, compelling several Chinese soldiers to run off to the area of the Chinese build-up. A group of Indian soldiers who chased them, crossing the Line of Actual Control (LAC), were held captive and released four days after Major General-level talks were held on both sides the morning after. Rough estimates indicate that we lost about 20 men, whereas PLA lost about 43.[3] Several of them succumbed to their wounds unable to survive the freezing temperatures overnight.

One of the main reasons for the building up of tension along the region is considered to be a new road: the Darbuk–Shyok–DBO Road, which India had built along one of the most remote and vulnerable areas along the LAC in Ladakh. Ladakh is inhospitable in terms of its weather conditions, its highest valley being 9,800 feet above sea level and cold desert temperatures touching about -20C during winters. Due to the climatic hostility of the region, it has largely been a peaceful area of the LAC. However, India's effort to build a several hundred kilometres long road in 2019 activated at Daulat Beg Oldi (DBO), the world's highest landing ground, which would connect to a high-altitude forward air base was a cause for suspicion among the Chinese. The worry was that the road could significantly boost India's capacity to move men and material quickly in case of conflict. China had also extensively developed its infrastructure along the India–Tibet frontier. Even before the Galwan skirmish, scuffles had occurred between the two sides at other disputed areas such as Gogra Hot Springs, Depsang Plains and south Pangong Tso lake, but the loss of lives had not been reported.

In order to keep the LAC area peaceful and to ensure no such deadly fights occur in the future, both countries undertook several rounds of talks between senior military officials and bilateral talks between diplomats. In the middle of a pandemic ripping through the world, the idea of the world's two most populous nations and the planet's two largest military forces at loggerheads with each other for weeks was very bad news, not only for both countries but also for the larger interest of humanity. Yet, India was not prepared to accept the territorial aggression which the PLA had been displaying akin to that in the South China Sea. In several of the disputed spots, the Chinese troops had inched closer and built temporary structures at patrolling points where the two countries had agreed not to engage. Though India was interested in peace and had made that abundantly clear to them in all global forums, it wasn't going to sit back and let its land be taken over by the Chinese. We were not going to be bullied this time around.

◆

## 30 JUNE 2020

INDIA | 2,20,493 ACTIVE CASES | 17,463 DEATHS

WORLD | 36,94,370 ACTIVE CASES | 5,72,879 DEATHS

The cases were on the rise, but India had managed to flatten the curve. The rise in cases was slow, gradual and the critical cases presenting themselves at hospitals were manageable due to the several infrastructure upgrades we had made over the last three months. However, a deeply eager Opposition along with its loyal ecosystem began to set a narrative that the government had flattened the wrong curve: the GDP curve versus the COVID-19 curve. Rahul Gandhi, best described by former president of the US, Barack Obama, as 'lacking aptitude or passion to master the subject'[4], motivated by media attention on the 'flattening the wrong curve' plot, tweeted a graph of a slow-moving Indian case-rise with a caption, 'frightening, not flattening.'[5] Close in line with President Obama's assessment, the infographic which he tweeted neither demonstrated fast-rising cases, nor a vertical caseload—something which we would have seen as early as May, had the lockdown not been announced, leading to mass deaths. As we may see further too, tweeting furiously with vim, vigour and venom would be the only familiar hallmark of Rahul Gandhi's political riposte to every issue he chooses to take up.

Mr Ram Sewak Sharma, the bureaucrat in charge of several major digital initiatives over the years such as Unified Payments Interface (UPI) and Aadhaar, had last month sought time to see the prime minister. Today, on 30 June, he was to finally meet with the PM to discuss how digitization could help India in its battle against the virus. He had retired from service several years ago but was brought back to head the Telecom Regulatory Authority of India (TRAI). A fine IAS officer with an educational background from University of California and subsequent doctorate from IIT-Delhi, he was one of India's go-to men for his expertise in data digitization and security. He had been planning the presentation he was about to make to the prime minister for months. There was no doubt in his mind that if a billion people had to be vaccinated in four to six months, then a 'digital vaccination certificate' would be required which could be used to allow friction-free movement as the country opened up. Ahead of time, he wrote in the first slide of his Power Point presentation: high digital coordination would be needed to achieve scale, save cost, increase economic value and avoid social issues.

He included his learning and experiences from Aadhaar in which he noted that within a year of launch, 1,500 empanelled agencies, 40,000 enrolment stations, 2 lakh trained operators and 15 lakh enrolments were all coordinated by the common digital platform put in place. In order to make the vaccination project a success, the government should be planning to achieve over a crore vaccinations per day, he opined. He proceeded to present a bunch of high-level ideas which included details on empanelment, necessary training, certification of providers and price discovery for vaccinating each person. He added ways to make payment at these empanelled locations and suggested pre-paid payment vouchers. He insisted that a large number of locations such as camps at community centres, mobile vans and so on must be activated instead of a few central places so as to avoid crowding and panic. He also suggested creating a National Testing and Vaccination Platform to orchestrate this entire effort. He added that other rules required in the domain would have to be factored in ahead of time: some people may not need to be vaccinated, so perhaps we should consider proving them with an 'Immunity certificate'; some people may not be eligible for vaccination due to age or pre-existing conditions, so we would have to identify these folks and exclude them from the vaccination programme; some vaccines may require multiple doses and the app created would have to be able to monitor this digitally per individual.

In his concluding remarks, Mr Sharma pitched to the prime minister that the government must invest in a scalable vaccination digital health infrastructure, as it would be critical for India to be self-reliant and resilient to absorb future shocks similar to COVID-19.

The prime minister shared his vision for COVID-19 vaccination with him, and technology formed its backbone. The PM wanted to ensure that the drive remained accessible, equal and neutral for every Indian irrespective of their class, caste, reach and financial status. According to the PM, the speed and scale of India's election process is a unique expertise that India has developed and there are very few countries that even come close. Using the same learnings and approach, India could create an important tool for vaccination. PM asked him to immediately get going and create a platform that could become a model for the world.

◆

## 3 JULY 2020

**INDIA | 2,36,836 ACTIVE CASES | 18,734 DEATHS**

**WORLD | 37,57,516 ACTIVE CASES | 5,78,433 DEATHS**

Three Corps Commander-level meetings had taken place following the Galwan Valley stand-off in which 20 Indian soldiers attained martyrdom. The last one as recent as 30 June was when both sides had decided to disengage troops in a phased manner. Both sides had been throwing accusations at each other holding the other responsible for crossing the poorly demarcated border and provoking the fight. Immediately after the clash, the prime minister, in a televised address had assured the Indians that Indian military was fully capable of defending our borders and that they had been given a free hand to take all necessary steps to protect the Indian territory. He had added that after the clash, no foreign soldiers were inside Indian borders and none of our territory had been lost or captured.[6]

However, in a surprise visit, in the early hours of the morning on 3 July, the prime minister accompanied by the Chief of Defence Staff (CDS) General Bipin Rawat and Army Chief M.M. Naravane landed at the Kushok Bakula Rimpochee airport at Leh and made his way after to a forward post in Nimu, Ladakh, at 11,000 feet.[7] The prime minister spoke to senior military personnel who briefed him on the Galwan clash along with activities at other points of tension. He then proceeded to visit the wounded soldiers, followed by a speech to uplift their spirits. A prime minister being present at a point of conflict hadn't happened in India's recent past, and not only did it boost the morale of the Armed Forces but also sent a tough message to the global community that India would not accept this expansionist attitude and would fight tooth and nail to defend its territory. His visit was also significant because at a time when most world leaders weren't travelling, the prime minister not only went to a forward base in Ladakh for the sake of the Armed Forces, even when his NSA was in isolation, but had also done so in the aftermath of Cyclone Amphan in West Bengal and Odisha a month ago.[8]

Following the visit, the Indian government was firm on its view that border tensions and bilateral relations would have to go hand in hand. Border tensions and clashes would not be looked at as stand-alone events with no effect on bilateral relations.[9] In a bid to display this line of thought, over the next couple of months, the Indian government took strategic policy decisions like banning several Chinese apps in circulation in India and also mandating disclosure of source of funds and prior government approval for foreign direct investments (FDIs) from border nations in various strategic sectors of business. While, on ground, the trade impact from that would not be major, the message that it sent out globally was strong, especially during a time when the world was holding China accountable for the spread of the pandemic and its irresponsible delay in alerting the WHO. In a post-COVID world, a supply chain rejig would likely follow India's stance on cutting down over-reliant trade relationships with China. In a situation where global supply chains would be recalibrated, India, empowered with the new atmanirbhar policies and a powerful labour force, would appear to be a rather attractive destination conducive for global business interests. To reiterate, in a recent comment in *The Australian*, former Australian Prime Minister Tony Abbott, noted, 'The answer to almost every question about China is India. With the world's other emerging superpowers becoming more belligerent almost by the day, it's in everyone's interests that India take its rightful place among the nations as quickly as possible.'[10]

# 13

## VACCINE DEVELOPMENT

**15 JULY 2020**

**INDIA | 3,31,387 ACTIVE CASES | 25,047 DEATHS**

**WORLD | 45,30,879 ACTIVE CASES | 6,56,269 DEATHS**

Over the last several weeks, officials from the Department of Biotechnology and the Biotechnology Industry Research Assistance Council (BIRAC) had been working closely with manufacturers of about 15 Indian vaccine candidates routed through discussions via the VTF. Determined not to stall a single candidate due to the unavailability of funds, they pumped in hundreds of crores of rupees in several of these companies at various stages during clinical and pre-clinical trials. They also offered technical support like making available clinical trial sites across the country, managing three immunogenicity assay laboratories and three animal challenge facilities.

All the way back in April, when Oxford University had arrived at a successful vaccine candidate, they tied up with several manufacturing companies around the world for scaling up production; SII being one of them. SII is the world's largest vaccine manufacturer in terms of volumes and was an early player in raising thousands of crores in order to develop and scale up vaccine production. However, several countries, especially the wealthier nations began an ugly race for vaccine hoarding, preordering significantly more doses than needed with multiple suppliers. In an effort to stop 'vaccine nationalism', the WHO along with Gavi, a Geneva-based organization and Coalition for Epidemic Preparedness Innovations (CEPI) created a joint fund called COVAX. The fund would carry the mandate to secure two billion vaccine doses out of which 92 million would be for low- and middle-income countries and the other billion for wealthier nations capable of shelling out money. To take forward this initiative, SII signed a licence with British-Swedish drug maker AstraZeneca and Oxford University to produce one billion doses, out of which 400 million were to be delivered before the end of 2020.[1] These doses would be reserved exclusively for low- and middle-income countries and half a million of them would go to India each year. Oxford University and AstraZeneca had already begun Phase I and II human trials in the UK way back in April 2020 and had progressed to Phase III trials in May. Just last month, in June, they had begun Phase III trials in Brazil and Phase I/II trials in South Africa as well.

As per best scientific practices, bridge trials are crucial in understanding how a potential vaccine candidate works on the local population, considering varying issues of ethnicity and genetic variations. They are especially important early on to observe adverse effects, before the vaccine has been safely administered on a large scale across a wide range of ethnicities. Considering this, if SII had to apply for emergency use authorization in India, it would have to conduct these trials and furnish the outcomes, despite its partner companies having conducted trials elsewhere in the world. In view of this, the ICMR extended ₹11 crore worth of financial assistance to SII to conduct bridge trials in India in addition to the help provided in recruitment of 1,600 candidates for the trials.[2]

Bharat Biotech's vaccine candidate Covaxin, which was being jointly developed with the ICMR, had also published positive results from its pre-clinical trials and had begun Phase I trials in the country. Phases I and II of the trials generally observe for mild and adverse effects in a limited number of people against a placebo vaccine. ICMR provided ₹35 crore to Bharat Biotech for the trials on 25,800 participants.[3] The Zydus Cadila vaccine was also provided ₹10 crore to initiate and facilitate human trials.

Vaccine development process is long and complex around the world. Typically, it takes about a decade to research, develop and test a new vaccine. However, the fact that the scientific community came forth to produce not just one, but several vaccine candidates, while adhering to best practices, is absolutely commendable. The three vaccine candidates in India which looked promising at the moment were based on different scientific theories. Bharat Biotech's Covaxin is based on an inactivated virus platform. An inactivated pathogen does not multiply and cannot cause disease but is capable of producing an immune response in the body, thus training the immune system to fight the virus and preparing the body sufficiently for future protection. In order to achieve this, a strain of the virus is inactivated using chemicals and converted to a safe immunogen and administered with an adjuvant (a substance used to improve the immune response) in multiple doses. This is one of the more traditional platforms on which several vaccines for other pathogens have been developed successfully in the past.

SII's Covishield is based on a viral vector platform. The SARS-CoV-2 virus is studded with proteins which it then uses to enter human cells. Covishield works by targeting these proteins by using double stranded DNA. The vaccine adds the gene for the coronavirus spike protein to a modified virus derived from a chimpanzee adenovirus which can enter human cells but can't replicate inside them. On being injected, the adenoviruses latch on to the proteins on the cells' surface from which they are engulfed. Once engulfed, they release the DNA into the nucleus of the cells from which the gene for the coronavirus spike protein can be read by the cell and copied into a molecule called mRNA which further leads to formation of spikes which can be recognized by the immune system and generate an immune response. This platform has been under research for years and was only recently approved for an Ebola vaccine made by Johnson & Johnson. Using a DNA strand makes the vaccine more tolerant and the adenovirus' tough protein coat helps protect the genetic material inside. This means it is less fragile than those based on RNA platforms, doesn't need to be frozen and has a longer shelf life when refrigerated at 2–8 degree Celsius (normal refrigerator temperature), making it logistically easier to transport and store in a vast country like India.

The Zydus Cadila vaccine, on the other hand, uses a new technology platform called DNA plasmid. It uses small rings of DNA or plasmids containing genetic information which is carried to the cells in order to make 'spike proteins', which can be used to penetrate the cells and generate an immune response. Since it is based on DNA, it is also stable at higher temperatures and doesn't need to be frozen, making logistics easier. This is also a needle-free vaccine with less adverse side effects, making it safer for administration in children. The vaccine can also be manufactured in laboratories which are Biosafety level I versus those based on inactivated virus platform which need Biosafety level III manufacturing units, thus making it relatively easier and cheaper to achieve large-scale production quickly. On approval, this would be the first vaccine in the world to be accepted under the DNA plasmid technology platform, a rather proud first step for India.

Gennova, an Indian company, had also reached advanced stages in the development of their mRNA-based vaccine. If successful, it would be India's first indigenous mRNA vaccine, further reducing our dependence on international manufacturers.

In a conversation, Mr Sanjay Singh, CEO of Gennova, had said to me, 'I had written my first email to the GoI regarding Gennova's efforts to create an mRNA vaccine in March 2020. Immediately after, the GoI asked us to show proof of concept and once we were able to demonstrate reasonable success, we were given ₹25 crore as seed funds to buy machinery and raw material.'

♦

## 12 AUGUST 2020

INDIA | 6,52,127 ACTIVE CASES | 47,484 DEATHS

WORLD | 57,15,499 ACTIVE CASES | 8,32,376 DEATHS

Considering that by now there was significant visibility on the availability of vaccines, a new group called the National Expert Group on Vaccine Administration for COVID-19 (NEGVAC) was constituted with Dr Paul and secretary of MoHFW as co-chairs. Members included representatives from five state governments: UP, Maharashtra, Tamil Nadu, Madhya Pradesh and Assam, representatives from AIIMS, technical experts, representatives from the National Technical Advisory Group on Immunisation, secretaries from the Ministry of External Affairs, Department of Expenditure, Department of Biotechnology, Department of Health Research, Department of Pharmaceuticals, and the Ministry of Electronics and Information Technology. Essentially, NEGVAC was constituted in order to find solutions for vaccination implementation on a large scale. They'd go on to decide priority groups, when to open up vaccination for the younger individuals, make protocols on which comorbidities would be considered for eligibility in priority groups, provide solutions for cold chain logistics for vaccine deliveries and ensure availability of associated medical equipment required like syringes, needles and such. For instance, it is this group which first conceived of a need for an IT platform to aid the vaccination drive following the prime minister's advice. They later passed down the mandate to the Empowered Group to upscale one already in place—Electronic Vaccine Intelligence Network (eVIN), which was then converted to CoWIN with significant upgrades. Essentially, NEGVAC acted like a body for practical churning on all issues which were likely to come up in India's vaccination journey.

As mentioned above, conversations with vaccine manufacturers were now handled by NEGVAC. With several vaccines around the world making progress and showing encouraging results, pre-orders were rolling in. By mid-August, the wealthy nations had begun to pre-order many vaccines in quantities far more than required for their populations. The US had secured 800 million doses of at least six vaccines in development, with an option to purchase around one billion more. The UK, becoming the world's highest per-capita buyer, purchased around five doses of various vaccines for every citizen. The EU nations were buying vaccines as a group and Japan too locked down millions of doses of vaccines for itself. This resulted in potential vaccine manufacturers already packed to capacity with orders from wealthy nations for doses which may not even be used and as a result other countries were left scrambling to secure doses even for vulnerable groups.[4]

While NEGVAC continued its engagement with foreign manufacturers, it became clear that Moderna and Pfizer were not willing to spare the kind of large quantities required by India within the time frame we were looking at: late 2020, early-mid 2021. On the contrary, they were willing to offer measly doses at expensive prices—ranging from $20–25. Despite that, NEGVAC continued to hold talks with them in order to work out a way to procure as many doses as possible and also pushing the possibility of a technology transfer model so that we could manufacture the volumes required domestically. With Sputnik, too, which was jointly developed by the Russian Direct Investment Fund and Gamaleya National Research Institute of Epidemiology and Microbiology, they began discussion on procurement of doses, leading to an advanced discussion on transferring technology to an Indian manufacturer in order to achieve scale. On similar lines, they also began to hold discussions with Johnson & Johnson, who was also in the process of developing a single-dose vaccine candidate which also led to similar conclusions—that unless we would manufacture it locally, the doses which they were willing to spare were very limited. All in all, by this time it became absolutely clear to the members of NEGVAC that if India had any chance to vaccinate its population in a relatively short time frame comparable to large, developed nations, we would have to become self-sufficient and run our own programmes with minimum reliance on importing vaccines.

◆

## 11 SEPTEMBER 2020

### INDIA | 9,57,854 ACTIVE CASES | 78,087 DEATHS

### WORLD | 63,58,014 ACTIVE CASES | 10,08,805 DEATHS

With the changing need in management of the pandemic, the originally formed 11 empowered groups were reconstituted into six: mostly clubbing functions of two groups into one. Empowered Group (EG) 1, headed by Dr Paul, would look into medical infrastructure and COVID-19 management plan. EG2, headed by the secretary of the Department for Promotion of Industry and Internal Trade, would work on ensuring the availability of essential medical equipment and augmenting human resources. EG3, headed by Amitabh Kant, would be responsible for coordinating with the private sector, NGOs and international organizations for COVID-19 response. EG4, headed by the secretary of Department of Economic Affairs, would be responsible for managing economic and welfare measures. EG5, led by the secretary of Information and Broadcasting, would be responsible for handling information, communication, public awareness, public grievances and data management. And lastly, EG6, headed by the secretary of Home Affairs, would look at strategic issues related to COVID-19 management.

◆

India saw cases peaking at about 90,000 new cases per day in September. However, India, confident in its capacity building of healthcare infrastructure and availability of essential supplies, continued to open up businesses to revive the economy. The last quarter, April to June, had seen a 7 per cent contraction in comparison to the same quarter in the previous year, 2019, reaching the point of technical recession. However, since the country began to unlock in June, several economic indicators began to show encouraging growth markers in merchandize exports, GST collections, digital transactions value, automobile sales and such. By September, data across multiple sectors was suggestive of noticeable recovery. Observing signs of improvement, the government increased its expenditure more specifically in capital spending. Comparing it with capital spending in October 2019 which was ₹137.6 billion, the government almost doubled its expenditure by spending about ₹315.2 billion. Nearly half of its capital expenditure went towards transport infrastructure building activities. The Ministry of Railways scaled up its capital expenditure to a whopping ₹81.8 billion, 176.3 per cent higher than the spend in October 2019. The Ministry of Road Transport and Highways had been scaling up its expenditure ever since July 2020 when the economy reopened. It spent a massive ₹70.4 billion in October 2020 as compared with just ₹670 million in the same month last year. During the first half of financial year 2020–21, it awarded ₹472.9 billion worth of projects to construct over 1,330 km of road length which was 60 per cent higher than the same time last year. Likewise, the Ministry of Housing and Urban Affairs spent about ₹20.3 billion as against a low ₹987 million last year in October. Transfers to states and UTs by the Centre for capital expenditure increased to ₹63.6 billion as opposed to a 10 times lower monthly transfer of ₹6.4 million in FY 2019–20.[5]

We should also note that the government spending on its flagship MNREGA increased by a robust 75.9 per cent to ₹105.1 billion in comparison to October last year. Back in June, the prime minister had suggested to officials across departments that,

> We must focus on boosting employment and livelihood opportunities for the migrants who have returned back to their respective states. Government expenditure should be planned to build durable rural infrastructure and providing modern facilities like internet connectivity in villages. I urge you to carry out skill-mapping exercise in each district in order to tailor government assistance. Through

the Garib Kalyan Rojgar Abhiyaan, [the] government will very much assist the above exercise by implementing about fifty thousand crores worth of projects within a hundred and twenty five days in a hundred and sixteen districts of the six large states in which migrants were returning.

Taking into account the prime minister's directions and vision, several states conducted the skill-mapping exercise, even before the migrants were discharged from the mandatory 14-day quarantine. To their pleasant surprise, many of them concluded that most returned workers were highly skilled in their respective domains and knowledgeable of verticals of the production chain. In response, states began to form district-level committees of officials who would assist in providing space, procuring machinery, raw material sourcing, organizing funds and conducting training workshops so as to help small-scale, self-sustaining industries start up. Several success stories have emerged out of this model and several new industrial hubs have now developed.[6]

To note, government expenditure on the main subsidy items of food, oil and fertilizers rose steeply by 90 per cent amounting to ₹291.9 billion in October 2020. These numbers are suggestive of the government's intent to spend on projects which had the potential to lead to more job creation, thus compounding the yields. In other words, adopting the modified barbell strategy, as soon as the economy began to show signs of recovery August 2020 onwards, taking into account on-ground feedback, the government increased its expenditure in sectors which yielded multiplier effects on growth. As a result of these targeted efforts, GST collections crossed ₹1 trillion for the first time in eight months resting on strong growth markers such as reduction in unemployment rates to pre-COVID levels, a strong NIFTY index higher than that of the previous year, industrial activity picking up and substantial improvements in port traffic, railway freight traffic and electricity generation.[7] After two consecutive quarters of economic contraction, the country's GDP entered into positive territory in the last quarter of the fiscal year and foreign reserves remained at an all-time high, suggesting that India was heading towards a very encouraging V-shaped economic recovery.[8]

◆

## 28 OCTOBER 2020

INDIA | 6,02,473 ACTIVE CASES | 1,21,341 DEATHS

WORLD | 90,76,624 ACTIVE CASES | 12,67,661 DEATHS

Elections in the state of Bihar were scheduled at the end of the month where the BJP in alliance with the Janata Dal (United) was seeking to retain power facing opposition from the coalition of the Congress and the Rashtriya Janata Dal (RJD). Way back in the month of June, Bihar's chief electoral officer H.R. Srinivasa had chaired an all-party meet to discuss safety measures which would need to be adopted leading up to the upcoming polls. While the BJP was prepared to take the virtual route for all its rallies, the opposition parties were very uncomfortable with the idea of cancelling in-person rallies citing that they didn't have the kind of resources the BJP did in order to ensure deep penetration of virtual meetings. This was after Union Home Minister Amit Shah had held a very penetrating virtual rally watched by at least 40 lakh people in which the party was believed to have pumped in tens of crores of rupees.[9] An RJD MLA had said, 'We do not have the resources and even workers to enable Tejashwi Yadav to address a large number of party workers. It is an uneven battle.'[10] The Congress meanwhile said that it was against completely banning traditional modes of campaigning. Congress leader B.P. Munan had said at the all-party meet, 'After all, how does one reach out to a population, which has no access to smartphones or the internet?'[11] Abandoning all virtual modes of campaigning, leading up to the elections, for several weeks all political parties held massive physical rallies attracting huge crowds with hardly anyone wearing masks or observing social distancing. While the flouting of COVID-19 rules alarmed the doctors of the sharp downturn in the fight against the virus it could take, Bihar miraculously managed to keep COVID-19 cases under control.[12]

Concurrently, in another large democracy like ours—the US—town halls, big rallies and conventions were being regularly held in the run-up to the national presidential elections scheduled in November 2020. Expectantly, they were being accompanied by huge spikes in COVID-19-positive cases in the destinations of the political rallies. By this time, about 50 countries in the world had gone ahead and held elections at various levels during the pandemic with varying levels of protocols and election management. While we saw a seven-day average in cases increase in some countries such as Singapore, Dominican Republic, Croatia, Serbia, Belarus and others, some, like South Korea, Sri Lanka and Iceland, were admirably able to keep their cases down.[13]

# 14

## ECONOMIC STIMULUS

**12 NOVEMBER 2020**

INDIA | 4,85,019 ACTIVE CASES | 1,29,536 DEATHS

WORLD | 1,20,88,604 ACTIVE CASES | 13,90,276 DEATHS

A slew of new stimulus measures were announced by Finance Minister Nirmala Sitharaman under the Atmanirbhar Bharat Package 3.0. Riding high on the success of the Garib Kalyan Rojgar Abhiyaan and increase in MNREGA uptake, the Atmanirbhar Bharat Rojgar Yojana was launched. This was intended to incentivize creation of new employment opportunities during the COVID-19-recovery phase in which the Union government would pay the employment provident fund contributions on behalf of the employees and employers for organizations employing up to 1,000 individuals. She also provided for an additional ₹10,000 crore for the PM Garib Kalyan Rojgar Yojana. The emergency credit line scheme which offered collateral-free loans to MSMEs and individuals for business purposes was extended until March 2021. In order to offer a significant boost to economic growth and domestic employment, the finance minister announced the approval of the Production Linked Incentive Scheme in 10 sectors in addition to the three sectors already approved earlier at the cost of ₹51,355 crore—critical key starting materials, drug intermediaries and active pharmaceutical ingredients and manufacturing of medical devices. In addition, another ₹18,000 crore was sanctioned under the Pradhan Mantri Awas Yojana (PMAY) in order to revive the housing and real estate sector. The additional funds would help to ground about 12 lakh houses and complete the construction of about 18 lakh which would help create job opportunities to over 78 lakh individuals and increase steel consumption by 25 LMT and cement by about 131 LMT. She also announced a reduction in performance security on contracts to provide relief to those in the construction and infrastructure sector and setting up of an infrastructure debt platform to provide project financing in the future. An amount of ₹10,200 crore was pumped in towards capital and industrial infrastructure for domestic defence equipment production, creation of industrial infrastructure and towards green energy initiatives. Finally, ₹900 crore were set aside for the Department of Biotechnology under 'Mission COVID Suraksha' for R&D of COVID-19 vaccines in India.[1] The ₹900 crore was further provided to five vaccine candidates in advanced stages of clinical development to help augment production facilities. Bharat Biotech and three public-sector manufacturers were provided grants under this to upgrade and purchase infrastructure and technology for vaccine production. Bharat Biotech was also given out a chunk of these funds to specifically enhance their production facility in Bangalore so that the company could roll out 10 crore doses per month by September 2021.

◆

Speaking of vaccine development, never before has India incubated companies by engaging in proactive risk financing on a scale as enormous as this. The model of an 'entrepreneurial state' was envisioned by the prime minister and subsequently achieved with the prime objective to inoculate all Indians as soon as possible. Ever since Indian manufacturers had begun to show success in vaccine research, the project occupied a special place in his heart. He was determined to make the model a success, thus setting an example for decades to come, not just in vaccine research but in other important sectors as well. All in all, the prime minister placed his bet on India's domestic manufacturers versus yielding to pressure by international vaccine companies.

Not only had adequate financing been arranged, but the GoI also cleared roadblocks and were instrumental in strengthening end-to-end systems in vaccine development, manufacturing and distribution processes which are typically highly complex, multistage processes. For instance, 11 Good Clinical Practice (GCP)-compliant clinical trial sites had been established, with each site having access to a cohort of 50,000 to 1 lakh healthy volunteers who could be tracked for long periods of time in order to facilitate human trials. Five of these sites were equipped to also carry out seroepidemiology studies which would provide critical information to estimate the spread of the virus in certain communities so that specific, localized policies could be planned. In addition, 35 clinical trial sites in hospitals were also set up to ensure that no time was lost in recruitment and carrying out of trials.

By this time, SII and Bharat Biotech were in advanced stages of Phase III clinical trials and their data was looking solid. NEGVAC engaged extensively with them in real time, along with others such as Zydus Cadila to chart out production capabilities and set achievable vaccination goals. NEGVAC's vaccination strategy was based on two components: the information coming in simultaneously from the manufacturers that vaccine availability would be limited in the first six months due to restrictions in their capacities. Even if capacities were ramped up, which NEGVAC and the GoI did finance, output would not increase overnight. It would take three to four months at the bare minimum to set up additional capacities. At this point, the input from NEGVAC to the PMO, after consultations with SII and BBIL was that by the end of August 2021, around 60 crore doses may be available: about 47 crore from SII and 13 crore from BBIL. The second component in the strategy was to plan who to inoculate on priority such that 30 crore high-risk individuals who had the maximum chance of mortality could get some level of protection before the second wave hit the country. Healthcare workers followed by frontline workers and senior citizens would have to be high up on the priority list once the vaccine drive roll-out began.

NEGVAC was also in close conversation with Pfizer, Moderna, Johnson & Johnson as well as Sputnik. However, it became clear early on that unless we adopted a technology transfer model and began to manufacture large doses of the vaccines within the country, the amount these companies could spare was extremely insufficient in comparison to our demand. Pfizer was willing to give us about 50 million doses and Moderna only about 7.5 million.[2] To top that, Pfizer and Moderna didn't want to conduct bridge trials in India, were quoting a very high price per dose ($20–25) and expected full legal indemnity.[3] In addition to that, the cold-chain logistics for safe transportation of mRNA vaccines was going to be a huge challenge for us. Despite these negatives, NEGVAC was in pursuit to procure the technology and transfer it to an Indian company which would manufacture the vaccines locally. Pfizer denied the request at the time, noting that technology transfer could only take place after the pandemic phase was over and the regular supply phase had begun. This was rather strange, since they had already committed to transfer technology to a Chinese firm called Shanghai Fosun Pharmaceutical.[4] Also, the clauses in the contract which they were making countries sign were very problematic to say the least—not only could countries *not* hold them liable for bad batches of doses but also had to indemnify them against adverse effects, supply delays or even total failure to supply. Even more frightening were clauses which prevented countries from introducing any potential drugs which would emerge as a cure for COVID-19 before Pfizer received authorization. To top this, countries would have to pay in full the cost of ordered doses regardless of authorization or delivery delays or a quality problem. In the event they failed to do so, it would be considered as breach where no domestic law of the land would hold and the jurisdiction of the courts of New York would have the power to acquire current and future sovereign assets of the purchasing country until all dues—for the vaccines as well as all legal fees—were paid.[5] In fact, alarming reports later surfaced about how Pfizer failed to reach a deal with Brazil and Argentina because the company engaged in 'high-level bullying' during negotiations to come to a deal. They attempted to hold developing Latin American countries to ransom by asking them to put up federal bank reserves, embassy buildings or military bases as guarantee against the actual cost of the vaccines and also future legal cases stemming from adverse effects of their vaccines.[6]

At the same time, NEGVAC connected Dr Reddy's Laboratories in India to Russian Direct Investment Firm and Gamaleya to commence adaptive Phase II/III clinical trials for the Sputnik V vaccine. Adopting a technology transfer model, Dr Reddy's would mass-produce and distribute the vaccine in India. Interestingly, Dr Reddy's has never manufactured vaccines and not only did NEGVAC successfully connect them to the Sputnik team but also ensured that Dr Reddy's tied up with six Indian companies to further pass on technology to manufacture Sputnik.

Similarly, Johnson & Johnson, in partnership with Biological E in India, had also begun Phase I/II trials in the country on a technology transfer model. In this case too, since the technology platform that Biological E used was one which would attack the receptor-binding domain (RBD) subunit—a crucial step in the process of how the infection spreads in the body—the required raw materials needed to be imported. Not only did the GoI, through NEGVAC, facilitate the import of these, but also placed an advance order worth ₹1,500 crore with the company which would be adjusted later on delivery of the doses in order to provide them critical financial assistance to purchase the required raw materials. Following the initial ₹25 crore of seed fund, Gennova, which was manufacturing India's first mRNA vaccine, was provided over ₹100 crore to further upgrade facilities, purchase raw material and conduct Phase III trials.

As soon as the vaccines became available, NEGVAC began to simultaneously plan the logistics of their equitable and correct distribution, with minimal wastage. Innovative technologies and digital trackers would have to be used while relying on some of our tried-and-tested measures of vaccine distribution. eVIN portal, an indigenously developed technology system which was capable of digitizing vaccine stocks and monitoring the temperature of the cold chain through a smartphone application, was planned to be upgraded and repurposed. eVIN was already being used in 12 states and was created in order to support the GoI's Universal Immunization Programme by providing real-time information on vaccine stocks and storage temperatures. Cold chain handlers were provided eVIN-enabled smartphones which would allow for digitization of vaccine inventories when they would enter net utilization for each vaccine at the end of every immunization day. These entries would simultaneously be uploaded on a cloud server to which programme managers at district, state and national levels had access to via an online dashboard which they could further use to replenish diminishing stocks. In addition, SIM-enabled loggers could be attached to cold chain equipment with capacities to capture temperature information through digital sensors placed in the refrigerators every 10 minutes. In case of a temperature breach, the logger alarms would send SMS and email alerts to the respective managers and technicians, inciting a quick response, thus saving vaccines from going bad. Over 17,000 people were already trained to use the eVIN technology, which meant that it could be scaled up easily and rather quickly.[7] It was e-VIN which would later become CoWIN after significant technological interventions with user interfaces. In line with the prime minister's directions in June 2020,

CoWIN was conceived to satisfy a need for a digital health ID to ensure that no Indian got left out from the vaccination process. They concurred that management of such a technological backbone would have to be handled by a separate expert team outside of NEGVAC.

Furthermore, NEGVAC had also brainstormed on the list of the initial recipients of the vaccine based on the WHO's recommendations which would include three crore people with maximum risk exposure. One crore doctors and two crore healthcare workers, central and state police forces, home guards, Armed Forces, municipal and Asha workers would be inoculated on priority.

◆

## 28 NOVEMBER 2020

INDIA | 4,54,231 ACTIVE CASES | 1,37,647 DEATHS

WORLD | 1,37,83,062 ACTIVE CASES | 15,54,518 DEATHS

Over the past several months, the prime minister had been hearing upbeat news about various Indian vaccine manufacturers and their noteworthy developments in putting India as a frontrunner in the race for COVID-19 vaccines. Now that several of the vaccine candidates were in the final stages of trials, he wanted to personally visit the teams, the scientists and the experts who were about to play a life-changing role in the life of all Indians, and perhaps, even in many other countries around the world. No amount of gratitude and encouragement was enough for these warriors, but he wasn't one for sitting it out. As a science enthusiast, so much so that he brought the Ministry of Science and Technology under him in the recent Cabinet expansion, he just had to visit these facilities, understand the manufacturing process and see for himself. Both his advisors also point out that he has a knack for sifting through scientific information which is ever-evolving and squeezing out the critical takeaways, a job which they say is a very difficult one for a leader.

There was one other thing occupying the prime minister's mind, 'Would a population accustomed over the years to receive and trust foreign-made vaccines be able to accept an Indian one?' Perhaps his visit to the facilities would also lend authenticity and become a trust-building exercise. India could not afford vaccine hesitancy at his point in time. Ahead of the visit, the PMO had tweeted, 'As India enters a decisive phase of the fight against COVID-19, PM @narendramodi's visit to these facilities & discussions with the scientists will help him get a first-hand perspective of the preparations, challenges & roadmap in India's endeavour to vaccinate its citizens.'[8]

On the morning of 28 November, the prime minister boarded an Indian Air Force (IAF) flight from New Delhi to Ahmedabad followed by a quick chopper ride to his first destination at Zydus Biotech Park in Changodar, Gujarat, to review Zydus Cadila's candidate ZyCoV-D. He was warmly welcomed by the Patel family following which Chairman Pankaj Patel, his son and joint managing director at Zydus Cadila, Sharvil Patel and their chief scientist briefed him on the technology platform on which their vaccine was based. If approved, it would be the first DNA plasma vaccine in the world, making a momentous contribution to the scientific community. They also briefed him about how the vaccine which was intradermal would be administered via a painless patch versus a needle syringe. They demonstrated a wide gamut of pharmaceutical products such as anti-viral drugs including remdesivir which they were working on and offering to combat COVID-19. After the briefing, they escorted the PM on a tour of the production unit and demonstrated the nitty-gritties of the manufacturing process for the vaccine. Since it was a packed trip, the PM immediately boarded the chopper back to Ahmedabad airport from where he boarded the IAF plane, had a quick in-flight lunch and took a short car ride after deplaning at Hakimpet IAF airbase, to the Bharat Biotech facility in Genome Valley in the Shameerpet area of Telangana's capital city Hyderabad.[9]

Reaching the Bharat Biotech facility at about two in the afternoon, he was welcomed by Chairman and Managing Director Krishna Ella, his wife and Joint Managing Director Suchitra Ella and their chief scientist. The team gave him an overview of the company including details on how they had been making rotavirus vaccines and supplying them to low-income countries. They broke their briefing down in four parts.

In the first part, they discussed the roll-out of their current vaccine candidate, Covaxin, jointly developed by ICMR, which was based on an inactivated virus. The second part that they discussed was the development, trial and approval of their nasal vaccine. They were very hopeful about this vaccine as it would provide sterilizing immunity. To understand what that meant, let's bring in some scientific context here. The COVID-19 virus is known to heavily target cells in the lungs. When a standard vaccine is administered, it first enters the lungs after which, depending on the technology, generates an immune response. Although they effectively prevent severe disease and death, offering substantial protection against the virus, they are not 100 per cent effective at blocking infection from entering your body. However, in the case of an intra-nasal vaccine, it would target the nasal mucosal cells offering a big boost of immunity to your upper respiratory tract and the lungs. This would mean that not only would you not get infected since your upper respiratory tract would be protected, but you also wouldn't be able to infect others. Intra-nasal vaccines may offer significantly better protection also because they closely mimic the way the virus naturally infects humans, i.e., through the mucosal membranes of the nose and upper airways.

Mr Ella informed PM Modi that due to the limited case studies and requirements in the past, the testing protocols for such a vaccine weren't robust. He requested for support from the GoI and the MoHFW to expedite these procedural requirements, so as to speed up testing and development of their nasal vaccine candidate. (Six months on, by August 2021, they had already entered Phase II trials and were hopeful of robust data on the vaccines' safety and efficacy.)

The third component of their discussion was about production capacity constraints at their Genome Valley facility, which was capable of producing only about one crore doses per month. They informed the prime minister of their Bangalore facility, which could be repurposed to make about four to five crore doses per month and also requested for quick approvals and assistance so that production could be ramped up in time. In addition, they discussed with the prime minister a larger production augmentation plan which would include transferring technology and upgrading various public-sector manufacturers in order to achieve scale. With this information provided to the prime minister, it became clear that while they would be able to produce a large number of doses in 2021, the production would be pointedly back loaded wherein a disproportionately large number of doses would be produced in the latter half of the year. (Since then, a lot of action has taken place: inter-ministerial teams have visited them and more capacity-building exercises have been carried out where four more manufacturers were on boarded.) Within the next five months, ₹65 crore was provided by the GoI to Bharat Biotech to augment their Bangalore facility. Haffkine Bio-Pharmaceutical Corporation Ltd in Mumbai was provided ₹65 crore to build capacity to produce two crore doses a month when functional. Indian Immunologicals Limited in Hyderabad was also provided ₹60 crore and Bharat Immunologicals and Biologicals Limited was supported with a grant of ₹30 crore to manufacture about 1.5 crore doses per month. In addition, Gujarat Biotechnology Research Centre tied up with Hester Biosciences and Omnibrx acquired technology from Bharat Biotech to produce about two crore doses per month.

The prime minister spent some time with the entire team of scientists at Bharat Biotech since they were quite enthusiastic to meet him and took a tour of the facility where he was explained the step-by-step production process. By 4.00 p.m., he left the facility—greeting the enthusiastic crowd that had gathered outside to see him—for Hakimpet airbase, from where he was scheduled to fly to Pune.

By 5.15 p.m., the prime minister had arrived at the Pune airbase, from where he boarded a chopper to make way to the manufacturing facility of the SII, covering a distance of about 10 kilometre. At SII, he was greeted by Chairman Cyrus Poonawalla, his son and CEO Adar Poonawalla and Adar's wife and executive director, Natasha Poonawalla. After being given a tour of the facility, the team expressed its confidence in ensuring adequate supplies and how it was looking forward to rising to the occasion to supply vaccines to India and the world. By November, SII had stockpiled about four crore doses, confident of Phase III trials yielding positive data and had majorly augmented their production unit with an ability to produce over 40 crore doses by July 2021. In an effort to assist SII to further ramp up production, the prime minister committed to provide advance funding to the tune of ₹1,200 crore for about six crore doses. Mr Adar Poonawalla later confirmed, 'I used these funds to further ramp up my infrastructure and purchase raw materials and machines at a premium cost, so that India could receive the vaccines in the shortest possible time.' By the time the meeting concluded, the prime minister had spent more time than was scheduled in his three-city visit. Unfortunately, due to take-off restrictions around sunset and delay in his schedule, he couldn't board the chopper and had to make the journey back to the airbase from where he was scheduled to fly back to New Delhi, by car, taking much longer than planned.

In the case of all the three companies, in response to requests for assistance in timely regulatory approvals, the prime minister made it abundantly clear to them, 'We are in the midst of a once-in-a-century pandemic. The GoI will ensure that there is no red-tape and no hold-up due to delay in bureaucratic processes. The government rather will work with you as a facilitator to quicken the process so that safe and effective vaccines can get to the people in the shortest amount of time possible.'

As the prime minister's visit concluded, the PMO sent out an official release highlighting his experience,

> The scientists expressed joy that the Prime Minister met them face to face in order to boost their morale and help accelerate their efforts at this critical juncture in the vaccine development journey. He expressed pride in the fact that India's indigenous vaccine development has progressed at such a rapid pace so far. He spoke on how India is following sound principles of science in the entire journey of vaccine development, while also asking for suggestions to make the vaccine distribution process better. The Prime Minister stressed that India considers vaccines as not only vital to good health but also as a global good, and it is India's duty to assist other countries, including the nations in our neighbourhood, in the collective fight against the virus.[10]

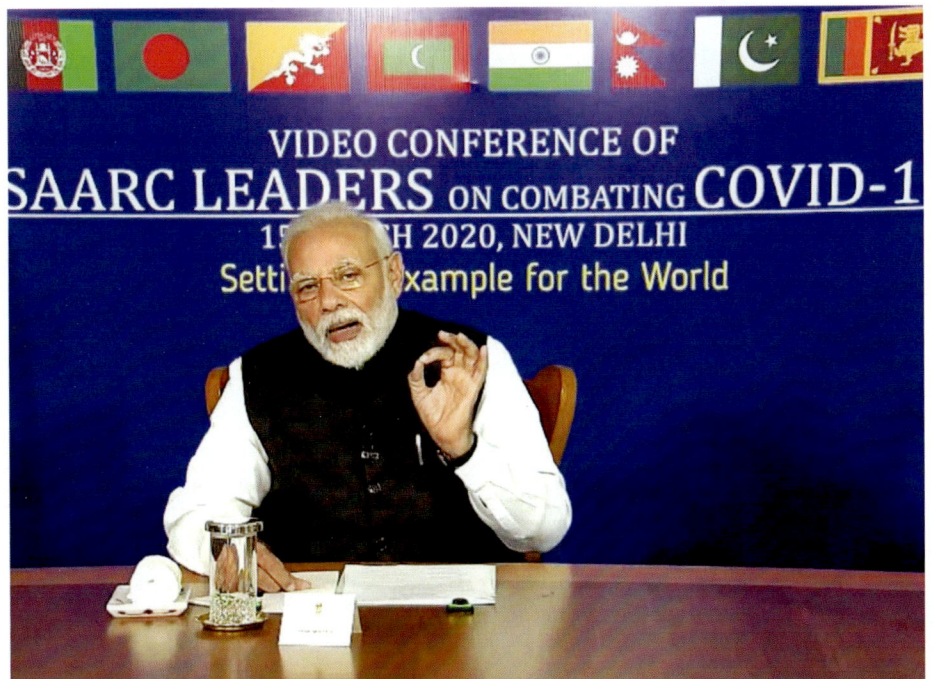

At the video conference of SAARC leaders on combating COVID-19 in March 2020 where Prime Minister Narendra Modi proposed setting up a COVID-19 emergency fund with an initial contribution of $10 billion from India which could be utilized by any SAARC nation for combatting the pandemic

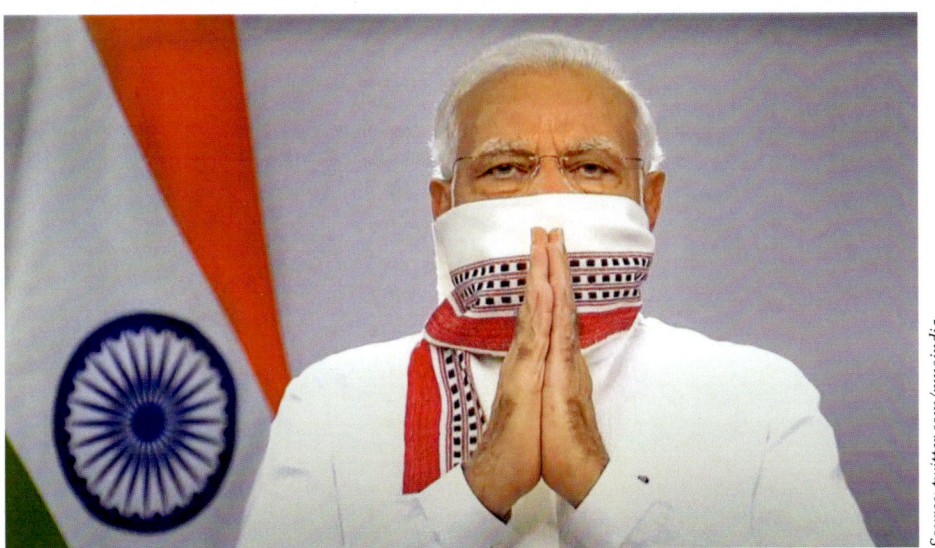

Prime Minister Modi wears a cloth face cover during a national televised address in April 2020 to promote mask usage

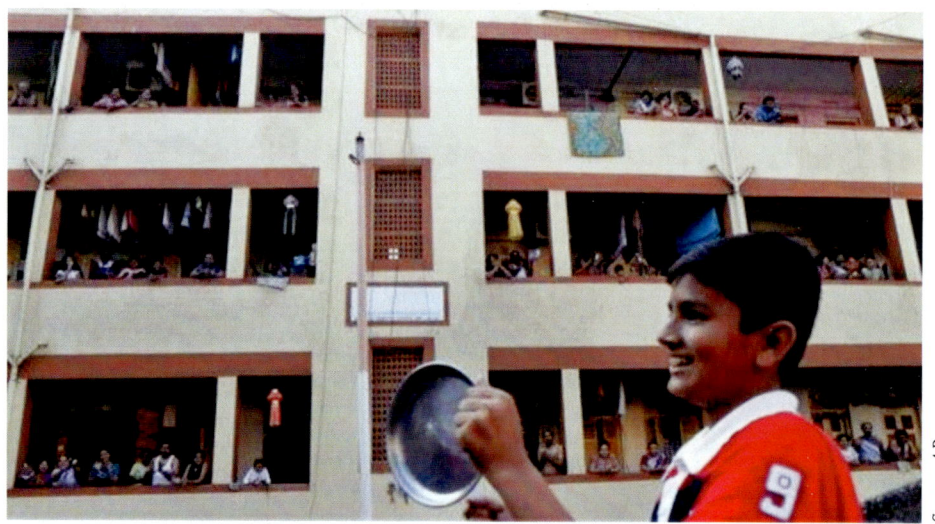

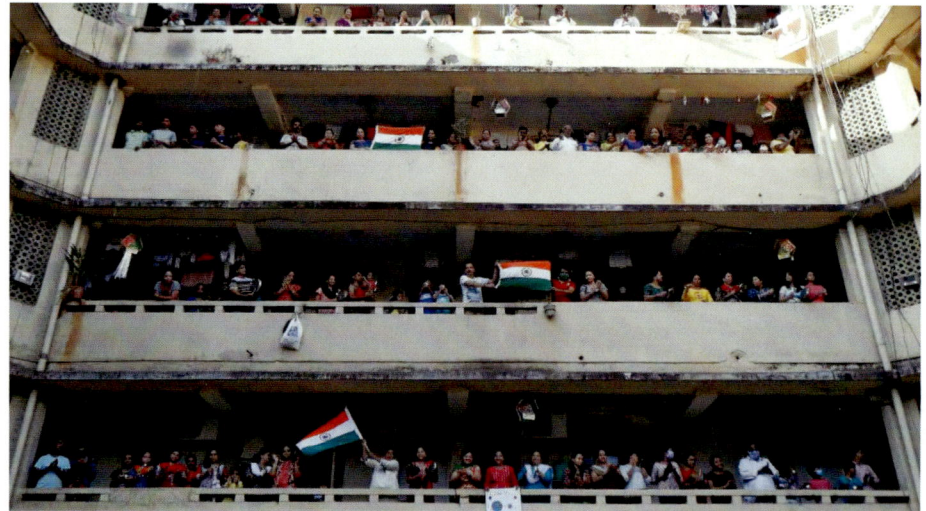

On junta curfew, a 14-hour curfew, people clapped and banged utensils from their balconies as a gesture of gratitude for healthcare and frontline workers, following the prime minister's call to action

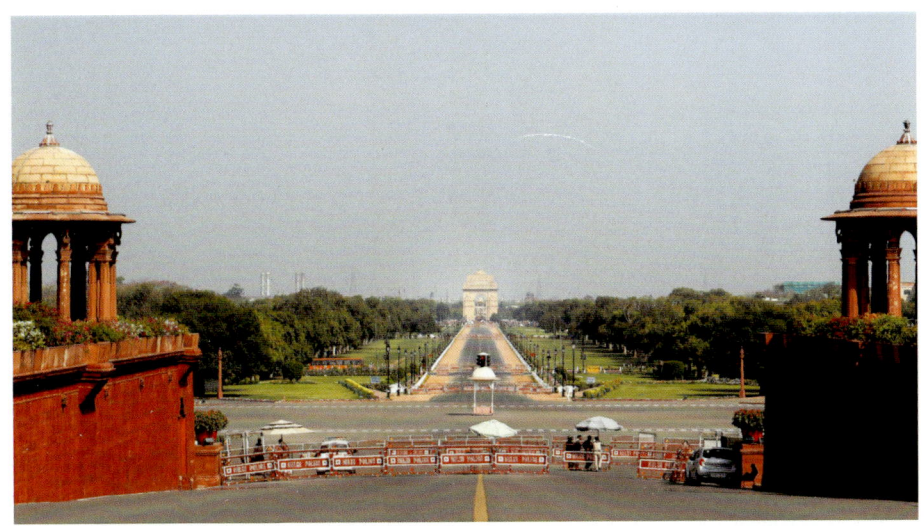

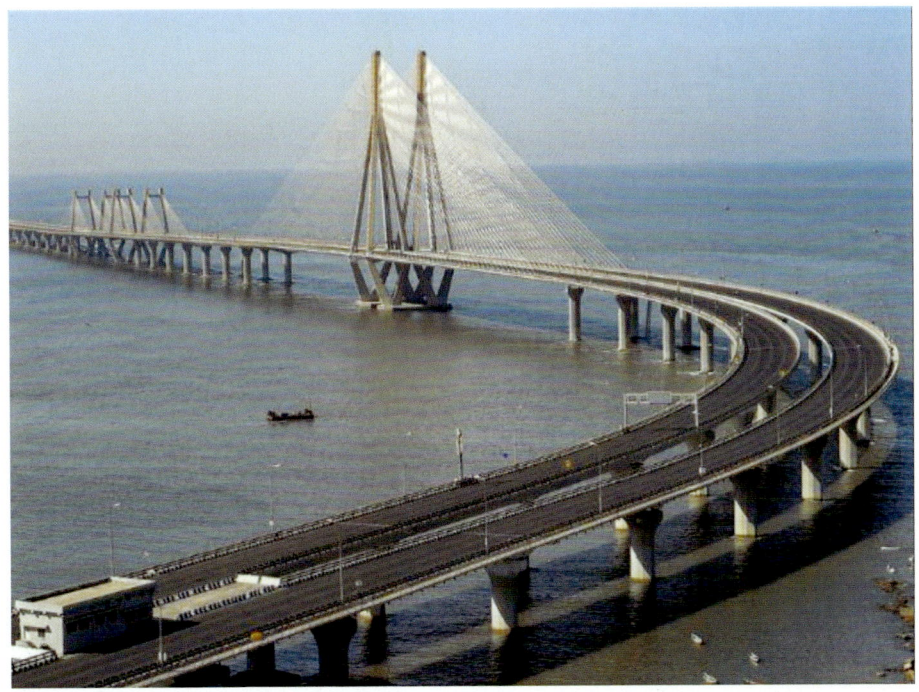

Raisina Hill in New Delhi (top) and the Bandra–Worli Sea Link in Mumbai (bottom) bear a deserted look after India goes into one of the strictest lockdowns in the world

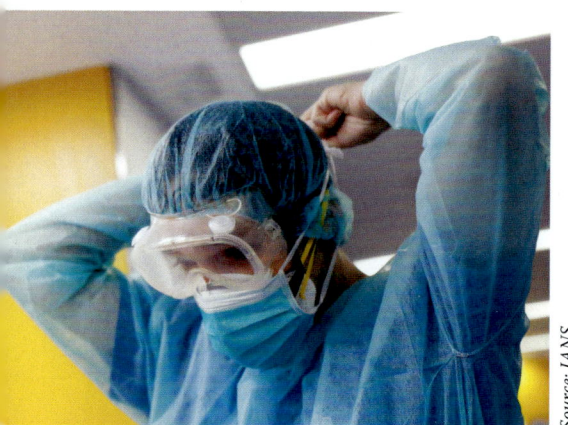

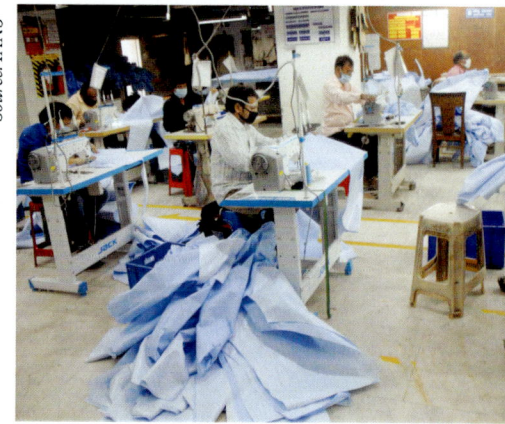

Source: IANS

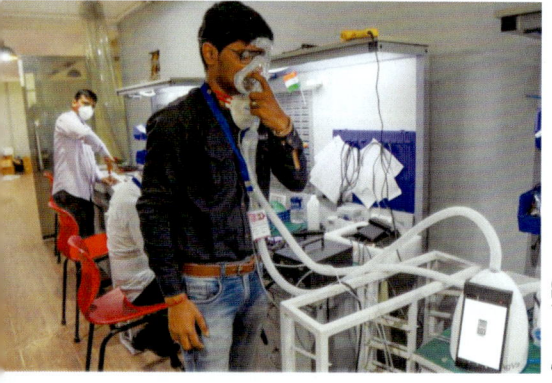

Source: AFP

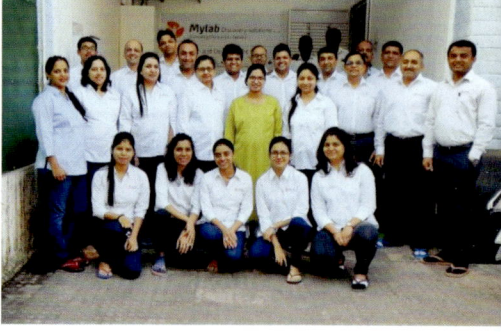

India achieves self-sufficiency in the production of N95 masks, PPE kits, COVID-19 test kits and ventilators in a matter of months

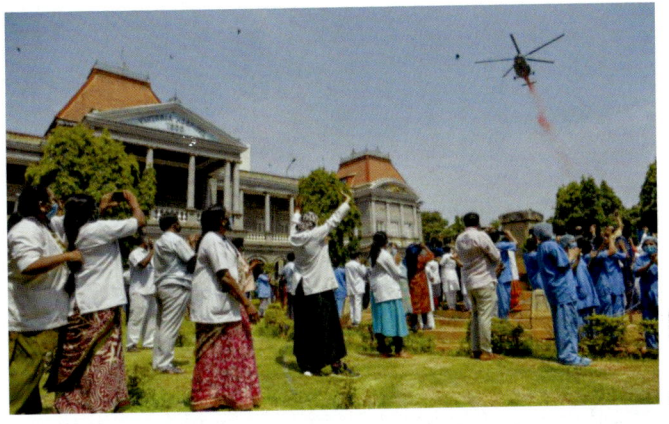

Indian Air Force helicopters offer salute to healthcare workers and doctors by showering flower petals during a countrywide fly-past exercise

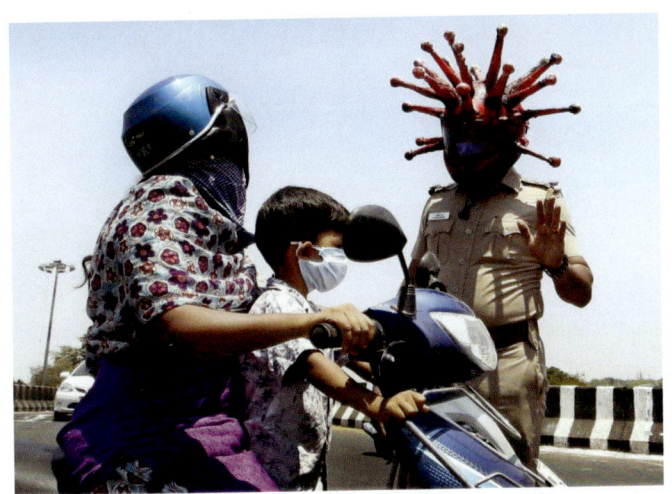

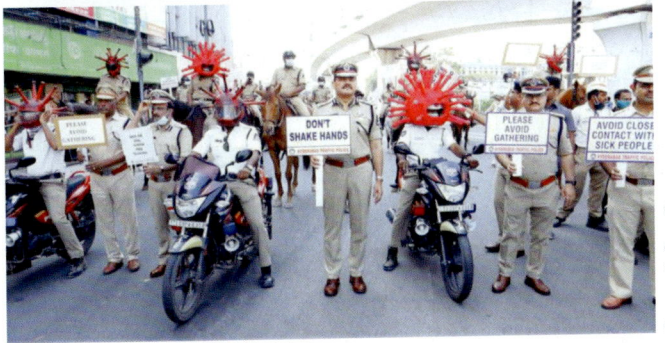

Police officers help to spread awareness about the novel coronavirus and enforce lockdown

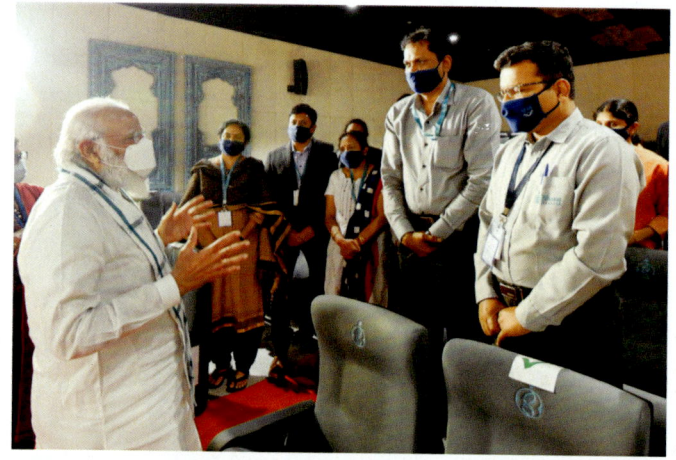

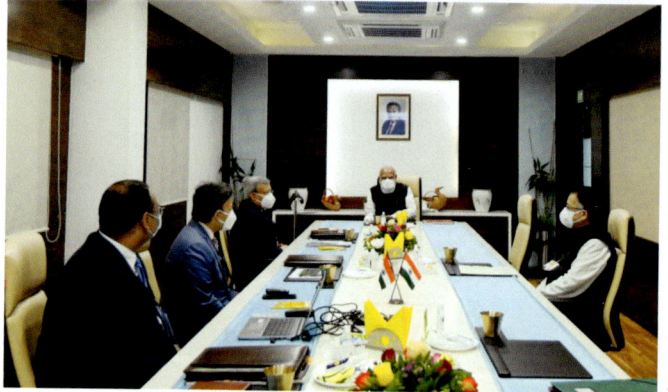

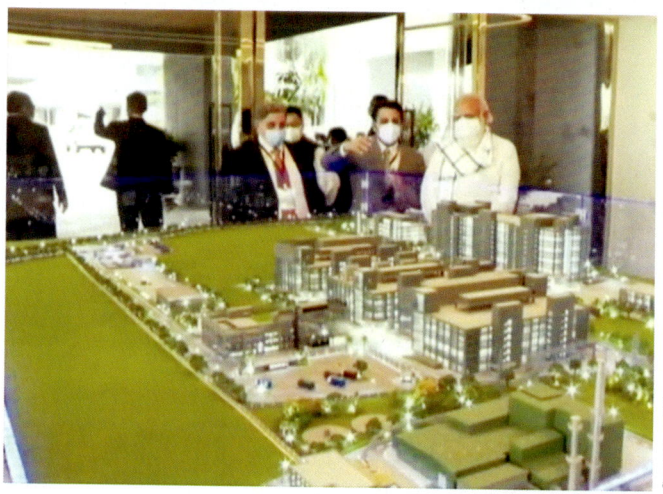

The prime minister visits Zydus Cadila, Bharat Biotech and Serum Institute of India in November 2020 to inspect and understand the vaccine manufacturing process and progress

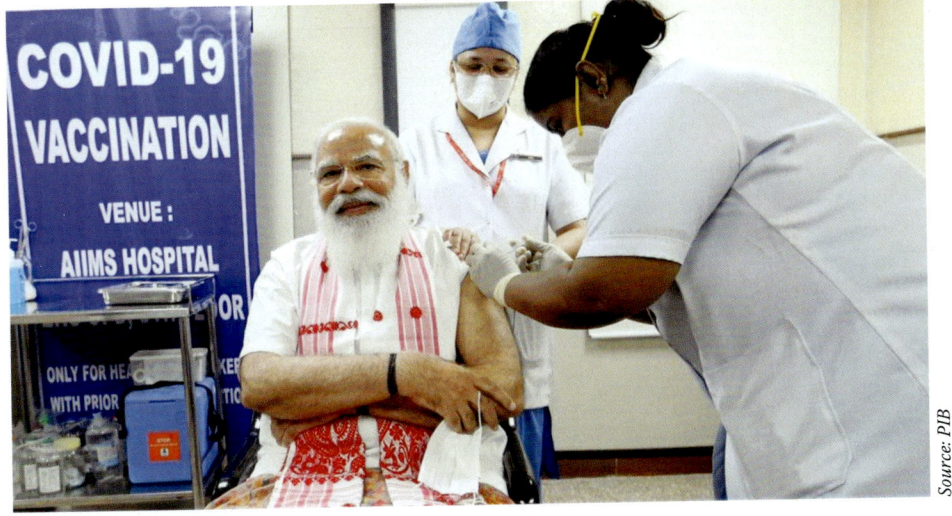

Prime Minister Modi takes the first shot of Covaxin, India's indigenously developed COVID-19 vaccine, on 1 March 2020

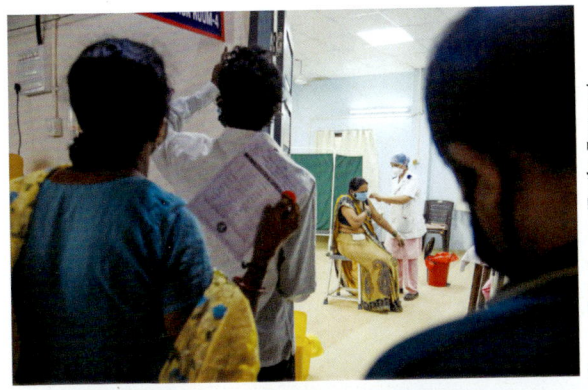

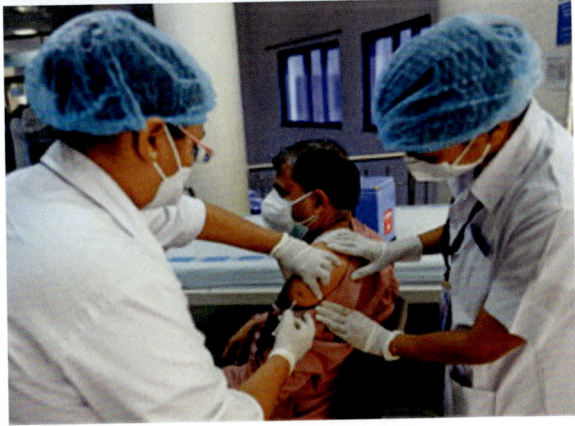

India runs the world's largest and most successful vaccination drive

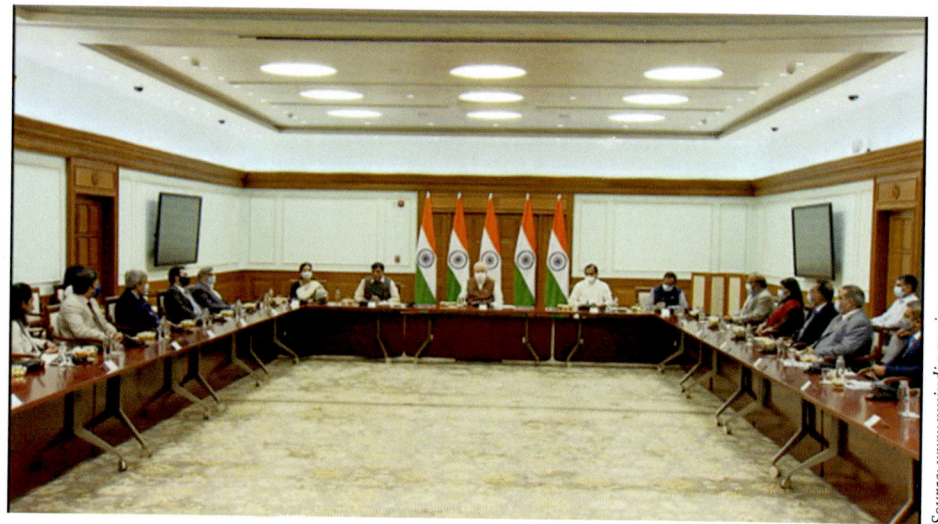

PM Modi holds a review meeting with vaccine manufacturers in October 2021

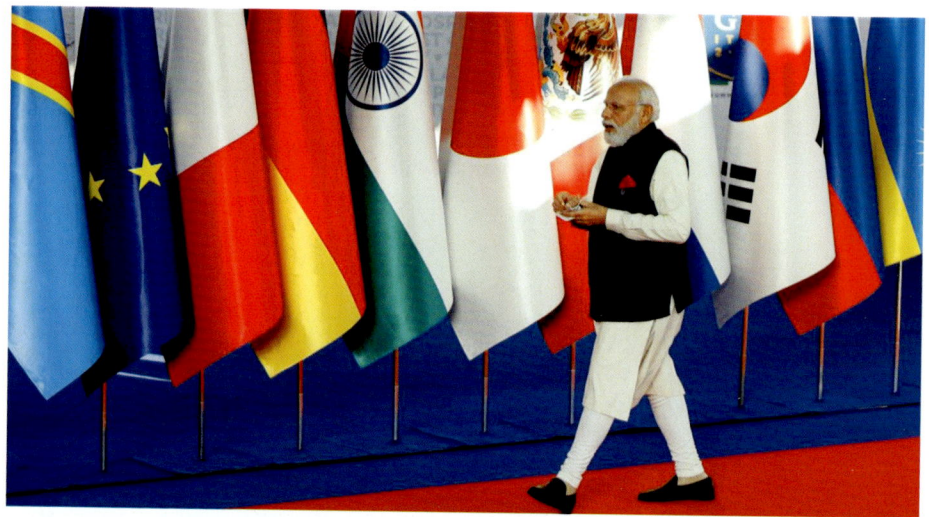

At the G20 Leaders' Summit held in Rome, in October 2021, PM Modi commits to over five billion COVID-19 vaccine doses by the end of 2022

## SECTION 2
## SECOND WAVE

## 15

## FARMERS PROTEST AND THE VIRUS MUTATES

**3 DECEMBER 2020**

INDIA | 4,15,935 ACTIVE CASES | 1,40,161 DEATHS

WORLD | 1,39,12,137 ACTIVE CASES | 16,09,735 DEATHS

In the parliament session of September 2020, three bills viz. the Farmers' Produce Trade and Commerce (Promotion and Facilitation) Bill, the Farmers (Empowerment and Protection) Agreement on Price Assurance and Farm Services Bill and the Essential Commodities (Amendment) Bill were passed by both Houses following which they received the President's assent and acquired the status of laws.[1] Over the course of the next many months, the passage of these laws would become a political boiling point attracting protesting groups who were accused by some people as being responsible for the advent of the second wave of COVID-19 in India.

Indian agricultural policies, central and state, have over the years been based on food security concerns, i.e., adequate availability of food and strengthening the ability of citizens to access it. The aforementioned bills were long-pending reforms which would provide choices to farmers to sell agricultural surplus at lucrative prices and an opportunity for barrier-free, interstate exchanges in new trade areas and digital spaces. The bills would open up the agricultural sector to involve private players, thus improving competition and forcing the government-regulated Agricultural Produce Market Committees (APMCs) to become more efficient, which in turn, would improve price realization. However, as soon as the bills were passed, several groups of farmers' unions began to protest against them.

To put these bills in context, we'd need to look at the problems that have plagued the agricultural sector in India for decades. Agriculture contributes about 20 per cent to India's GDP, down from almost half of the GDP contribution in 1991. The primary reason for this has been disproportionate growth in other sectors and services due to deregulation and delicensing as a result of which they have now stormed ahead. Despite this, Indian political will thus far, hadn't been strong enough to open up the agriculture sector, perhaps due to possible political repercussions, a display of which came to be witnessed once the bills were passed. About 87 per cent of all farmers in the agrarian sector are small and often landless. These farmers are poor and produce very little additional produce which can be sold in the market to generate income, i.e., marketable surplus. They are usually net buyers of food grains and often work as labourers on land owned by rich farmers to supplement their income. The rich landowning farmers act as moneylenders and suppliers of seeds and fertilizers to these small farmers in the locality. They also play a disproportionate role in the functioning of the local APMC, thus creating an elaborate ecosystem to exploit the smaller farmers. All in all, since the richer farmers produce excessive marketable surplus, they are usually the prime beneficiaries of increases in the minimum support prices (MSP)—a guaranteed price offered by the government on produce. The new laws not only retain the APMC and MSP systems but also create a parallel system of private markets in order to expand the supply chain and negotiating capacities of the small farmers, thus protecting them from the malpractices of the rich farmers' and traders' nexus which control APMCs. The laws also open up the opportunity for contract farming, reducing price volatility for the farmers and eliminating last-minute negotiations after harvest as in the case of MSP.[2]

However, some groups of farmers from the northern states of Punjab and Haryana, which account for the largest beneficiaries of produce procurement under MSP by the government via its agency the FCI, possibly became insecure about the fact that the FCI may gradually scale down procurement targets bearing an impact on their earnings. They also became worried that the PDS allotments may eventually move to the direct benefit transfer system, cutting out trader middlemen. PDS allotments account for over 80 per cent of FCI's outflows, benefitting wheat and paddy growers the most. The primary demand of the protesting farmers' unions was to make purchase of all crops at MSP rates mandatory, changing the structure of grievance redressal systems and cheaper access to storage facilities—most demands which the government was willing to agree on and accordingly amend the laws.

However, despite assurances to include the demands in the rules, given during the round of talks with three Union Cabinet ministers on 13 November, the protesting farmers banded under various unions and began to march towards New Delhi with disproportionately large amounts of ration and fully equipped vans and trucks with air conditioners, generators and high-amp connectors.[3] Fearing that they were going to stay put for the long haul, considering the sowing season for Rabi crops had just concluded and they now had about two months to kill before a round of insecticide spraying on the fields, the Haryana government ordered the state police to stop the protesting farmers in their tracks. India was still inching out of the first wave of COVID-19 infections and could not let super-spreader events like these take us back in our fight against the virus. Violence broke out between the Haryana State Police and the farmers who were travelling on tractors and trolleys, breaking police barricades set up along the way. Under the Epidemic Diseases Act, the police mandated to control large crowds used tear gas and water cannons to stop them.[4] Despite their efforts, the farmers continued onwards and by 30 November, over two to three lakh farmers had converged at various border points around New Delhi.[5] Union Home Minister Amit Shah requested the farmers blocking the border points to move to Delhi's Burari ground following which the Centre would hold discussions with the farmers on their demands.[6] Rejecting the appeal from Shah, the farmers continued to stay put at the borders, pressing for permission to protest at the more central location, Jantar Mantar in Delhi.[7] At the sites of congregation, no COVID-19-appropriate behaviour was followed. Over the next couple of months, all rounds of dialogues between the government and the farmers' unions remained inconclusive, with the latter unwilling to discuss anything or dismiss the protests until the laws were repealed.[8] Originally, the main point of contention between the government and farmers remained the MSP as the latter believed that the laws would lead the Centre to eventually dismantle the MSP system, leaving them at the mercy of large corporates. The government in all rounds of talks held with them continued to assure them that the MSP regime would remain unaffected.[9]

The Supreme Court intervened, offering to set up a neutral panel of experts, bringing in a stay order on the laws until the panel concluded its report.[10] In all disregard for the law of the land, the protesting groups refused to budge from the borders and protesting sites. Images of them organizing movie nights and exquisite pizza parties at the protesting sites began to do the media rounds, leaving many wondering about their motives and source of funds.[11] Neither were they willing to have a dialogue with the government, nor were they respectful of the Supreme Court's judgement, which is the highest law of the land. In fact, about 10 months later, in October 2021, the Supreme Court once again reprimanded the protestors, 'We have stayed the farm laws. There is nothing to be implemented. What are the farmers protesting about? No one other than the court can decide the validity of the farm laws. When that is so, and when farmers are in court challenging the laws, why protest on the street?'[12]

In Indian politics over the years, the poor farmer is often used as a symbol of vote-bank appeasement. Images of farmers out in the cold, sleeping in their tractors, created a hot political atmosphere for the Opposition to take strikes at the Modi government. The BJP ally in Punjab, the Shiromani Akali Dal, walked out of the NDA as soon as the bills were passed in Parliament. After all, if they hadn't, they'd have to risk their core vote-bank, considering the fact that most protestors were from Punjab. The Congress and other regional parties in the Opposition labelled the laws as anti-farmer and demanded that the government repeal them immediately.[13] Interestingly, many of these parties had promised in their manifestos that if voted to power, they'd bring in similar reforms in the agro-sector. To offer context, it is important to note that agriculture policy is a state subject and agriculture is in the state list under the Constitution. Entry 33 of the Concurrent List provides the states powers to control production, supply and distribution of products of any industry, including agriculture. This means that each state would have the power to stop these laws from being implemented in their respective states if they wished to. Also noteworthy is that several states already had many of these mechanisms introduced in the Centre's new laws in place for years. For instance, Maharashtra, since 2000, under the Congress and NCP regime, had been issuing licences to corporates to purchase goods from farmers outside of the APMCs. The Congress had included in its 2019 national manifesto that if brought to power, it would abolish the APMC system. Sharad Pawar, former Union agriculture minister during the UPA regime and president of the NCP, in his autobiography had advocated for direct access to private markets for farmers and doing away with APMCs.[14] He had even written to several chief ministers in his capacity as the Union agriculture minister in 2010 to seek their support to 'encourage the private sector in providing competitive marketing channels in the overall interest of the farmers'.[15] But when it came to collecting political brownie points by piggybacking on the protesting farmers, all these opposition parties took a complete U-turn and made the protesting farmers guinea pigs to achieve their political motives.

To drive my point home that the Opposition created a slugfest out of a non-issue, let us consider an example of when the former prime minister Manmohan Singh heading the UPA government in 2004 had said,

> We need a second green revolution, making use of modern advances [...] For that we need to revitalize India's research agricultural system, India's extension system, India's credit system. The more we commercialize our agriculture, the more our farmers need access to commercial inputs and that was a modernization of our agriculture credit system. There are other rigidities because of the whole marketing regimes set up in the 1930s which prevent our farmers from selling their produce where they get the highest rate of return. It is our intention to remove all those handicaps which come in the way of India realizing its vast potential as one large common market.[16]

In fact, when Prime Minister Modi spoke in the Rajya Sabha on these bills, he responded to the former prime minister's comments, 'Manmohan Singh talked about it but Modi is having to do it now. Be proud.'[17]

Scarily, the crowd at the protest sites was rolling over the upcoming months, which meant that several folks chose to return to the villages and sent over other members of their families. What this catalysed was a spread of the infection to rural parts of the states of Punjab and Haryana, where the bulk of the protestors came from. A close look at COVID-19 case data from Punjab demonstrates that the declining of the post first-wave curve halted its downward trend by January 2021 and turned into a flat line for a month after which it began to rise sharply. Notably, genome sequencing of several samples at the time from Punjab, Haryana and Delhi were attributable to the Alpha variant (B.1.1.7 strain) which originated in the UK.[18] One must also keep in mind that the second wave didn't really begin when the number of cases started rising, but rather when the preceding, declining trend of the curve of the first wave ended. A closer look at district-wise data of areas where most of the protesting farmers came from in Punjab and Haryana shows similar declining trends from the first week of January 2021. On further observing curves on a graph plotting case numbers in various states, it becomes amply evident that the rise in cases began in Punjab and Haryana weeks before it began in Maharashtra, which is popularly believed to be the state which started the second wave of COVID-19 infections in India.[19]

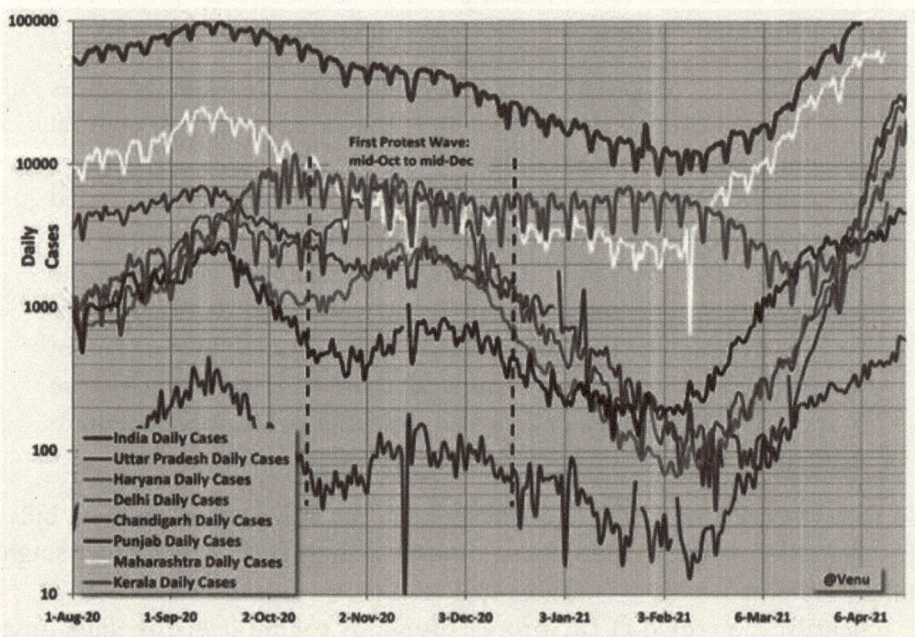

*Figure 15.1: India: Wuhan Epidemic Data*

Source: Venu Gopal Narayanan, 'Data Story: Did the "Farmers' Protest" Cause the Second Wave of Covid-19 in India?' *Swarajya*, 11 May 2021.

Persuaded by political strategists, several sections of the media worked in overdrive to lash out at the government and brand it as anti-farmer. A sympathy wave was carefully crafted for the Rahul Gandhi-led opposition parties by positioning them as sensitive and pro-farmer leaders. The problem with this strategy was that Rahul has been visible mostly on social media platforms. In no way does his persona seem like someone who'd be at natural ease amidst groups of commoners. On the contrary, he comes across as a dynast, who prefers to be surrounded by others like him—only to step out of that group for political photo-opportunities and media interactions. It is my firm and humble belief that keeping him hidden from public view at most times is a deliberate strategy— after all, he is gaff-prone and tends to fumble while speaking. So, keeping him somewhat sheltered is the best tactic that his political pundits can adopt. Adding to his woes are his sympathizers in the party and media who overcompensate and go rather overboard. His party's spokespersons also come across as loose cannons. Thus, for the prime minister and his party, it makes most sense to just stand back; let all the world's camera lenses focus on Gandhi's light-and-sound show. Many top forlorn and despondent leaders from the Congress and other opposition parties see eye-to-eye about the politically comfortable position that the prime minister usually finds himself in due to lack of Gandhi's credibility; that there is no need to eliminate someone who is already in self-destruct mode. Gandhi truly is BJP's greatest asset, they say.[20]

After the ebbing of the first wave, the central government had begun to give more autonomy to the states and UTs to use guidelines developed by the GoI during the first wave and implement them in their respective regions to the best of their wisdom. So naturally, with the Delhi government lay the jurisdiction of controlling crowds at the protest sites. However, they chose to turn a blind eye despite a surge in COVID-19 cases and harp on the back of the popular anti-establishment media narrative that was taking shape. It was all too spicy an opportunity for them to let go of. Neither did they attempt to dismiss the crowds, nor did they carry out a respectable number of tests at protest sites. They didn't bother to put in a mandatory quarantine rule for rolling protestors either. Despite assurance from the central government that the farmers' demands would be taken care of followed by intervention by the Supreme Court, the farmers refused to budge unless the laws were repealed—no negotiation, no dialogue. In this case, the central government was left with no choice but to use force to dispel the crowds, in the larger interest of the health of the population. However, with an already anti-farmer media label quickly building up, imagine the reputational damage of images of the Armed Forces dismissing crowds of farmers circulating in the media would have done? All in all, this was a double-edged sword, if the GoI didn't act to dispel the protestors, the virus would get an opportunity to spread unchecked and if it did act by bringing in the Armed Forces, the media would be ruthless building a narrative of police brutality being used against peaceful, protesting farmers.

◆

## 9 DECEMBER 2020

### INDIA | 3,75,137 ACTIVE CASES | 1,42,684 DEATHS
### WORLD | 1,42,52,240 ACTIVE CASES | 16,75,358 DEATHS

On 4 December, Pfizer had applied to the Central Drugs Standard Control Organisation (CDSCO) to seek approval for emergency use authorization of its vaccine candidate after it had secured such clearances in the UK and Bahrain. SII and Bharat Biotech too applied in the following days to come, after which CDSCO scheduled an expert committee meeting on 9 December to review all the three applications. In the meeting, Pfizer failed to submit to the DCGI any adequate data and details required for a decision to be made on the approval process. They sought more time for making a presentation before the committee.[21] It seemed like they came to the meeting only to demonstrate that they were ahead of the rest and intimidate competition, but didn't seem very serious about getting the emergency use authorization from the DCGI at that point in time. They weren't supplying bulk vaccines to European countries yet and hence didn't have adequate data on the effect of the vaccine on ethnicities other than those in the US who had received their shots either.

In the 9 December meeting, the subject expert committee constituted by the CDSCO asked SSI to submit updated safety data of phases II and III clinical trials carried out in India as well as immunogenicity data from the clinical trial in the UK in addition to the outcome of the assessment of the UK's Medicines and Healthcare products Regulatory Agency for grant of emergency use authorization. Bharat Biotech had only submitted the interim data from Phase I and Phase II trials and was asked in the same meeting to submit safety and efficacy data from the ongoing Phase III trials in the country in order to be further considered for the approval.[22]

♦

While India's active caseload was consistently on the decline since its peak in September, several countries of the world were being hit by a second wave of infections. The UK was particularly seething from the rapid surge of the second wave seemingly brought upon by a new strain of the coronavirus—Alpha variant (B.1.1.7), which was more transmissible and fatal, compelling the UK government to announce a slew of new sweeping restrictions.[23] As mentioned earlier, several positive samples from Delhi, Punjab and Haryana at the time were attributable to this variant.[24]

To keep a close watch on this and other probable variants and mutations, India set up a network of 10 government laboratories called the Indian SARS-CoV-2 Consortium on Genomics (INSACOG). Private laboratories, although capable, were disallowed to carry out genome sequences on samples in order to ensure that a certain testing standard was maintained on sequencing. There was also a stringent protocol which needed to be followed for sample collection and analysis in order to put the data in a set which would make sense epidemiologically. Let me elaborate, as of October 2021, while India had the capacity to sequence over 1,00,000 samples, the challenge was not the capacity to test, but rather procedural. Sequencing is not just sequencing; connecting the dots so that data can be analysed to make contextual sense is more important. In order to carry out genome sequencing effectively, end-to-end tracking and follow-up with each patient giving their sample is required. In India's case, capacity restrictions are not the bottleneck. Getting samples which are tagged with correct metadata including details and clinical symptoms of the associated individuals is a mammoth task in a country like ours, where the system is already fatigued and overwhelmed.

It is INSACOG's efforts in December 2020 which yielded conclusions that several positive samples from north India were caused due to B.1.1.7 strain (Alpha). A cause for worry.

# 16

## THE WORLD'S LARGEST VACCINATION DRIVE

**1 JANUARY 2021**

INDIA | 2,51,255 ACTIVE CASES | 1,39,084 DEATHS

WORLD | 1,60,77,452 ACTIVE CASES | 19,45,918 DEATHS

The special expert committee of the CDSCO convened to discuss the proposals submitted by Bharat Biotech and SSI for their respective vaccine candidates: Covaxin and Covishield. No proposal from Pfizer had come through and they remained absent from the meeting as well. For a vaccine to be given approval, three types of data sets need to be looked at: safety data, immunogenicity data and efficacy data. Safety data analyses mild and adverse effects of the vaccines on a large number of people. Immunogenicity is the antibody response generated in individuals as a result of the administered vaccines. To comprehend efficacy data, we need to first understand how it is calculated. As part of the trial, the vaccine is administered to a large number of people, after which the number of infected people among the vaccinated group versus the number of infected from the placebo group are compared after a certain number of infections occur; which then tells us how efficacious the vaccine is. This is a time-consuming process, because a minimum number of events need to occur, i.e., people need to be infected, the study needs to be unwinded, and vaccinated and placebo groups need to be compared. There is no way to predict how much time it may take for those predecided number of events to take place.

In the case of SII, the firm had adequate safety, immunogenicity as well as efficacy data from their UK study which enrolled over 20,000 participants.[1] Their candidate (AZD1222) had received emergency authorization from the UK government on 30 December 2020.[2] SII also presented an updated data sheet of their ongoing bridge trials in India on a cohort size of 1,600 participants, based on which they were granted the authorization for emergency use by the DCGI.

Bharat Biotech's trials, on the other hand, included a much larger cohort of about 25,000 participants, out of which over 22,500 were already enrolled including folks with comorbidities. While they presented strong safety and immunogenicity data among the enrolled participants, they were not in a position to present the entire efficacy data during the 1 January meeting. To arrive at it, the whole trial would need to be complete and in their case 130 events (COVID-19 infections) would have to occur. Only after they'd have occurred would the scientists be able to unwind the trial and look at how many of those 130 were from the vaccinated group and how many were from the placebo group to fully calculate how efficacious the vaccine was. However, they did submit safety and efficacy data on non-human primates, followed by interim data on 40 events and then on 80 events.

The genome sequencing reports which had come in from Indian samples mostly in the northern parts of the country, regarding the presence of the Alpha strain (B.1.1.7), which was responsible for UK's second wave, were of great concern. Despite demonstrating an impressive efficacy rate of 91 per cent on the original strain after two doses were given 8–12 weeks apart, the government anticipated that there might just be a chance that Covishield may not be fully effective on the Alpha strain or any future developing variants. Since Covishield is based on a spike protein technology platform, where a part of the virus is injected to generate immune response, its effectiveness may be impacted if that particular part of the virus mutates. Covaxin, on the other hand, is based on an inactivated virus technology platform which means that it would be able to demonstrate effectiveness against new mutations as well. A couple of studies have also pegged Covaxin's effectiveness to be higher as compared to other vaccine candidates based on the same inactivated virus technology platform, like China's Sinopharm.[3] While there was just one variant of concern in January 2020—the Alpha variant, in addition to the original strain—there really was no way to ascertain that there were no other, more fatal variants in circulation or to come in the foreseeable future. Based on all of these developments and considerations, the DCGI made the decision to go ahead and grant emergency use authorization to Bharat Biotech's Covaxin as well.[4]

The Opposition attacked India's decision to approve the vaccines, with several of its leaders questioning their authenticity. Anand Sharma, MP of the Indian National Congress, said to the media regarding Covishield, 'The DCGI statement is puzzling and the government must reveal the final data of global efficacy trials and the final trials in UK which has been shared officially by UK's MHRA following a government-to-government agreement signed between the two countries which should be put in the public domain to avoid any confusion on the proven efficacy of the vaccine.'[5] As deputy leader of the Congress in the Rajya Sabha, one would expect Sharma to have the wisdom that India would not and should not need to sign any agreements with governments of other countries to validate the safety of its own vaccines which had gone through the process of conducting rigorous bridge trials in the country and were to be Made in India. To add fuel to the fire and undermine the credibility of our vaccines, Shashi Tharoor of the Congress also continued the rhetoric, 'Covaxin has not yet had Phase 3 trials. Approval was premature and could be dangerous. @drharshvardhan should please clarify. Its use should be avoided till full trials are over. India can start with the AstraZeneca vaccine in the meantime.'[6] Tharoor, as an active MP, had to have been clearly aware of the dangers of emerging variants and also very familiar with the proficiency of our scientists compounded with the urgent needs of keeping the country safe. The interim data submitted by Bharat Biotech was solid. The technology platform which their vaccine was based on has proven its safety in other vaccines for decades. There was no need whatsoever, at such a critical juncture with the second wave of the virus looming that the Covaxin approval should have been postponed. However, Tharoor chose to politicize the vaccine approval instead of being supportive in what would take India on the centre stage in the world order and end up saving millions of lives. The devil lies in the details, they say; notice how Tharoor carefully avoided mention of SII in his tweet. This is not an oversight. It is deliberate—so as to give off the impression that AstraZeneca is not an India-made vaccine. Repeated wordplay like this is an often-used ploy to create or change the course of a narrative towards desired goals and Tharoor is the undisputed master of the craft of diplomatic wordplay. Meanwhile, Akhilesh Yadav, chief of Samajwadi Party, a regional political party in UP, also in the Opposition, tweeted, 'We have full confidence in the wisdom of our scientists, but none in the BJP's unscientific ways of banging vessels and BJP's unpreparedness to fight the pandemic. We will not take the BJP's political vaccine. Once our government comes to power, we will inoculate people free of cost.'[7] Just to explain how much disruption ludicrous statements like these cause, let me take you through a study in which Dr Shamika Ravi at Brookings Institute was monitoring vaccination rates in various districts in UP. They found that the districts which had the least vaccination uptake were indeed those in which Akhilesh's Samajwadi Party had tremendous influence.[8] Perhaps recognizing the potential negative public health impact of this and its poll consequences in 2022, six months later, his father and founder of Samajwadi Party, Mulayam Singh Yadav, had to publicly take the Covaxin jab to reverse the damage. Following which, Akhilesh too made a U-turn over his earlier remarks and noted that he too would get vaccinated with Covaxin.[9] However, back to his unscientific proclamations, about half a year later when he took to the streets to campaign for poll-bound UP, he confessed that he hadn't taken the second dose of the vaccine since he had had COVID-19 and didn't think it necessary to take the second dose.[10] Similarly, social media was heated up with a fractured debate; the Opposition's ecosystem attacked the government and the ruling BJP on catalysing approvals for the vaccines by discrediting the wisdom of the top scientists who made data-based decisions. The BJP retorted with its party president J.P. Nadda tweeting,

> Time and again we have seen whenever India achieves something commendable—that will further public good—the Congress comes up with wild theories to oppose and ridicule the accomplishments. The more they oppose, the more they are exposed. Latest example is the COVID vaccines. To further their own failed politics and nefarious agendas, Congress and other Opposition leaders are trying to cause panic in the minds of the people. I urge them to do politics on other issues, they should avoid playing with people's previous lives and hard-earned livelihoods.[11]

Other leaders from the BJP and their social media loyalists also defended the government's decision and called out the Opposition leadership for trying to spread fear and vaccine hesitancy. The Opposition's effort to dent the vaccine credibility made a larger dent to the country on the international stage. When Bharat Biotech applied for Emergency Use Listing from the WHO, the latter took an unusually long time in granting it. Krishna Ella, Bharat Biotech's chairman, a few weeks after WHO's approval in a Times Now Conclave, expressed his frustration with the Opposition ecosystem by saying,

> The way anti-things happen, that has hurt us more. If someone wants to take on the political system they can take on different angles, but not on the healthcare issues. When Prime Minister took the vaccine, immediately they said it's a BJP vaccine, it's a Modi vaccine. All sorts of synonyms. I want people to realise instead of criticising just ask us, we will tell the truth. But making own opinion that hurt us very badly. The negative things said put the WHO too in an awkward position. They wanted to be doubly sure and reviewed our vaccine much more intensively. We are scientists, we don't understand the politics. We are the only vaccine in the WHO who've gone through so much scrutiny.[12]

◆

## 16 JANUARY 2021

### INDIA | 2,09,158 ACTIVE CASES | 1,53,368 DEATHS
### WORLD | 1,83,23,340 ACTIVE CASES | 21,46,252 DEATHS

Two weeks following the approval for the emergency use authorization of Covishield and Covaxin were spent in preparing adequate distribution of the available stockpiled vaccines to all states and UTs so that India's vaccine drive could commence. The first phase of the drive would cover doctors, nurses, frontline workers like the police, the Armed Forces and other healthcare workers—totalling to about three crore people. The GoI would pay the cost of the vaccines in full for this group. The prime minister flagged off the vaccine drive, after which he tweeted, 'On 16th January, India takes a landmark step forward in fighting COVID-19. Starting that day, India's nationwide vaccination drive begins. Priority will be given to our brave doctors, healthcare workers, frontline workers including safai karamcharis (cleaners).'[13]

Meanwhile, even before the first phase of the drive kicked off, the government had begun to plan the second phase of inoculating those over the age of 50 and those with comorbidities over the age of 35. An important part of the planning was the need to set up a robust digital backbone for it. The government planned to introduce an app which would have four modules: user administrator module, beneficiary registration, vaccination and beneficiary acknowledgement and status update features. The app would be called CoWIN (COVID Vaccine Intelligence Network). It would be able to automate allocation of the vaccination session by using the Aadhaar number, send out SMS reminders of vaccination appointments and QR Code-enabled digital certificates. Although the general public would only be able to self-register once the vaccination drive opened up for Phase II, for Phase I, the CoWIN ecosystem would already have in its database the entire list of the Phase I recipients.

In early January, Cabinet Secretary Gauba telephoned Ram Sewak Sharma, who had now retired from the civil services after over five decades to come in for a meeting with PM Modi. The prime minister had asked him to come on-board to help build CoWIN, perhaps as a follow-up to the presentation that Sharma had made to him back in June 2020, in addition to his contributing role in NEGVAC—a job that Sharma was thrilled to take up. While in NEGVAC, Sharma was instrumental in leading the process of converting eVIN to CoWIN. On the same day, the Empowered Group on Vaccine Administration, with him as a convener, was created in order to ensure that necessary decisions could be made swiftly without any process hold-ups. On 14 January, in the meeting with the prime minister, the PM reiterated to him that a solid, secure and highly efficient product would have to be created. Encouraged by the boost, tech experts and developers got together under a team led by Sharma, to create a platform which would go on to become the backbone of the largest vaccination drive in the world. One of the primary concerns was the security of the data. This platform would be used by every single Indian which would mean that their details would be available on the platform, making it absolutely essential to protect the data. Hence, the team concluded that the platform would have to be built on the principles of 'privacy by design'.[14] This design feature would entail that only the bare minimum relevant data from each individual would be collected, that no data would be used without consent of the individuals, the use of the data would be limited to the specific purpose for which it was collected and lastly, notice would be provided to each individual about where their data was being used.[15] The data input would be encrypted and non-downloadable, ensuring minimum amount of threat to the possibility of hacking. With these principles in place, the final product was created with four interfaces. The first is the citizen interface, the dashboard which individuals would be able to view in order to register for vaccinations. The vaccinator interface would be available for hospitals and vaccination centres both public and private, in which they would be able to upload information on vaccine stocks and vaccination capacities. The third interface would publish updated lists of vaccination centres along with timetables on a real-time basis. The last interface would once again be a citizen interface for individuals to download QR-coded vaccination certificates. When domestic travel opened up after the first wave, RT-PCR negative test reports were made mandatory by several state governments to furnish at airports and state borders. People began to forge their names and dates via apps such as Adobe Photoshop instead of taking an RT-PCR test, voiding the benefits from such a policy intervention.[16] QR-coded certificates would eliminate the stymieing arising out of similar mischief in vaccine certificates.

Many countries around the world which had begun vaccination drives had created their own systems which could keep track of vaccinated individuals as against vaccine stock availability while also be able to provide proof of vaccination. As economic activities and international travel would increase when the world emerged out of the pandemic, it would become imperative for individuals to show proof of vaccination. For this purpose, the international community had begun to consider the idea of a 'vaccine passport'—a document which contained an individual's full record of vaccination. Such an idea seemed great in theory if all countries had equitable access to vaccines. However, when put in practice, it would be hugely discriminatory to smaller nations which weren't able to get hold of enough vaccines for even their frontline workers. Several months later, during the 47th

G7 summit (11–13 June 2021), when the vaccine passport idea was discussed, India's official stand was to oppose such a mechanism, as it would promote further inequality between the wealthier and poorer nations.[17] However, while our official stand was opposed to using a vaccine passport, if proof of vaccination became mandatory to be able to undertake international travel, a QR-coded proof of vaccination for Indians would certainly provide for easier integration into the vaccine passport mechanism around the world. As predicted, by October 2021, several countries had opened up travel and while it took activation of several diplomatic channels by the Indian government to facilitate recognition of the CoWIN certificate, they were successful in ensuring that our certificates stood ground around the world.

At the summit, the prime minister also pressed for text-based negotiations for a temporary patent waiver for COVID-19 vaccines—an idea that resonated strongly with the participating leaders and the UN General Secretary, António Guterres. A TRIPS (Trade-Related Aspects of Intellectual Property Rights) waiver would highly benefit middle- and low-income nations to access vaccines. As early as October, India and South Africa had approached the World Trade Organization (WTO) to seek temporary waiver on parts of the agreement on TRIPS.[18] While initially the President Joe Biden-led US government was opposed to the idea, months later it finally came around in the interest of speeding up vaccination drives equitably worldwide.

Placing our bets where our word was, and in an effort to ensure that all countries had equal access to vaccines, we began our vaccine diplomacy programme 'Vaccine Maitri'. Ever since India had begun to plan its vaccination process, the prime minister had been of the firm opinion that unless everyone was safe, no one was. This meant that unless the whole world had equitable access to vaccines, the pandemic would not go away. Having led the country from dependant to supplier status for medical essential equipment such as N95 masks, PPE kits and ventilators as well as several medicines crucial in the fight against COVID-19, the prime minister was certain that India would live up to being 'the pharmacy of the world' even when it came to vaccine supplies. Unlike other western countries which engaged in vaccine nationalism displaying their power, India, true to its nurturing soft-power character, engaged with the rest of the world as a provider—fulfilling other's needs, alongside looking after its own.

In addition, our vaccine manufacturers had pre-decided agreements with select nations to provide a certain amount of doses in exchange for the raw materials that they would provide. It was important to adhere to these as well. By the third quarter of 2020, Adar Poonawalla, CEO of SII, had raised over ₹10,000 crore from COVAX and advances for orders from several other nations in exchange for providing timely, requisite doses of Covishield. In order to honour those agreements, SII would need to export vaccines while simultaneously supplying them domestically. Diplomatically, it was also in the best strategic interest of the Indian government to help out nations in times of such a global crisis. Poonawalla also raised an interesting point at a later date in 2021 when I spoke with him,

> Look, very early on in the pandemic, I decided to raise stakes to secure India. I tied up with various organizations to come up with a vaccine which had three important components: technological ease of production, one which wouldn't require cold-chain transport and a product which was cost-effective and affordable for middle- and low-income countries. Tell me, what is the value of ₹250 today? That's the cost of my vaccine. Based on these, I raised money early from international network so that I could get a head-start in the production process and secure India as soon as possible. Look at the speed with which we raised infrastructure! SII supplies to over 150 nations worldwide. Many of these markets have only recently opened up to the Indian pharmaceutical industry, which benefits us as a whole. In order to retain our supply chains in those markets—even from a security standpoint, the vaccine export initiative by the Indian government was absolutely critical.

All in all, we began to provide our neighbouring nations and other key partner countries with vaccine doses—both Covaxin and Covishield. Several of those beneficiary nations were able to initiate their vaccine drives because of receiving vaccines from India.

◆

## 26 JANUARY 2021

**INDIA | 1,77,119 ACTIVE CASES | 1,53,368 DEATHS | 80 LAKH VACCINE DOSES**

**WORLD | 1,83,02,463 ACTIVE CASES | 21,46,252 DEATHS | 4.68 CRORE VACCINE DOSES**

While India was making steady progress in its vaccination drive, several noteworthy political developments were taking place too. Protesting groups veiled under the ambit of farmers protests against the new farm laws had intensified their presence at five border points of the national capital: Singhu, Tikri, Ghazipur, Palwal and Shahjahanpur. The crowds were large and unruly. No COVID-19 protocol in sight. No consideration for their own or national safety. When asked about the fear of the virus by the news channel cameramen, they'd say, 'The new laws will kill us, COVID-19 might not.'[19]

Seventy-one years ago, on this day—26 January—India's Constitution came into effect, making us the world's largest democracy. Each Republic Day, we celebrate this remarkable achievement in democratic self-governance with an elaborate five-kilometre-long parade in the national capital displaying India's military prowess with tanks, weaponry and precision marching by the Armed Forces and the world's dignitaries joining our top leadership along Rajpath to view the spectacle. The parade begins near the Presidential Palace, passes through India Gate and winds up at the Red Fort.

This year, keeping in mind COVID-19-appropriate protocol, the parade was planned to be shorter, culminating at the National Stadium versus the Red Fort, with smaller marching contingents and fewer cultural performances. Only 25,000 spectators along the three-and-a-half kilometre stretch were to be permitted as opposed to over one and a half lakh every year.

Earlier in the week, the protesting farmers' unions under their umbrella body, Samyukta Kisan Morcha (SKM), had sought permission to hold a tractor march in the national capital, coinciding with the Republic Day parade. They assured the Delhi Police that they would take routes which would not interfere with the Republic Day parade and the tractor march would remain a peaceful affair. On 24 January, the Delhi Police gave them permission to hold this tractor march on 26 January, falling short of providing a time frame to complete the march. Farmers' unions interpreted this communication lapse as a march which would be allowed to go on in the national capital from anywhere between 24 to 72 hours beginning on 26 January. The Delhi Police put security arrangements in place by barricading the routes on which they wouldn't be permitted. For their rally, which had permission to mobilize only 5,000 tractors, over two lakh tractor-trolleys had planned to enter from the five border points and cover over a hundred kilometres.[20]

The week before, two rounds of talks were held between the central government and the farmers' unions but had yet again remained inconclusive. Many of the unions were accepting of the government's proposal to put the implementation of the laws on hold for 18 months and make further progress in deliberations. However, they were silenced and disallowed from discussing their satisfaction with the government's proposal in the media. Out of the 32 unions from Punjab, over 15 wanted to accept the government's proposal and call off the protests in an open vote which took place in their union leaders' meet.[21]

Although the rally was only permitted to start after the Republic Day parade, the protestors in violation of the guidelines started early. What was promised to be a peaceful march quickly began to turn violent when confrontations between the Delhi Police and protestors broke out because the latter diverged from the permissible routes. The rogue protestors attacked police busses and broke barricades, almost running over several men in uniform on duty trying to stop them. In response, the police used tear gas and batons to control the unruly crowd.[22] The SKM proudly declared, 'We have broken the barricades, we have our tractors, people are marching, some leaders are also on horseback…thousands of farmers have already reached the capital. Outside the Delhi police headquarters tear gas and batons were used, protestors also attacked the police buses stationed there.'[23]

High-speed tractors rammed down multiple police barricades which were put up to stop the crowd making its way towards the Red Fort. Protestors on horsebacks used weapons like swords, kirpans and fursas to attack the policemen who attempted to stop them. In response to the violence, which went out of the Delhi Police's hand, Home Minister Amit Shah deployed paramilitary forces. About 400 policemen suffered injuries. Despite all efforts to stop the rioting mob, several hundred reached the Red Fort, where they climbed on the ramparts, mounted poles and hoisted a yellow flag with an emblem in the centre which some groups believe was the Nishan Sahib (religious Sikh community) flag while others confirm it to be a Khalistani (extremist Sikh separatist group) flag.[24]

After the episode it became clear that the protesting movement at the borders of New Delhi was no longer one which prioritized farmers' concerns, but one which had deep-vested interests to unsettle peace in the national capital. The SKM distanced itself from the violence claiming that anti-social elements took over their planned march. Several unions, especially those who were satisfied with the assurances from the government, began to return to their villages. Seeing that the movement was losing steam quickly, the leader of SKM, Rakesh Tikait, shed some tears appealing to the protestors to stay put, breathing life into the protests. In order to take control of the law-and-order situation and avoid a repeat of the events which took place on 26 January, the internet was cut off for a few hours at the protesting sites along the borders of the national capital.

What picked up steam, however, was the media narrative to slander the prime minister and his government. In fact, parallel to the protests losing steam, some sections of the media were fully fired up. Despite the brazen acts on Republic Day, these sections weren't able to untie their blindfolds and wake up to the fact that the movement no longer remained a debate on issues that the farmers were facing. Anti-national, anti-farmer groups had hijacked the protests with an underlying agenda to keep it going as long as possible, and create as much noise as possible. In a week after the deplorable acts on Republic Day, celebrity pop-singer Rihanna tweeted a picture of farmers on a tractor with a question, 'Why aren't we talking about this?#FarmersProtest.'[25] Interestingly, in a matter of minutes, her tweet was retweeted and replied to by several popular people around the world with a clear leaning towards the other side of the ideological line than from the one the current establishment comes from.[26] Global climate activist Greta Thunberg too retweeted Rihanna's tweet attached with a 'toolkit' comprising actions which one could take to support the protestors. Some of the prescribed actions such as organizing protests outside the closest Indian embassy, media house or government office and creating a social media storm on pre-decided dates[27] were clearly aimed to disturb peace within the Indian society. The fact that she deleted this toolkit later stating that it was still being updated by folks on ground was even more suspicious. Popular pornographic actors like Mia Khalifa also got involved in the social media activism siding with the protestors.[28] Several journalists, writers and editors of publishing businesses in India who carry an anti-government imprint took forward the narrative ignited by these international celebrities, turning a blind eye to the extremists' hijack. An interesting pattern began to emerge; freelancing journalists in India tied up with international media outlets and started regularly flushing out content which took forward the narrative painstakingly built by the Opposition. To cite an example for this, a Canada-based, Indian-origin poet and influencer with millions of followers who writes on issues of body image and female sexuality hosted an Instagram Live session with a journalist, Rana Ayyub, a serial critic of the prime minister who had also been making recent appearances on several international media outlets with a single agenda to paint the Modi government as Islamophobic and incompetent.[29] On further investigation by the New Delhi Police, revelations appeared that this poet regularly upholds and defends the activities of an organization called the Poetic Justice Foundation[30], a pro-Khalistan outfit, which played an active role in putting together the toolkit posted by Thunberg.[31]

It later came to light that Rihanna was paid $2.5 million by a public relations firm, Skyrocket. Greta Thunberg is one of the directors of Skyrocket, which also appears to have direct links to Poetic Justice Foundation.[32]

Twitter became overactive with influencers who pushed the same narrative on a daily basis, many of them new employees of the five lakh social media warriors newly hired by the Congress.[33] In a few months, the narrative, instigated regularly by leaders of the opposition parties, became so banal that citizens began to see through the agenda and stopped responding to the paid-for stories. As it no longer tugged at people's heartstrings, the Opposition lost interest and slowly let the issue subside, by beginning to use this network on a new issue.

The most damage that this episode did was that it possibly took India back several steps in its fight against the virus. As mentioned earlier in the book, case curves in Punjab and Haryana had begun to plateau and halt their downward trajectory. Samples from these states which were sent for genome sequencing revealed that 20 per cent of all samples cases were from the Alpha variant of the virus which had pushed several countries like the UK and Spain into the grip of a deadly second wave of COVID-19 infections.[34] Painfully, after a slew of such undesirable events, 10 months later in November 2021, the prime minister announced that in the interest of the nation, he would initiate parliamentary proceedings to repeal the farm laws since his government wasn't able to on-board all sections of the farming community. He added that he still believed in the reformative power of the laws but he would work with all groups to find an agreeable piece of legislation, in the hope of ending the protests.[35]

# 17

## THE SECOND WAVE AND KUMBHA MELA

**14 FEBRUARY 2021**

INDIA | 1,40,217 ACTIVE CASES | 1,56,872 DEATHS | 84 LAKH VACCINE DOSES

WORLD | 16,434,660 ACTIVE CASES | 25,38,664 DEATHS | 9.9 CRORE VACCINE DOSES

Meanwhile, doctors across the state of Maharashtra were noticing a sudden rise in COVID-19-test positivity rate amongst patients they were attending to during their daily practice—a majority of these patients were asymptomatic and would have gone undetected had they not presented themselves at clinics for non-COVID-related medical attendance. They began talking in hushed circles about the possibility of a looming wave. At around the same time, oddly, three districts in the state of the Vidarbha region—Amravati, Akola and Yavatmal—began to see a steep spike in the number of new infections. Amravati and Akola began to register an average of 1,000 new infections daily causing an alert in the state government machinery.

The Maharashtra COVID-19 Task Force set up in the early days of the pandemic by Chief Minister Uddhav Thackeray's government was closely evaluating the evolving situation. The experts in the task force were very well expecting a second wave; however, they had thought that it would have occurred in December 2020 or January 2021. They advised the Health Department to send samples from these high-caseload districts for genome sequencing without further delay. By the third week of February, samples from Amravati, Yavatmal and Satara showed a common mutation which was different from the original strain of the virus but not similar to the ones recently found in the UK, South Africa or Brazil. To make matters worrying, the strain found in samples from Amravati was one that escaped antibodies which was later flagged as a 'Variant of Concern' and came to be known as the Delta variant or B.1.617. On ground, it was showing signs that it could be highly transmissible and cause deadly infections in the younger population as well. Whether it was evading vaccines too was yet to be seen. The mutation from Satara was a completely new one too, and researchers who conducted the genome sequencing couldn't find any body of literature to verify or predict its behaviour.[1] Almost like an exploding time bomb, Amravati and Yavatmal were recording 50 per cent positivity rates within days.[2] The Centre was keeping a close watch on the developments. Dr Shashank Joshi, Padma Shri awardee and member of the Maharashtra COVID-19 Task Force, noted in a conversation with me, 'What was unusual was that during the first wave, we saw that if one member of the family tested positive for COVID-19 and the other members took abundant precautions, the spread of infection to them could be avoided. During February, in Amravati, Akola and Yavatmal we were seeing that almost all members of the family were testing positive together. Even before genome sequencing was done, we suspected that this change in behavioural pattern could be due to a highly transmissible mutation.' Dr Paul went a step further to explain the role of mutants in viral transmission, 'We would like to underline the fact that we do not see attribution of mutant strains to the upsurge of the infection being seen in some districts. But this is work in progress and we will continue to watch the situation with full responsibility. The behaviour of the mutants is being constantly and closely watched in the country and when we are doing sequencing, we are not just looking for these strains, but also looking for an abnormal shift in virus character.'[3] That's the thing with mutant strains, you can't really foresee its clinical impact on the general population unless it is out there, spreading. And by then, it is already too late to take any precautionary measures because the wave is upon us. The Maharashtra government ramped up its testing in the high-positivity districts and imposed fresh curbs on movement.

Kerala, too, had turned into a COVID-19 hotspot, with over one-fifth of all cases in India concentrated in the state. A month earlier, in January, in Kerala, the Alpha variant had been detected in several samples of UK returnees[4] and controlling the highly transmittable variant had become challenging for the state machinery. As mentioned earlier, at the time, Alpha variant was also found in samples of folks testing positive in northern parts of the country: Delhi, Punjab and Haryana. What seemed to have compounded the problem was that since daily new cases were at their lowest points in India, people had let their guards down. COVID-19 protocol wasn't being strictly followed or enforced by governments. Relaxations had been given to resume travel, activity and social events. It was perhaps this intermingling of undetected COVID-19-infected persons—some of whom were attributed to the original strain, while some were due to Alpha—which provided a fertile host for the pathogen to proliferate and evolve into a more fatal variant like the Delta.

By March, the Maharashtra government had managed to bring down the positivity rate in the high-impact districts to about 12 per cent. However, a new disturbing trend of the virus spreading to semi-rural areas began to appear. Just like in Maharashtra, transmissible variants were also spreading rapidly in other parts of the state and country. Since most cases were asymptomatic, the initial spread remained largely undetected. To give you another example, let us take Delhi's case. The Alpha variant was so quick in its propagation that in January it had just begun to get detected in the genome sequencing samples in Delhi. By February, about 20 per cent of all positive samples in the Delhi NCR region were attributable to it and by March that percentage had increased to 40 per cent. Parallel to this, let us look at the speed of the Delta spread. Towards the end of February, 5 per cent of samples from Delhi were due to the Delta variant, in March that percentage had increased to 10 per cent. By April, when one in every three people were testing positive for COVID-19, over 60 per cent of positive cases in the region were caused by the Delta variant. A team of scientists from the Institute of Genomics and Integrative Biology that did extensive studies on the Alpha and Delta variants observed, 'While much more remains to be done, three takeaways for now are: Delta (B.1.617.2) is more transmissible than Alpha (B.1.1.7), there seems to be greater immune escape and reinfection, and fully vaccinated breakthroughs were disproportionately due to Delta.'[5]

All signs pointed towards a possibility of the next wave upon us. This wasn't a surprise. In September 2020, the Dr Paul-led empowered group had presented its report to the PMO. It looked at how India would need to prepare to deal with this increased caseload now that a second wave was inevitable and that India would likely see peaks of about three lakh cases a day as compared to the 90,000 cases per day which the country witnessed at the peak of the first wave. One of the main reasons why the Dr Paul-led empowered group concluded the inevitability of the second wave, close on the back of the peak of the first wave was because countries around the world were experiencing second waves with peaks higher than the first wave. In the 1918 flu pandemic, the second wave had killed more people than the first. They thus concurred, 'The more the infections in the first wave were suppressed early on, the more likely we were to get a recurrence at some point. Calculating the rate of recurrence of the second wave based on the impact of artificial measures like lockdowns used for suppressions of infections during the first wave was a very difficult challenge.' To elaborate, if the peak of the first wave was kept artificially low, there would inevitably be a second wave. India's placement to face the second wave would be calculated by considering the amount of people inoculated with our approved vaccines in addition to the amount of population with immunity after the first wave. However, with the virus mutating, the two unknowns which remained like dangling knives on our heads were: there was no way to predict the timing of the impending wave due to the unknown nature of the new variants and that there was no way to ascertain the extent of fatality they would cause. However, back in September 2020, when Dr Paul had presented his Group's report, the PMO had sanctioned ₹200 crore from the PM CARES fund, for installing 162 dedicated Pressure Swing Adsorption (PSA) medical oxygen generation plants in public health facilities. Ninety-two were planned to be ready by March, 59 by April and the rest by May 2021.

◆

## 1 MARCH 2021

**INDIA | 1,68,665 ACTIVE CASES | 1,58,396 DEATHS | 1.22 CRORE VACCINE DOSES**

**WORLD | 1,47,01,140 ACTIVE CASES | 26,68,765 DEATHS | 15.19 CRORE VACCINE DOSES**

The day began with the prime minister leaving from his residence for AIIMS in Delhi, where he was scheduled to take the first shot of Covaxin. Today marked the day when India had opened up its vaccination drive to cover people over 60 years of age or those over 45 with comorbidities. The prime minister waited his turn for a month and half since the country began vaccinating frontline and healthcare workers, refusing to take the vaccine out of line. Since February, leaders from the Opposition and their ecosystems had begun to question as to why the prime minister had not taken the vaccine when other world leaders were making a beeline in their respective countries to get the shot on priority. The prime minister's stance on this was clear. He had said in his video conference with the chief ministers on 13 January, three days before the vaccine drive began, 'No politician, even by mistake, will not take the vaccine during the first phase because the first right on the vaccine is for frontline and healthcare workers.' Not only has the prime minister shown personal disdain for entitled folks during his tenure, but has also passed several policy decisions which reject the VIP culture—widespread in India. Hence, not allowing politicians to cut the vaccine queue was in line with his demonstrated school of thought. Naturally, as a politician, he would lead by example, and wait his turn for the vaccine too. However, the fact that he was not taking the vaccine was being woven into media stories about how his actions were fuelling vaccine hesitancy and helping the Opposition build up on its questioning the credibility-of-Indian-vaccines narrative. In later months of the vaccine drive, during an interaction with the prime minister, he had said:

> There was no question of me taking the vaccine in January. Equality has been the cornerstone of our vaccination drive. If I would have cut the line as the prime minister of the nation, so many more individuals with privilege would have thought it was ok to do so too and that they'd get away with it. In the truest sense,

the fundamental thought behind creating a platform like CoWIN was also to ensure equality—that a technology platform would not discriminate on the basis of rich, poor, class and such other factors and treat all individuals equally in assigning slots for jabs. In fact, for very vulnerable individuals like the handicapped who may have difficulty accessing documents, we created a system where they'd only need their Unique Disability ID to get the vaccine. We even put together an SOP early on for vaccination of folks who don't have any kind of photo ID whatsoever—like nomads, saints, seers, ascetics, inmates, homeless and such groups. I was clear from the very beginning that no discrimination should be done in the process of vaccine administration and that every individual in the country would be entitled to receive the vaccine. As for the criticism on the credibility of the vaccine, it is now abundantly clear, as India makes such commendable headway in her vaccination drive of having administered over a billion doses—that Indian vaccines are of superior quality with due credit owed to our best scientific minds and competent manufacturers.

◆

Apart from Dr Paul's Empowered Group 1 report submitted in September 2021 predicting three lakh cases at its peak for the second wave, no scientists in the world had raised any alarms or predictions for the speed, nature and timing of the second wave in India. In fact, in February 2021, with states raising alarms on the mounting costs of maintaining COVID-19-related infrastructure, the experts in the Group had advised states and UTs to undertake careful de-escalation with specific criteria requirements to be met. However, they also advised caution in their report that the nationwide sero-survey carried out in December 2020 showed that 75 per cent of the Indian population was still susceptible and the contagion could make resurgence anytime. This basically debunks the theory that the opposition parties and some sections in the media spread like wildfire that the task force didn't meet even once in 2021 during the peak of the second wave which engulfed the country a few months later. They basically implied that because our scientists in the task force didn't meet, they couldn't advise the government on the imminent second wave. There are two points I want to clarify here: there was no need for the original Dr Paul-led VTF to meet since they had essentially offloaded their responsibilities to NEGVAC, EG1—the empowered group on emergency management plan and strategy, EG4—the empowered group on vaccination (all three helmed by Dr Paul) *and* the most recently constituted EG on vaccine administration chaired by R.S. Sharma. Second, the ICMR-constituted NTF, co-chaired by Dr Bhargava and Dr Paul, met seven times between 1 January 2021 and 15 March 2021, details of which can be found on the ICMR website for those who would like further details on the agenda of their discussions.

Now, let us consider what other scientists studying and following India's COVID-19 journey were saying at the time: Indian media's favourite epidemiologist Washington D.C.-based Dr Ramanan Laxminarayan, at the Center for Disease Dynamics, Economics & Policy, had said in the early months of 2021, 'India suffered through a lot and because it suffered through a lot, it's reached the other shore now. I don't see the prospect of a second wave in India. If it does happen, it will likely be a modest one.'[6] Similar echoes were sounded by Bhramar Mukherjee at the University of Michigan, 'There is a human barricade for the virus. By the end of March 2021, we should see a very slow, steady decline in cases.'[7] Dr V. Ramasubramanian of Apollo Hospitals had also said, 'Probably the severity of the second wave would be much milder because 60 percent of our population is younger. The second wave would be far milder than what the US and UK are witnessing. We are seeing a surge in several states, but it will not be as severe as the first one and would be shorter and fizzle out sooner.'[8] Dr Shahid Jameel, director of the Trivedi School of Biosciences at Ashoka University, had also noted, 'India's first wave was quite broad. The peak was not very sharp. As a result of that I think India may not have, what we traditionally call, a second wave. This is entirely my hypothesis.'[9] Dr T. Jacob, virologist and former professor at CMC Vellore, had commented that, 'The coronavirus epidemic seems to be nearing its end and is likely to transition to the endemic phase in a month or two.' Dr Rahul Pandit, director of Critical Care Medicine & ICU at Fortis and member of Maharashtra COVID-19 Task Force, had also failed to predict of Mumbai, which did bear the heavy brunt of the second wave, stating, 'Mumbai is slowly approaching closer to the end of the pandemic. There are several pockets in the city that have already developed herd immunity.'[10] None predicted that in a couple of months India will be engulfed by the wrath of the virus. Even the Congress party leaders thought on the same lines. In an article written by P. Chidambaram on 10 January, his first line was, 'The pandemic seems to be on its way out, but not gone yet. The vaccine seems to be on its way in, but has not yet reached households. The one thing that has remained unmoved is controversy.'[11]

◆

Possibly encouraged by the smooth experience from Bihar and from other parts of the world in addition to the scientists' opinion of the country reaching some kind of an endemic stage, the Election Commission (EC) had scheduled assembly elections in five states starting end of March and running in multiple phases all the way until the end of April. As discussed earlier in the book, even before the Bihar elections, the EC had held an all-party meet to consider substituting traditional modes of campaigning with e-rallies. While the BJP had already hopped on to the idea with the home minister having held successful e-rallies already in the state, the idea was heavily opposed by all opposition parties including the Congress. Eventually, the EC had to cave and allow physical rallies to take place. During the upcoming polls as well, all political parties held huge rallies in all five states going in for the polls: Tamil Nadu, Assam, West Bengal, Kerala and Puducherry with zero effort to substitute them with e-rallies. With the ruling Trinamool Congress government led by Mamata Banerjee for two terms wanting to retain power and the BJP intending to make large inroads in the state, West Bengal became a political battleground. For reasons outside the scope of this book, it was crucial for the BJP to acquire a solid footing in the state which had very little presence of the party up until now. West Bengal shares a very porous border with Bangladesh, Bhutan and Nepal and a general belief is that a lot of undocumented immigration takes place through it, bringing problems of smuggling of illegal substances and unwanted miscreants. On top of that, corruption and misgovernance had been plaguing the state for decades, obstructing large investment and economic progress to bring it at par with the other large Indian states.

Political atmosphere during the campaign remained charged up, with parties inviting huge mask-less crowds to their rallies. The prime minister too held several rallies which attracted massive crowds. Top leaders of all competing parties participated in extensive campaigning across the five states. These political rallies which saw absolutely no COVID-19-appropriate behaviour being followed turned into super-spreader events. The new mutations found breeding grounds and endangered the country's fight against the virus. Naturally, the already rising graph of COVID-19 cases acquired speed, quickly reaching a point that overwhelmed the country's healthcare systems.

The political rallies, especially those conducted by the prime minister, received great ire. Despite all political leaders campaigning, it was the prime minister who the people held accountable and rightfully so, since he is India's premier leader. They blamed him for being callous and taking his eye off the COVID-19 fight. In retrospect, to be fair, the EC should have postponed polls during a sniggering wave of the pandemic. And if it did go ahead with the polls, with meticulous planning for crowd management, it should have set stringent restrictions in place for campaigning and rallies which *all* parties should have adhered to. But, the speed at which cases rose, it was also difficult for anyone to predict the extent of cases. Also if elections were postponed, would President's rule have been accepted by all parties in all poll-bound states? All parties, in the spirit of Indian unity, should have suspended physical rallies, keeping in mind that it was still *us* against the *virus* and not *you* against *me*. However, in a deeply fractured political atmosphere, where it was unimaginable to have competitors sit across the table and take decisions in the larger interest of the nation, this was an unrealistic expectation to have!

◆

**11 MARCH 2021**

INDIA | 1,99,273 ACTIVE CASES | 1,59,454 DEATHS | 2.10 CRORE VACCINE DOSES

WORLD | 1,43,40,314 ACTIVE CASES | 27,60,017 DEATHS | 20.62 CRORE VACCINE DOSES

Meanwhile, almost simultaneously, in Haridwar (Uttarakhand), the Kumbha Mela was scheduled to be held through the months of March and April. The Kumbha Mela is the largest religious gathering on earth which takes place every 12 years in sync with every full revolution of the planet Jupiter (Brihaspati in Indian astrology). It is held to celebrate the Hindu myth of *samudra manthan*—the churning of the cosmological ocean by the gods and demons to secure *amrit*, the nectar of immortality. The congregation is marked by four main holy dips (Shahi Snan), which take place through the duration of the mela, along with a celebratory gathering and discourses by saints. The holy dips are considered as soul-cleansing exercises for Hindu seers, a path to absolve one of past sins. The congregation, apart from being attended by Hindu pilgrims from across India and the world, is also attended by sadhus (saints) who belong to the 10 monastic orders called *akharas*. These seers live in remote caves and only step out for the Kumbha Mela, which is usually held on a rotational basis, every three years in four sacred tirthas (river-bank cities): Prayagraj, Haridwar, Ujjain and Nasik. Attendees also include ascetics (Naga Sadhus), some of them militant ascetics, who are devoted Shiva worshippers. Tradition has it that it was them who controlled and managed the Mela until 1801 and would fight for the privilege of taking the first snan, which conferred upon them power and status. Even today, visuals of ash-covered Naga sadhus and other members of the Juna Akhara, the largest monastic order racing down the banks into the water carrying tridents are a common sight. Also common are visuals of tens of thousands of ascetics, some dressed in saffron robes, some nude and covered with ash, with wild dreadlocks riding on horseback, or in golden seats on elephants. Conch blowing, gong beating and loud drumming usually accompany this dramatic entry of the akharas.

The new Uttarakhand chief minister Tirath Singh Rawat decided not to cancel the event despite the raging pandemic and proceed with a shorter, less attended one. The Uttarakhand government was confident that it would be able to manage reduced crowds and ensure that COVID-19-appropriate protocols were followed. For this, it had deployed about 15,000 police personnel, several CCTV cameras and drones for surveillance. Sanitizer stalls and hygienic changing rooms which would undergo regular sanitization were installed as well. All travellers entering the Mela were required to upload a negative RT-PCR test taken up to 72 hours prior in order to get an entry pass. The time of snan was also limited to one and a half hour for each akhara. However, despite their best preparations, the waves of people arriving were too overwhelming for the government to ensure that COVID-19 protocol was followed. Within days, the city of Haridwar and neighbouring areas became COVID-19 hot spots with a surge of cases. Seven Hindu saints and over 300 pilgrims tested COVID-19 positive within a week of the beginning of the festival.

Pictures of huge crowds immersing themselves into the river for the shahi snan took over television news channels, front-page stories and social media. Several people began to question as to why the festival was allowed to take place at all. As much as it is within the rights of citizens to ask this question, the fact is that cancelling a huge religious gathering, which is a matter of utmost faith in several religious groups, is easier said than done. Just a few weeks later, a revered seer Swami Avdheshanand Giri Maharaj, in an article, emotionally expressed his frustration with the narrative. He said,

> As saints, we normally refrain ourselves from writing in the public domain on issues of policy and current discourse, but the way the discourse has been systematically vitiated in the last few weeks has compelled me to write this. The way the Kumbha Mela has been maligned has deeply pained not just me but crores of ordinary Hindus. Our most revered traditions have become part of a political tug-of-war, and that too, as part of some pre-planned tool-kit? What crime have the saints, seers and crores of ordinary Hindus committed that they have to be so shamed and humiliated in their own country?

He went on to say, 'First, the Kumbha mela is a millennia old tradition and the decision on time and date is taken by saints and seers based on astrological predictions.'[12]

Now, can you imagine restricting ascetics who only venture out of their caves, where they meditate for years on end, from performing what they consider the supreme act of cleansing for their soul? What kind of counter-reaction would it have generated? Would they have stayed put or would they have barged through police barricades despite the ban on the event and dipped into the holy waters? In such a situation, how would the police personnel have stopped the raging ascetics? Would the situation have gone out of hand? These were difficult but pertinent questions which the Uttarakhand government possibly had to consider when the decision on allowing a smaller, restricted Kumbha Mela was made. To their credit, they did manage to keep the attendance of devotees significantly limited over the three most important days of the festival as compared to previous years, as evidenced by key mobility indictors such as occupancy figures for all hotels in the district, vacancies in registered parking lots, cell phone presence accessed from mobile towers and passenger traffic from all vehicles and trains to and from Haridwar. For instance, on 14 April this year, the day of the Shahi Snan, only 12 lakh devotees took the holy dip as compared to 1.8 crore in the previous Shahi Shan in 2010. Local governments have a tendency to often exaggerate numbers, perhaps to demonstrate that they are capable of handling large footfalls. That seems to be precisely what happened in this case too. They initially claimed attendance numbers which they had to retract by calculating actual attendance figures after the High Court came down heavily on them. Inflated numbers presented by the local administration in conjunction with the skilfully shot visuals by crafty media persons gave off an impression that the Kumbha Mela was flooded with people and the authorities were showing off their management skills. However, due to the powerful visuals presented by predisposed media, the local government came across as completely tone deaf to the COVID-19 situation in the country.

Second, as Swami Avdeshanand Giri Maharaj also expressed, even in other countries, religious sentiments were duly considered; in Germany, for example, Chancellor Angela Merkel reversed her decision to enforce a lockdown to accommodate Easter gatherings in 2020.[13] In Israel, after over a year of lockdown restrictions, a religious festival which drew thousands of ultra-Orthodox Jews went out of hand, resulting in mass stampede that led to over 45 deaths and over 150 injuries. Both are pertinent examples which demonstrate the need for governments to carefully consider deep-set religious belief systems which form the fabric of that particular society.

A few days after the second snan held on 12 April, the head of Mahanirvani Akhada, Mahamandaleshwar Kapil Das died due to COVID-19. Despite this, the ascetics and seers were not making any official commitments to withdraw, possibly due to revered religious processes being paramount for them as compared to loss of their own lives. As the infections began to submerge public health systems in the area, undercutting all government estimates, the prime minister eventually had to step in to request the head of the Juna Akhara, Acharya Mahamandaleshwar Avdheshanand Giri, to withdraw from the Kumbh in greater public health interest. After the prime minister's appeal, the Juna Akhara wound up their activities and pledged to observe the other two snans symbolically. Taking Juna Akhara's example, the other akharas followed suit.

However, the damage done in terms of the infection spreading unchecked, the lives lost to COVID-19 and the public outrage on seeing images of millions grossly violating COVID-19 protocols was irreparable. While we saw similar events taking place in Israel, Easter events in Germany and other parts of the world, the media projection of the Kumbh was specially hateful and criticism for the government for allowing such an event even more repugnant. On the global stage, at a time when Hinduism is fast gaining popularity as one of the most tolerant and peaceful religions especially amongst the 'woke generation', the far-Left sections of the media seemed to go out of their way to paint the Kumbh as an abhorrent ritual responsible for the second surge of the virus in the country. Slowly but surely, the Hindu way of life—yoga, Ayurvedic remedies to boost immunity, vipasana getaways and karmic consciousness—are gaining increasing popularity amongst an overtired Gen Z looking for a way to escape the click-bait media-induced anxiety. The fact that Hinduism does not forcefully convert, is tolerant and allows flexibility to follow the path one connects with seem to attract millennial folk—an occurrence upsetting other dominant, extreme religious groups worldwide. The angles of the pictures shot at the Kumbh and the accompanying narratives written for pieces which would be widely circulated globally were put together with a clear mocking tone for the Hindu way and customs. The stories were braggadocio and overhyped with an apparent ridicule for the Modi government that promotes them.

In contrast, a Muslim cleric's funeral in UP saw tens and thousands of unmasked people in attendance just a week after the Kumbh.[14] However, that episode warranted barely any mention in media outlets.

Likewise, in the last week of March when Punjab had India's highest COVID-19 mortality rate and was witnessing a rapid surge in cases, thousands of Sikh devotees gathered in the city of Anandpur Sahib to celebrate the Hola Mohalla festival. Media houses reporting from ground found that neither any COVID-19 protocols were being followed in the festival grounds nor inside the premises of the main gurudwara, Takhat Sri Kesgarh Sahib.[15] The president of the Sikh Gurdwara Parbandhak Committee (SGPC), an organization which manages Sikh places of worship, quashed the government's proposal to ask devotees to present a negative COVID-19 report before entering the festival and further said that it will not suspend any religious congregation.[16] Despite this, there was barely any media outcry or bashing of the Sikh traditions among voices which seemed quite vocal in expressing their reservations about the Kumbha Mela.

Several comparisons were made in the media about the handling of the Tablighi Jamaat episode and that of the Kumbha Mela. In both events, the prime minister chose not to use force to disburse the crowd and instead appeal to the religious heads, either himself or by deputing Doval in the case of the Tablighi episode. In both episodes, he gave the states the first right to manage the situation using their law-and-order machinery; intervening only when it went out of hand of the respective state's leadership. Once again, when only after his intervention the Kumbha Mela concluded ahead of time, it became clear that in order to run a complex country like India, rife with various religious beliefs with varying levels of intensity, it was crucial to take all religious leaders into confidence. As mentioned earlier in the book too, some of these relationships that the prime minister has painstakingly built over the years, since his days as Gujarat CM are often on display, whereas at other times, they are more concealed in nature.

## 17 MARCH 2021

**INDIA | 2,52,748 ACTIVE CASES | 1,60,384 DEATHS | 3.06 CRORE VACCINE DOSES**

**WORLD | 1,44,82,166 ACTIVE CASES | 28,15,397 DEATHS | 25.34 CRORE VACCINE DOSES**

The prime minister held a video conference with all the chief ministers alerting them to be vigilant in view of the swiftly rising cases in several districts of the country. Driving the seriousness of the situation, he said,

'70 districts of the country have witnessed 150 percent rise in the last few weeks. We need to stop this emerging "second peak" of Corona immediately. If we do not stop this growing pandemic now, then a countrywide outbreak can occur. I urge you all to take quick and decisive steps.'[17] He noted that COVID-19-appropriate behaviour was not being followed and that local and regional governments had gotten negligent in forcing adherence to mask usage. He urged the chief ministers to address these governance problems at regional levels. The fact that we had done reasonably well in combatting the virus up until this point should not turn into slackness. He advised the chief ministers that while the people should not be brought into panic mode, they should incorporate experiences of dealing with the first wave in the strategy of controlling the impending one. He also advised them that special attention should be given to strengthening the 'referral system' to boost contact tracing activities and also the 'ambulance network' should be immediately fortified especially in smaller cities. Raising alarm on the emerging mutants the prime minister said, 'We need to identify emerging mutants and assess their effects in order to appropriately strategize our response.' Before ending his directives to the chief ministers, he expressed concern over high rates of vaccine wastage in some states and asked the CMs to engage with local-level authorities to bring it down at all costs. He advised them to set up more vaccination centres so that vaccination rate can be increased as supplies increase and asked them to stay vigilant about the expiry dates of the vaccines.

In the entire period, from September to April, the Centre dispatched many advisories and teams to states with high caseloads to assist them in strategizing appropriate and timely responses to the surge of cases. From the time of the peaking of the first wave in September 2020 continuing through the second wave, the Centre sent a total of 75 high-level, multidisciplinary teams comprising public health experts and clinicians from reputable institutions to 22 states/UTs. Fifty-three of these central teams were stationed in 30 districts of Maharashtra, 11 districts of Chhattisgarh, nine districts of Punjab and three districts of Gujarat all the way until April 2021. In addition to constantly appraising the states of their findings and recommendations, the Centre also identified high-impact districts and reviewed COVID-19 response in them from time to time. In addition to these, over 25 advisories were sent to states between

September 2020 and April 2021, reminding them not to be complacent and to keep strict vigil regarding COVID-19-appropriate behaviour.

On 23 March, the Ministry of Home Affairs issued an advisory with updated SOPs for effective control of COVID-19 titled 'States/UTs mandated to strictly enforce Test-Track-Treat protocol, Containment measures, COVID-19 appropriate behaviour and SOPs on various activities.'[18]

# 18

## OXYGEN CRISIS

**20 MARCH 2021**

**INDIA | 3,09,664 ACTIVE CASES | 1,60,927 DEATHS | 3.71 CRORE VACCINE DOSES**

**WORLD | 1,46,74,406 ACTIVE CASES | 28,41,527 DEATHS | 26.57 CRORE VACCINE DOSES**

By the middle of March, the case trajectory, which is the seven-day average of new COVID-19 cases, had risen by 67 per cent across the country from the touching lows which saw less than 11,000 cases a day, just over a month ago. The plateauing trend in several states had replaced itself by a full-blown upward trajectory, marking a clear beginning of the next wave. Another pattern which emerged was the disproportionate rise in cases across the states. From the numbers at this point, five states appeared to have led the resurgence of the virus in the country where cases seemed to be rising twice as fast as the national average: Punjab, Maharashtra and Haryana. New Delhi and Madhya Pradesh followed with a significant gap in numbers. Punjab saw cases go up over 509 per cent from the deepest low point following the first wave—eight times the national average. Maharashtra saw the second highest resurgence of cases at 331 per cent from bottoming out after the first wave, closely followed by Haryana at a 302 per cent rise. While the tidal wave of cases in Punjab, Haryana and New Delhi could be attributed to the rolling crowds of protestors, Maharashtra's rise was possibly driven by the Delta variant discovered in February.

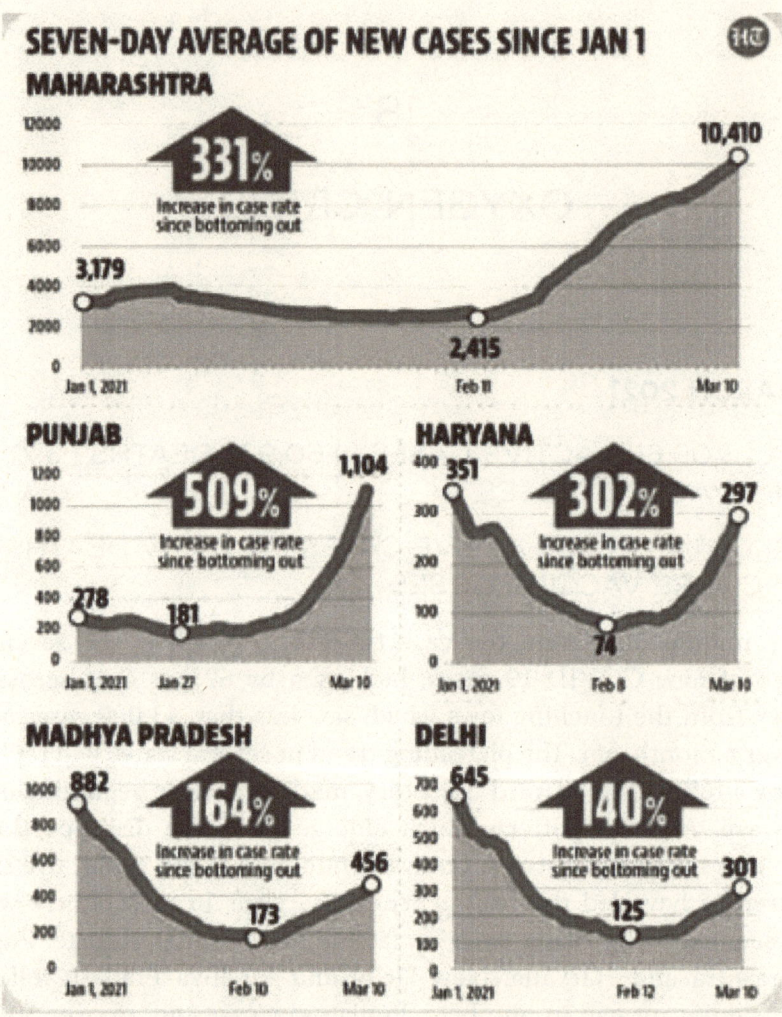

*Figure 18.1: Seven-Day Average of New Cases Since 1 January in Maharashtra*

Source: Jamie Mullick, '4 charts that show India's second wave has started,' *Hindustan Times*, 12 March 2021.

Other indicators had also begun to demonstrate that the country had entered some sort of a rapidly rising wave. Positivity rate had begun to rise sharply in several districts, especially in these high caseload states; 70 districts of the country witnessed 150 per cent rise in the last few weeks.¹ At its lowest point after the first wave it was down to about 1.6 per cent, whereas now, about 2.6 per cent of all samples collected were testing positive. As a general rule, an increasing positivity rate is a good barometer to indicate that cases in that community were set to rise in the upcoming days.

◆

## 27 MARCH 2021

### INDIA | 4,86,696 ACTIVE CASES | 1,62,730 DEATHS | 5.14 CRORE VACCINE DOSES

### WORLD | 1,50,77,877 ACTIVE CASES | 29,11,249 DEATHS | 31.64 CRORE VACCINE DOSES

Several states had begun to make adequate preparations for the looming second wave. 'Maharashtra, and more specifically Mumbai, bore the brunt of COVID—twice,' Dr Shashank Joshi would recollect after the ebbing of the second wave. He also said how they had in March, after detection of the Delta variant, begun to plan for supplies and essentials which would be required when the wave hits. As part of this, Dr Joshi explained how Maharashtra's COVID-19 Task Force took immediate measures and carried out oxygen audits in the month of March to estimate their possible oxygen requirement and decide SOPs for oxygen outflows during treatment of COVID-19 patients. He mentioned, 'During the first wave, we faced several challenges including a shortage of oxygen. This time we wanted to ensure that rationing of oxygen and accurate estimating of requirement was carried out.' On this line of thought, just a month after they started their oxygen audit exercise, they advised hospitals in the state to discontinue using high-flow nasal oxygen (HFNO) cannula and instead turn to non-invasive ventilation while treating COVID-19 patients.² HFNO machines typically are guzzlers of oxygen and can use up to 80 litres of oxygen per minute. Similarly, other states such as Karnataka[3] and Kerala[4] too set up oxygen audit panels in hospitals so that irresponsible oxygen wastage could be avoided.

Oxygen rationing wasn't a new, unheard-of concept in the global medical community. Ever since the pandemic hit the world, it was clear that to combat a virus that mainly affects human respiratory systems, oxygen would be a life-saving commodity. In the first week of January, the US had a record number of daily hospitalizations which required explicit rationing of oxygen, medical supplies and ICU beds. Authorities in several high caseload districts, for instance, the Los Angeles Emergency Medical Services Agency instructed emergency responders to limit the use of supplemental oxygen and just deny transporting patients who don't seem like they could be revived.[5] The Mayor of London too, had then warned, 'One in 30 Londoners now has coronavirus. We will run out of beds for patients in the next couple of weeks unless the spread of the virus slows down drastically. The occupancy of hospital beds is nearing 100%.'[6] The Alpha variant (B.1.1.7) seemed to have caused the vertical ascent of cases in the recent weeks and several media reports demonstrated the intense pressure that this kind of an explosion put on UK's National Health Service.[7] Just earlier in the year, two of Brazil's largest cities—Sao Paulo and Manaus—ran out of oxygen.[8] However, when Union Minister Piyush Goyal advised that state governments should ration oxygen and keep a check on demand-side management as the GoI worked to keep up and improve the supply,[9] there was an outcry. The Opposition's network went berserk, almost catatonic over Goyal's comment as if it was absolutely unheard of. Senior Congress leader and former Chief Minister of Madhya Pradesh Digvijaya Singh retorted, 'How stupid Piyush ji!! Oxygen demand is need based. How can it be kept in control? From day one all Doctors were saying that the only treatment of COVID-19 is through O2 supply. GOI failed to plan for emergency. As they have failed on all fronts to deal with COVID-19 virus.'[10] So much for intelligent political discourse in civil, parliamentary language!

◆

Just like when the virus was hitting us in March 2020, the prime minister had held video conferences with influential groups like radio jockeys, folks from the media and individuals from the private sector; he conducted another round of video conferences. His message was clear: to create awareness and prepare the people for a wave without instilling panic or fear. He requested them to issue continuous reminders on following COVID-19-appropriate behaviour and exercise caution. Aware of the increased fatality of the circulating variants, he also began to make calls to senior citizens including those from the Rashtriya Swayamsevak Sangh (RSS) family to enquire about their health and safety. For him, it was a way of connecting with his extended family and people who he had spent time with decades back. According to the prime minister, in conversations, his seniors not only gave him their blessings, but also feedback on what was happening in society and in their personal lives. This warmth is what kept him going in the tough times.

On 4 April, in a high-level meeting at the PMO which was attended by Principal Secretary Dr Mishra, Cabinet Secretary Rajiv Gauba, Dr Paul, Mr R.S. Sharma, PSA VijayRaghavan, Secretaries of Home, Health, Pharmaceuticals, Biotechnology, AYUSH and Dr Bhargava, the prime minister showed concern towards the alarming rate of growth of new cases. Maharashtra was contributing 57 per cent of all cases in the country, and Punjab and Chhattisgarh were contributing 16.3 per cent and over 7 per cent of all deaths in a seven-day average, respectively. It was especially concerning that the death rates were so high in Punjab and Chhattisgarh. In addition to these three states, seven others were contributing to more than 91 per cent of all new cases in the country. The prime minister asked, 'Why is the death rate so high in Punjab and Chhattisgarh? If one state is contributing more than half of the total cases of the country, we must investigate why along with sending them whatever help they require. Let us send central teams of public health specialists and clinicians to Maharashtra, Punjab and Chhattisgarh for assistance. For sustainable COVID-19 management, *jan bhagidari* is absolutely crucial; people's involvement at every level is paramount! For this, we must run a special campaign from April 6th to 14th for a week which will emphasize on 100 per cent mask usage, personal hygiene and sanitation.' The team informed him that although at this point the exact correlation between the mutant strains and the growth of cases could not be ascertained, the sharp rise could also be attributed to COVID-19 fatigue, a decline in compliance of COVID-19-appropriate behaviour and lack of implementation of containment measures at local levels. The prime minister was also briefed on the progress of vaccine development where production capacities of SII and Bharat Biotech were discussed along with efforts to ramp up production. He was also informed about the conversations of NEGVAC with foreign vaccine manufacturers and the outcome of those conversations. He grew concerned and informed his team that COVID-19 should be fought in a mission-mode approach in states and districts which were reporting high caseloads so that the efforts that we had made so far over the past 15 months wouldn't be squandered. Recognizing the need for transparency in the vaccination drive, he asserted that states and UTs must be informed of daily performance and their feedback should be taken from time to time so that appropriate timely changes could be made.[11]

Four days later, in a video conference with all the chief ministers, he reiterated the worrisome situation the country was heading in as it crossed the peak number of cases seen during the first wave. He directed the chief ministers to mindfully impose local curbs while initiating aggressive awareness campaigns to urge people to follow COVID-19-appropriate behaviour. He particularly stressed on the importance of micro-containment strategies instead of broadband lockdowns. He gave an example of night curfews in particular as an effective strategy around the world,

> Today, when India has developed all the resources required towards the COVID fight, it is now time to go through the test of our governance. Our emphasis should be on micro containment zones. Wherever night curfew is in place, the phrase 'corona curfew' should be used there so that awareness regarding coronavirus is maintained. Some people have this intellectual debate whether corona strikes at night. (It does not.) However, the imposition of night curfew has been an accepted experiment globally because it serves as a reminder to people that they're living in the Corona-era (to make them aware to keep following COVID protocol) while their daily activities are not affected to a large extent. It is best if 'corona curfew' starts at 9 PM or 10 PM in the night and goes on till 5 AM or 6 AM in the morning, so that other activities are not affected.[12]

Shekhar Gupta, editor of *ThePrint* and a long-time media personality, had tweeted, 'There's a new addition to the list of The Great Indian Absurdities. It is the latest competition among the states to impose night curfews to fight COVID-19. Only the Indian establishment could've conjured up a link between the virus & the night.'[13] Many, many others also expressed their opinions on similar lines. Perhaps they came from a place of scientific ignorance, being too involved in their bubble forgetting to look around the world to see what other countries had done and what had worked. South Korea, several European countries such as France, Italy and Belgium[14], heavy caseload states in the US[15] and Sri Lanka[16] were amongst the list of countries which had successfully imposed night curfews even during the first wave of the virus. It took another heavyweight personality like Kiran Mazumdar-Shaw to remind Gupta that even Britain had imposed such a policy measure.[17] While the prime minister gave out his reasoning behind night curfew, several individuals who had lived through disasters and wartime in India were particularly concerned that if millions of people lived in cities without jobs, food and very little or no savings, despair would set in and 'food riots' could become a very real possibility. The prime minister first eliminated desperation arising out of hunger by providing free food grains to every poor family. However, lack of income could still induce despondency. In an interview, former chief statistician and present chairman of the Standing Committee on Economic Statistics, Pronob Sen had expressed a similar concern reiterating, 'It (rioting) has happened before. It wouldn't be a new thing.'[18] If countrywide riots began, we simply didn't have enough police force to bring them under control. A night curfew would at the bare minimum demotivate folks from leaving homes so that those who did venture out could be easily controlled by the cops.

Moving on, the prime minister reminded the chief ministers that during the first wave, the country had successfully managed to bring down active cases from 10 lakh to 1.25 lakh. The same strategies which had worked last time would be effective even now and urged them to implement them in mission mode so as to prevent the peak from going up and bring it down quickly. He repeatedly stressed the need to ramp up testing and prescribed a target of 70 per cent RT-PCR tests, despite the fact that increased testing would obviously lead to higher positive numbers. He appealed,

> The only way out is testing. If the testing leads to a higher figure of positive cases, let it be. The states should not be judged just

because of the numbers. Therefore, this is my request to you to come out of this pressure and instead focus on testing. Even if there are more positive cases, let it be. Only then, we will be able to find a solution. If there is a need to increase shifts in labs (so that increased workloads can be better handled without compromising on the quality of sample collection and processing), then I think it should be done. As I said earlier, we have to put emphasis on testing in containment zones. Not a single person should be left without testing in the containment zones. You will see faster results.[19]

He suggested to the chief ministers to adhere to and pay proper attention to the SOPs which the Union Health Ministry had prepared for containment zones after a lot of research and experience. He also advised them to get hospitals in the states to join webinars organized by AIIMS Delhi in order to be fully aware of the National Clinical Management Protocols.

The PM also informed them that while the Centre was making efforts to increase the capacity of vaccine manufacturing to the maximum along with the development of new vaccines, it wasn't easy to increase capacities overnight. Hence, we would need to prioritize their use based on limited availability. He said,

The nationwide strategy was made only after discussions and consent from the state governments. I request you to focus on vaccinating all those who are above 45 years in the high focus districts on priority by keeping a check on vaccine wastage.[20]

He suggested running a dedicated four-day campaign 'Tika Utsav' to create awareness of the vaccine and try to get as many eligible folks vaccinated as possible, looking at it as a trust-building exercise in the people for the government's vaccination efforts.[21]

◆

Over the next week, the prime minister held extensive review meetings starting with one on the status of oxygen availability and supplies. In pre-COVID times, ordinarily India produced 9,000 tonnes of liquid oxygen each day, out of which 10–15 per cent went towards medical supplies and the rest was used in industries such as steel making.[22] India's demand of liquid medical oxygen (LMO) pre-COVID was about

700 tonnes per day, which increased to 5,700 MT per day during the first wave in August 2020.[23] As states began to demand larger quantities, the GoI had to think of options to not only augment the supply but also make arrangements for its transport. In April 2020 itself, the DCGI had issued orders to industrial gas manufacturers to be allowed to be given licences for manufacturing medical oxygen within 24 hours of application. Looking at the rising requirements of medical oxygen, the MoHFW issued an order with immediate effect to use LMO for medical purposes only. As a result of these interventions, the supply of medical oxygen increased from 1,250 MT to 8,914 MT in less than four weeks. Steel plants enhanced their daily production by reducing production of liquid nitrogen and liquid argon, cutting down usage of gaseous oxygen and decreasing safety stock from 3.5 days to 0.5 days, thus making available about 25,000 MT of LMO in their storage tanks. This resulted in increased LMO from them to 3,250 MT per day by 1 April and subsequently 4,000 MT per day by 10 May from their pre-COVID levels.

During the meeting, the prime minister was apprised of all the aforementioned actions, but he felt that more efforts would need to be made to augment production and subsequently supply. Focus was on the 12 high burden states of Maharashtra, Madhya Pradesh, Gujarat, UP, Delhi, Chhattisgarh, Karnataka, Kerala, Tamil Nadu, Punjab, Haryana and Rajasthan, where officials presented district-level data on the COVID-19 situation. The prime minister was also briefed on the mechanism which the states and the Centre was adopting while working together on projecting and estimating oxygen demand for the next fortnight—under which 4,880 MT of oxygen would go out to these states by 20 April, 5,619 MT by 25 April and 6,593 MT by 30 April. The prime minister directed the officials to make attempts to increase production capacities of the oxygen production plants. To ensure that there would be no issues in movement of tankers carrying oxygen, the prime minister advised that all necessary action including exemption from registration permits for interstate tankers and procedural road blocks must be cleared. If demand for oxygen increased drastically and the supply was matched, the prime minister pre-empted the need for additional tankers and cylinders which would be required concurrently. India currently had about 1,200 cryogenic tankers in circulation and if LMO demand went up so would the need for transporting equipment. Hence, based on the advice of the experts, the team made a decision to allow using nitrogen and argon tankers to transport oxygen which would take the number up to 2,000 and also permitted the use of industrial cylinders after due purging. The team was also was directed to make efforts to import tankers, for a bridge-gap arrangement.[24]

In the same virtual meeting, the prime minister was surprised to see two senior officials of the Department for Promotion of Industry and Internal Trade (DPIIT) present: Mr Guruprasad Mohapatra, Secretary of DPIIT and Ms Sumita Dawra, Additional Secretary of DPIIT. Only last week, they had both tested positive for COVID-19. Both officers had been frontrunners in ensuring scaling up of oxygen and ensuring timely distribution throughout the country. Due to the fact that they had to be physically present at work during a pandemic, DPIIT had arranged for regular testing of their officials. In the first week of April both had tested negative, but on 12 April, Ms Dawra had tested positive following which on 15 April, Mr Mohapatra also tested positive for COVID-19. However, further blood work and investigations revealed that Mr Mohapatra was already in the second week of the disease—the infection had evaded the earlier tests and he had gotten false negatives up until this advanced point of the infection. Mr Mohapatra had gotten considerably weak by the 16 April meeting with the prime minister, so much so that during the meeting, he sat cross-legged on the bed. At one point during the meeting, he tried to reach out to a copper water bottle kept at the side of the room and he had to struggle to get up and make his way to the bottle. Watching his condition, the prime minister asked, 'Guruprasadji, why are you in the meeting? I am surprised to see you; I know that you have tested positive. You must take time off and tend to your health.' Mr Mohapatra gestured to show his appreciation for the prime minister's concern and tried to say something, but his mic had an audio issue and what he said wasn't very audible. The next day, on 18 April, he was admitted to AIIMS, his condition worsening over the next month and unfortunately, on 19 June, he lost his life to the virus.[25] It is truly relentless service from bravehearts like Mr Mohapatra, who succumbed to the enemy while fighting for the rest of us which encapsulates the true spirit of India's fight against COVID-19.

♦

## 15 APRIL 2021

**INDIA | 15,68,138 ACTIVE CASES | 1,755,624 DEATHS | 10.23 CRORE VACCINE DOSES**

**WORLD | 1,68,41,005 ACTIVE CASES | 31,20,321 DEATHS | 48.51 CRORE VACCINE DOSES**

While on one end, India surpassed all countries in the world, barring the US, in the number of vaccine doses administered, on the other, on this day, we crossed two lakh daily cases just 10 days after clocking one lakh daily new cases.[26] The Dr Paul-led Empowered Group 1 had anticipated reaching peaks of two and a half to three lakh daily cases at the peak of the second wave, way back in September 2020 and the administration had prepared accordingly. They had also added in their September report that the pattern of the disease appeared to be an urban-concentrated one. Thus, cities were divided into five groups based on size and density; aggressive preparedness measures were undertaken in major ones such as Mumbai, Delhi and Bengaluru to be able to absorb 500 cases per million people per day. Any number significantly higher would quickly buckle our healthcare systems and create extreme shortages of medical supplies, ICU beds and oxygen. And that is exactly what followed. In the next seven days, by the third week of April, we crossed a grim figure of over three lakh new cases per day with no sign of the surge dying down[27], distributed unevenly with saturations in the northern and western states of the country. Most hospitals in the states which were hit hardest were filled to capacity with no beds to spare. From this point on, critically ill patients would have to be turned away. ICUs in hospitals were also maxed to capacity with coronavirus patients, all requiring oxygen support. This led to an even graver problem; these hospitals quickly began to run dangerously low on oxygen supplies, leaving it to the GoI to make additional oxygen allocations to states than planned.

While India had the capacity to meet the rising demand, it would require diverting most of the country's oxygen supply from industrial sites towards medical supplies.[28] A major problem however was that most of the steel plants were located in the eastern states of the country, from where it took anywhere between five to 10 days to transport the cryogenic tankers carrying LMO by road to the western and northern states, which saw high caseloads. This also meant that not only would it take long to transport the LMO to the states, but also that that many cryogenic tankers which were already in tight supply would be held up for as many days, as they would take the same amount of time to return for refilling. State governments began to make impractical requests. Maharashtra made a request to the Centre to fly them LMO via Air Force sorties.[29] LMO being highly flammable could not be transported by air, it would explode. The prime minister suggested to his team that if LMO couldn't be transported by air, empty tankers could surely be! On the instruction of the prime minister, the Indian Air Force stepped in to conduct sorties to lift empty tankers and transported them to the plants for refilling, thus cutting down travel time of bringing empty tankers back to the production sites. The final option to reduce total travel time was to transport LMO-filled tankers by rail.

However, the empowered group on logistics and supply (EG2) found that the height of the most tankers being used in India interfered with the height of rail over bridges and overhead equipment at several locations along the railway route. After an analysis of various tanker sizes in use, the Group found that only road tankers T1618, which had the height of 3,320 mm, could be used and that too only if they would be placed on flat wagons (DBKM), with a height of 1,290 mm. In addition, to prevent any hazardous events, route clearances would have to be taken and speed restrictions would have to be imposed along some sections on the routes, depending on overhead clearances. On 18 April, a successful trial was organized at the Boisar Railway Station along the Western Railway line in the Mumbai Metropolitan region where a loaded T1618 tanker was placed on a flat DBKM and all the required measurements were taken. The Oxygen Express took its first route on 19 April, as 10 empty tankers from the Kalamboli Railway Station in Maharashtra were sent to Vishakhapatnam and Jamshedpur for loading of LMO tankers and brought back successfully.[30]

A week later, the prime minister, still noticing a crunch in oxygen availability, in a rather off-beat pilot floated the idea if temporary COVID-19 care centres could be built around industrial units which produce gaseous oxygen of requisite purity, especially those closer to urban and high caseload areas. He was advised that many industries such as steel plants, refineries with petrochemical units, industries using rich combustion processes and power plants have oxygen plants that produce gaseous oxygen, which could be tapped for medical use. Five such COVID-19 care centres were set up as an experiment, which would make about 10,000 oxygenated beds available in a very short period of time.[31] He also noted the progress on 1,500 Pressure Swing Adsorption plants being established through the contribution of the PM CARES fund and other public-sector undertakings (PSUs) and directed the officials to fast-track their set-up as much as possible. Tough times call for innovation and with oxygen still falling short in several places, he asked if nitrogen plants could be converted to oxygen plants. He was informed that the only difference in the process of producing nitrogen and oxygen is the use of carbon molecular sieve (CMS) which would need to be replaced by zeolite molecular sieve (ZMS) along with some other doable tweaks. As per his usual style, the prime minister reached out to industry associations which identified about 37 nitrogen plants that could be converted to produce oxygen in a short time span.[32] On 18 April, following directives of the PM, the Union Home Secretary issued an advisory to states and UTs to take necessary measures to prohibit the supply of oxygen for industrial purposes in view of the surge in cases.[33]

◆

In yet another high-level meeting on 17 April, attended by Principal Secretary Dr Mishra, Secretaries of Home, Health and Pharmaceuticals and Dr Paul, the prime minister explicitly instructed that the entire national capacity must be utilized to ramp up vaccine production since collective vaccination was really the only way to emerge from the pandemic. He wanted an update on the status of the production augmentation of remdesivir and other medicines which were needed. While the GoI had already made efforts to increase remdesivir production from 27 lakh vials in January 2021 to an expected output of 74 lakh per month in May 2021, the prime minister insisted that the full potential of the pharmaceutical industry should be used to meet the rising demands of the hour of crisis. However, he advised that caution must be exercised while prescribing remdesivir and other medicines and the team must ensure that they are prescribed under approved medical guidelines. He was also of the opinion that a strict watch should be kept on their misuse and black marketing. Equally aware that hospitals were becoming overburdened, the prime minister directed that additional beds, temporary hospitals and isolation centres must be built on a war footing. Based on his instructions during the first wave, the DRDO had built a 500-bedded Sardar Vallabhbhai Patel COVID-19 Hospital in Delhi in a record time of 12 days. The facility had been restarted. Due to his intervention, in Lucknow too, a 600-bedded hospital was built in a matter of weeks by the DRDO. Similarly in Gujarat, a 900-bedded facility and in Bihar a 500-bedded facility was planned to be up and running in less than two weeks.[34]

To further explain the volatility of the situation on ground and how the entire government machinery—the Centre and states—worked in tandem with each other, to usher in life-saving solutions, it is important to note Iqbal Chahal, MCGM Commissioner's experience. On the intervening night of 17 April, when the city of Mumbai was logging over 8,000 new coronavirus cases per day, oxygen supplies in six hospitals in the city was on the brink of running out. Maharashtra's total installed oxygen capacity was about 1,200 metric tonnes, which included oxygen for industrial, COVID-19 and non-COVID-19 use. By the first week of April, the state had begun to consume 90 per cent of its available oxygen. That is when the state COVID-19 task force projected that within a week, oxygen consumption would increase to over 1,700 metric tonnes and arrangements to amplify supply would have to be made immediately. They requested the central government to allocate about 500 metric tonnes, which was approved. The oxygen was planned to be transported from Haldia in West Bengal to Mumbai, with a turnaround time of eight days. In the forthcoming days, Chahal noted,

> In the midst of these talks, on the intervening night of April 16-17, I was informed around midnight that six hospitals were running out of oxygen. There were 168 patients there… So, between 1 am and 5 am, we deployed 150 ambulances and brought these patients to our jumbo COVID centres. Fortunately, we had 3,600 empty beds, of which 850 were oxygenated beds. I was so relieved that no lives were lost. After the operation, I couldn't sleep at all, and around 7 am I sent messages to top functionaries of the Government of India, including the Cabinet Secretary, Home Secretary, Health Secretary… I sent another set of messages to top eight leaders of Maharashtra, starting

with the honourable CM. I said, this is not the end of the problem and this may happen again. Within 15–20 seconds, I had an incoming call coming from the Cabinet Secretary, Rajiv Gauba. He told me, tell me what you want... I said we have to import oxygen into the state. I told him that we can't manufacture oxygen at such short notice and that the turnaround time for oxygen coming from Haldia was around eight days... I worked under Gauba sir when I was joint secretary in the Ministry of Home Affairs... I told him that Reliance Industries was just 16 hours away from Mumbai, in Jamnagar, and oxygen tankers can come from there every night. He said that such an allocation cannot be made just for one city. I told him that he can allocate it to Maharashtra and I will make sure that it comes to Mumbai city only... And then 125 MT of oxygen was allocated to us from Jamnagar. The same evening, tankers started moving ...[35][36]

As a contrast to this experience, Maharashtra Chief Minister's Office (CMO), in response to dealing with the oxygen shortage in the state, announced on the same day that, 'Chief minister (Uddhav Thackeray) is trying to contact PM Modi on phone over shortage of oxygen and Remdesivir and he was informed that the Prime Minister is on Bengal tour.'[37] Several other opposition parties joined into this attack, fervently retweeting news articles quoting the CMO's statement. While petty politics of this nature was being played out, Chahal and the Union Cabinet Secretary were working out solutions to amplify Maharashtra's oxygen supply as evidenced by Chahal's aforementioned statements. The prime minister too, in the last week had chaired two comprehensive review meetings on the oxygen supply arrangements to the 12 high burden states (Maharashtra included) on 16 April[38] and 17 April[39]. Anyone who knows how the PMO of India works, especially a chief minister of a state, is well aware that a prime minister is never unavailable; he travels with a mobile office replete with a competent team and close aides along. However, the kerfuffle which followed in the media sensationalizing the prime minister's unavailability only with the intent to create a spicy story went on to demonstrate how baseless statements were made by senior political leaders who were completely ignorant of actual realities.

◆

## 20 APRIL 2021

### INDIA | 21,55,109 ACTIVE CASES | 1,84,032 DEATHS | 11.16 CRORE VACCINE DOSES

### WORLD | 1,72,93,478 ACTIVE CASES | 31,81,145 DEATHS | 52.22 CRORE VACCINE DOSES

The prime minister, in a televised address, expressed sympathy with the people who had lost their loved ones in the second surge of the virus in the country. He assured the people that the government was doing all that was possible to ensure that beds, oxygen and medical supplies were made available to meet the rising demands. He announced that vaccination would open up for folks over the age of 18 from 1 May which would likely contribute to resumption of economic activities. He specified that while his government was working to save every life possible, they also had to ensure that economic activities functioned smoothly. For that, he requested states to enforce strict lockdowns and close up economic activities as a final resort in the fight against the virus.[40]

During his speech, his facial expressions gave away the exhaustion that he was experiencing ramping up resources from every corner of the country to make ends meet for the people. Over the next couple of weeks as part of his outreach efforts to various contributing groups of people, the prime minister held meetings with leaders of the pharmaceutical industry[41], vaccine manufacturers, industrial producers of oxygen[42] and the nation's leading doctors seeking their cooperation to combat the wave; this was in addition to his regular review meetings with senior officials of the government and the Indian forces. To each of the attendees in these meetings, apart from showing deep gratitude for their contribution, he cross-checked current status, urged them to do the best they could and promised government assistance from the top. A close aide of the prime minister who was part of most meetings in the PMO during the second wave would later say,

> The prime minister is resolute. He would take continuous meetings during the second wave, one after the other, trying to get on top of issues as quickly as possible, tirelessly. But even for me, just being present in one strenuous meeting after the other, encountering one challenge after the other and going out of our way to find immediate

solutions was mentally draining. So, imagine how the prime minister must have felt knowing that 1.3 billion lives depended on him! He isn't someone who gets bogged down though, always ready to take a challenge head-on.

◆

A day later, on 21 April, a top 48-bedded private hospital in New Delhi (Sir Ganga Ram Hospital) had first flagged an SOS that they had about eight hours of oxygen remaining after which they would run out. This was followed by similar calls from other small and large hospitals in the area. Max Healthcare network of hospitals sought urgent intervention from the Delhi High Court after which the latter held a special hearing at 9.30 p.m. in which it reprimanded the Centre by saying, 'Beg, Borrow, Steal. It's your job to get oxygen.'[43] Sounds gut-wrenching, isn't it? The fact that the High Court had to step in and remind the Centre to provide oxygen which Delhi was asking for in the midst of a pandemic, was a story capable of tugging at the toughest heartstrings. However, to better understand the context, let us first understand what Delhi was asking for, whether that was a rational demand in itself to make during a raging second wave and if the Centre truly refused to supply the demanded quantity. The Centre had set up a real-time oxygen war room for monitoring movement and the supply of medical oxygen, which was essentially a virtual control room that the additional secretary-rank IAS officers from the DPIIT, Health, Home Affairs, Railways and Steel as well as dedicated officers from states/UTs were part of and monitored regularly. WhatsApp groups of officers from the DPIIT and dedicated senior IAS officers from states/UTs were also set up for ease of communication between the Centre and the states/UTs and for clarity on oxygen requirement, which was dynamic due to increase in the number of cases. These senior officers of the GoI and states/UTs shared information and problems for which immediate solutions were arrived at on a real-time basis, 24/7. Now, as of 15 April, Delhi had demanded 490 MT of oxygen, as evidenced by their communication on the aforementioned WhatsApp group and also placed on record in the Supreme Court. Within a couple of days, suddenly, they increased their demand to 700 MT. Taken by surprise, the additional secretary of the DPIIT spoke with the chief secretary of Delhi and they agreed that 100 MT, in addition to 490 MT, would be an agreeable extra, sufficient allocation.[44] However, despite that, Delhi continued to raise their demand of 700 MT in the High Court. Additional Secretary, DPIIT, Ms Dawra later confirmed on record in Court, 'I have not received any official message or call for more allocation [of oxygen] or message in [the] control room. They [the Delhi government] can ask for more and we can allocate more.'[45]

It is abundantly clear that officially the Delhi government had only raised a demand of 590 MT of oxygen, which the Centre had allocated. Despite that, perhaps only to shift the blame at the mismanagement of the oxygen, Delhi government went to Court saying that an oxygen shortage in the city was due to the Centre's refusal to allocate oxygen which they had demanded. An ingenious plan which worked to their advantage as the media lapped up the story. Videos of desolate folks running from pillar to post craving for oxygen in addition to the victim card which the Delhi government played seemed to have done wonders to shift the blame on the Centre for the oxygen shortage in the national capital.

The Delhi High Court came down on the Centre and ordered it to supply 700 MT of oxygen to the Delhi government daily and warned of contempt proceedings if it failed to do so.

To slightly rewind the situation, officers from the Centre were in touch with officers from the state governments of high-risk states right from the first week of April. The Centre would ask for estimates of requirement of oxygen for the next five, 10 or 15 days and plan allocation accordingly. But the Delta virus was a new beast, something which the world had not previously seen. The requirement of oxygen grew exponentially, which even the states themselves had not accounted for. With the exponential increase, previous calculations came undone. This led to the worst of politics being played out. Questions were raised on oxygen allocation as if no mechanism of officers was ever in place on this issue. Human psychology is such that we often need someone we can blame. Would it be right to blame states for not anticipating the future requirement of oxygen? Would it be right to blame the Centre for planning according to the requirements sent by states? This was a once-in-a-century crisis caused by an extremely unpredictable virus.

Some even blamed the Centre for over-centralizing control in the pandemic and states having to request the Centre for its share of oxygen.

But let us look at the counter scenario. Imagine if the Centre had said it would empower all states to manage their own oxygen. In such a hypothetical case, only some states would have managed to organize their own supplies while others would have had no source. Equitable or need-based distribution would be out of the question.

As soon as the allocation increased, Delhi came up with a new issue; that tankers carrying oxygen to Delhi were being blocked in UP and Haryana. On 22 April, in a press conference, Deputy Chief Minister of New Delhi Manish Sisodia noted that 'jungle raj' by the governments of UP and Haryana (both BJP-ruled states) was why Delhi was not receiving timely oxygen.[46] He blamed them for blocking and hoarding oxygen which was meant for Delhi. One of Delhi's primary vendors for oxygen supply was Linde India, whose plant is based in Faridabad, Haryana. Sisodia's charges were that the Haryana government was not letting the vendor release the tankers to come to Delhi. However, when media folks spoke with the collector of Faridabad, Dr Garima Mittal, she strongly negated Sisodia's accusations, 'I do not know where this news is coming from. Everything is fine. I don't know about the specific case of the hospital, but there is no issue here. All the tankers are leaving the state, there's no issue at all. Nobody has been stopped. There is absolutely smooth movement as has been going on. Oxygen supply will be as usual.'[47] Only a few hours after her response, Sisodia once again tweeted that supply had been restored.[48]

Even as the hearing was ongoing in Court, on 23 April, top officials of Sir Ganga Ram Hospital announced that 25 patients died because the hospital, which was filled to capacity, had to lower its oxygen flow to even critical patients due to shortage.[49] However, the chairman later announced, 'I would not ascribe the deaths to oxygen shortage. A large number of patients are in serious condition in hospital. But we are facing severe oxygen shortage.'[50] On the same day, even Jaipur Golden Hospital reported 21 deaths due to short supply of oxygen horrifying the country. But later, a committee formed to look into the reason of death of these patients concluded that the deaths which took place were not because of the lack of oxygen but because of 'respiratory failure.'[51] It further added in its report which was submitted to the High Court on 4 May that, 'almost all the patients were already very sick or critical, either from the time of admission or during the course of the hospital stay, even before the evening of April 23'.[52] In their statement to the court, they specifically conveyed their disappointment with the Kejriwal government, 'Yesterday a minister in Delhi Government said hospitals are raising unnecessary SoS. Please tell us, how many hours before deaths start happening should we call them? I was supposed to get 3.6 MT at 5 pm, but I didn't. The Delhi government's bureaucratic department has completely failed; they don't understand the supply chain and disrupt it. Let me deal with my supplier; let them not come in the way. Even offer of tankers were rejected by Kejriwal government.'[53] Strangely, the next day, the Delhi government issued an ad in the newspapers stating that they were short of tankers!

This didn't stop here. Chief Minister Kejriwal wrote a letter to Union Minister Piyush Goyal stating that the output of a major oxygen supplier to Delhi, Inox Air Products, was being diverted to other states and that his government was in no position to look for and sign on a new supplier at this critical point in time.[54] Hawkish, bright and difficult, I believe Kejriwal is the sort of man who can start a fight in an empty room. However, the chief of Inox Air Products Siddharth Jain wrote a letter to the Centre stating that the trucks carrying oxygen were having to 'travel an additional distance of 100 kms from their unit in Modinagar, UP to reach hospitals in Delhi because thousands of protestors still stationed at Singhu and Ghazipur borders were blocking them.'[55] In fact, he even attested to his statement in the High Court during the oxygen crisis hearing, 'When my truck leaves, it is working like a milkman. Our trucks are diverted midway. Why would I not want to give oxygen? It is my business. Nobody has complained except for Delhi hospitals. I wonder why.'[56] The protestors blocking the oxygen tankers were the same guys who just a few months ago had vandalized the city on Republic Day. However, politicians quickly realized that if newsbreaks began to appear showing these protestors blocking critical life-saving oxygen supply, it would be the end of public sympathy and they wouldn't be able to milk the cause of the protesting farmers for any further political gain. So, almost on cue, the Delhi Police began to escort incoming tankers from UP and Haryana to the hospitals providing them a safe corridor and protection from the protesters.

As the wave ebbed, Siddharth Jain said, 'Unlike other states, Delhi was not arranging for logistics to call for the oxygen to the state, instead just complaining. It is not the union government's job to pick up the oxygen and deliver it to end locations. It is not their job to go to Odisha, pick up the oxygen and come to Mumbai and pour it in a tank. What do the states exist for? What is their job? It is the job of the state to go and organise the logistics and go and get the allocated product.'[57]

Meanwhile, several media channels busted a black-marketing racket in Delhi where a cylinder of oxygen was selling anywhere from ₹15,000–1 lakh. Oddly, the police either had no idea of this or were choosing to ignore it until the Delhi High Court pulled up the Delhi government for keeping no record of where the oxygen coming to them was being diverted.[58] In response to the Bench, the Delhi government's excuse presented by their Senior Advocate Rahul Mehra was, 'The government has found itself in an unprecedented situation and that it was "learning".'[59] The Court further observed that the controls imposed by the state government were leading to hoarding of cylinders and also noted that a substantial quantity of oxygen was supplied to gas re-fillers, but there was no mechanism or account for further supplies that they made to hospitals or nursing homes. Further, the Court also observed that Seth Air Supply, which was also one of the vendors for oxygen supply to the Delhi government, was not given a formal order to supply. The Court noted, 'We are surprised. Seth appears to be a rather big supplier. They are holding 20 MTs of liquid medical oxygen but they do not form part of your order. There seems to be something fishy. It cannot just be an oversight. Why are they not part of your order? You are crying you do not have oxygen but the vendor does not know whom to supply.'[60]

In addition, citing orders from the Delhi government to hospitals asking the latter to ensure that each patient that presents themselves at the hospital must be provided with oxygen and medical supplies within 15 minutes, the Bench reprimanded the Delhi government stating, 'You are completely out of sync and you do not know what the ground reality is. You do not know how hospitals are coping with the situation—what is the inflow of people, shortage of oxygen and medicine, doctors and paramedics. Why do you come up with these orders? We do not understand. You think you have discharged your duty by issuing this kind of order and the public will be happy that the government has issued this kind of order? Let us tell you this is nothing but a paper exercise.

You are just satisfying your own conscience probably.'⁶¹ Concluding the hearing, the Court asked the Chief Secretary of Delhi Vijay Kumar Dev to hold a meeting with oxygen suppliers, re-fillers, hospitals and nursing home immediately to work out a distribution plan.⁶²

◆

Under such tense circumstances, the prime minister held a video conference with chief ministers of high-burden states on 23 April, urging them to aggressively adopt trace, track and treat mechanisms to put a halt to the rising surge of cases. He noted that about 70 districts in the country were witnessing a rise of over 150 per cent cases and urged them to take quick and decisive steps to stop the emerging second peak of COVID-19. He further insisted that states increase their RT-PCR testing and carefully follow the SOP for surveillance of contact of travellers coming from abroad. He further directed the states to continue to spread awareness of COVID-19-appropriate behaviour and strictly enforce it amongst people.⁶³ Parallely, Union Home Minister Amit Shah too held a review meeting and gave directives to various authorities to augment supply of oxygen for medical purposes. An expert group especially formed for the purpose was directed to optimize and rationalize the allocation to states and UTs. Additionally, the Ministry of Home Affairs wrote to all states and UTs to ensure that adequate security was provided to oxygen-transporting vehicles and accordingly make provisions for exclusive corridors for transportation. The MoHFW too continued to engage with states from time to time in order to guide their response to the wave of infections. With high caseload states, they engaged on a one-on-one format to provide any and all possible assistance to them.

Proficient at playing the victim card, Kejriwal broadcast a section of the video conference between the prime minister and the chief ministers of a dramatized appeal he had made with folded hands to the prime minister to direct all chief ministers to allow smooth movement of oxygen tankers coming to Delhi. Telecasting a live conversation with the prime minister was a clear breach of protocol and the prime minister had to pull him up during the conversation, 'Let me say something, this is strictly against our tradition, our protocol… that a chief minister is running a live telecast of an in-house meeting. This is inappropriate and we must refrain from doing so.'⁶⁴ ⁶⁵ Oddly, Kejriwal raised points of airlifting oxygen and bringing in oxygen via the oxygen express trains with no knowledge that the former was already being done and for the latter, the Delhi government had placed no request with the Union government to do so yet. The wily move seemed to be a manoeuvre to steer away the conversation from what other chief ministers were doing in their respective states to one that would place the blame for Delhi's woes on the Centre.

Despite the Delhi government's mishandling of the oxygen distribution and management, allowing it to be traded in the black market unchecked, the Delhi High Court warned the Centre that if it doesn't provide 590 MT of oxygen to Delhi daily, it may consider initiating contempt proceedings.[66] In fact, the Delhi High Court directed the Centre to show cause as to why contempt proceedings should not be initiated against it for failing to comply with its order on the supply of oxygen to Delhi. Meanwhile, Delhi was not able to lift even its allocated quantity of oxygen and Kejriwal, in a video conference, announced that they would import 18 cryogenic tankers from Bangkok and 21 ready-to-use oxygen plants from France with the help of the Indian Air Force, if the Centre permits.[67] Immediately, the GoI agreed to let the Delhi government use the services of the Indian Air Force for the same. However, six months in, the Delhi government hasn't been able to import a single tanker or oxygen plant. On the flip side, many states such as Andhra Pradesh, Telangana and Odisha had made arrangements beforehand in conjunction with their top oxygen suppliers and imported tankers in a long-lease mechanism.

The Centre then moved the Supreme Court against Delhi High Court's show-cause notice of contempt[68], which then came down hard on them holding them in contempt if they failed to provide Delhi's demanded 700 MT oxygen every day—even as they took cognisance of the fact that Delhi may have mismanaged oxygen supply and distribution. They came down heavily on the Delhi government stating, 'We want you to convey a message to the highest authority that there should be a sense of cooperation with the Centre in this humanitarian crisis. We don't want political bickering at the time of crisis. Politics is at the time of elections. There has to be a sense of cooperation. A spirit of dialogue. Saving lives is the priority.'[69] The Court constituted a 12-member National Task Force, convened by the Cabinet secretary, to formulate a methodology to achieve the goal of scientific, rational and equitable distribution of oxygen to the states.⁷⁰ Inspired by Delhi's demand, several other opposition-run states also began to flag oxygen shortages. Oxygen allocation made to states by the Centre was based on the formula which took into account current cases along with availability of hospital infrastructure including ICU beds. If states did not reveal real case numbers, naturally allocations would not be sufficient. Once again, quoting MCGM Commissioner Iqbal Chahal becomes pertinent to make my point clear. In an interview, he was asked who was to blame for the oxygen crisis plaguing the country to which he replied,

> The GoI should not be blamed at all (for states facing an oxygen shortage). If anybody has to be blamed, it is states. I'll tell you why. As far as Maharashtra is concerned, we have been very honest with the figures. We were putting out figures of over 60,000 new positives every day, when the whole country was laughing at us. Many states of India were not even ready to admit how many cases they had. How does [the] Centre allocate to them? One of our neighbouring states had 6,000 cases when we had 60,000 cases. But I'm sure if they had tested properly, they would also have 60,000 cases... Now, how does [the] Centre allocate them equal amount of oxygen like us? So, when states have only 1,000 or 2,000 cases, their allocation will be very poor. If allocation is poor, people are going to suffer...⁷¹

While the Centre eventually did supply the 700 MT of oxygen demanded by Delhi after 2 May, it lay unused for many days since tankers sat idle as oxygen tankers in hospitals were full and thus were haphazardly diverted to other hospitals which they weren't meant for without even informing them. Allotment of re-fillers for hospitals was changed frequently, thus creating uncertainty and confusion due to which hospitals were unable to get their oxygen cylinders refilled in time, thus often resulting in oxygen shortage at these hospitals.⁷² On some days, it was even returned to the suppliers.⁷³

To understand why Delhi's demand was rather overestimated, it is essential to put the numbers in perspective by taking a close look at Mumbai's case study. When Mumbai had a similar caseload (approximately 90,000 active cases) as New Delhi in the month of April, it required only about 245 MT⁷⁴ of medical oxygen versus Delhi's constantly increasing demands of 700 MT, 900 MT and eventually 1,200 MT.[75] To get to the root of the problem, the Supreme Court set up a five-member subgroup which conducted an oxygen audit after the Centre ramped up its supply to meet the amount Delhi asked for. The audit revealed that the average stock of oxygen across hospitals in Delhi was about 1.4 times of the daily oxygen requirement, with some hospitals holding on to over four to five days of stock. This meant that Delhi was also holding on to the tankers carrying LMO for a longer period of time; some taking as long as 36–54 hours to empty, thus impacting the national supply chain. At a later date, on 23 June, the media leaked findings of the interim report by the Supreme Court-constituted oxygen audit committee which was headed by AIIMS Chief Dr Randeep Guleria. The report found that,

> There were significant errors made by the hospitals in the data that they were reporting. Initial summing up of oxygen consumption claimed by the hospitals (1140 MT) was about 3–4 times higher than what was the expected consumption (289–391 MT) using formulae for the established bed capacity for these hospitals. It was noted that some hospitals had claimed extremely high oxygen consumption with very few beds, while others had shown high negative consumption values that could not be justified. The claims appeared to be erroneous, leading to extremely skewed information and adjustment for both extremes resulted in more realistic values. It was thus recognised that there was a problem with the quality of data being generated for calculating oxygen requirement and capacity building was needed to gather correct data.[76]

The Delhi government had shown that the actual consumption reported by hospitals was 1,140 MT per day. However, after 'correction' of the error, the oxygen requirement fell to 209 MT. The report further noted that hogging of more oxygen than needed during a national fight, where many other states were also in need of oxygen led to their supply getting affected.[77] When the report emerged, Kejriwal tweeted in Hindi, 'My fault was that I fought for the breath of 2 crore people. When you were [Prime Minister Narendra Modi] busy campaigning for election, I was burning the midnight oil to arrange oxygen. People have lost their relatives due to oxygen shortage. Please don't lie, they are feeling bad.'[78]

He left out the part mentioning that shortages were made to appear due to lack of efforts, planning on part of his government and black marketing!

What kind of a government-hospital-black market syndicate was being run to create a fake alarm of oxygen shortage, demand much more than required by getting hospitals to grossly overestimate need and make the excess disappear into the black market so that there would still be shortages?

While this episode played out for months in the media, Indians were paralysed with shock that such politicking would play out at the cost of their lives. Who would take responsibility for deaths which occurred in states other than Delhi because Delhi lapped up their share of oxygen due to error in calculation?

In the time of an unprecedented national crisis of this nature, many states stepped up to the challenge and made several positive alterations to keep lives safe. Some states like Andhra Pradesh and Telangana imported cryogenic tankers on a long-term lease, some like Maharashtra, Karnataka and Kerala put out oxygen audit reports to prevent wastage of oxygen, some like Odisha, which had surplus oxygen production,[79] went out of their way to send out oxygen to others and some like Kerala and Tamil Nadu[80] adopted a 'triage centre' model to direct patients to appropriate medical care so that those who didn't require oxygen wouldn't be unnecessarily put on it. But Delhi's response to a crippling second wave was absolutely underwhelming and complacent. One of their largest suppliers, Siddharth Jain, who ended up supplying 2,700 MT of oxygen at the peak, would later state in an interview,

> India manufactured 6,000 to 7,000 tonnes of product. In peak one, it required only 3,000. We believed we were good. Nobody expected this (rise in O2 demand) in such a short period of time. By the peak of the second wave India's requirement was at 9,000 tonnes. For a country to increase its oxygen production by 30%, in one month, is unprecedented. Oxygen is manufactured only in 70 locations across India but the consumption of oxygen happens in over 7000 places across the country. More than the production of oxygen, the supplying of oxygen was a major hurdle because in some cases, oxygen was being transported over 1,500 kilometres one way.

He added, 'This additional 2,000 tonnes a day that the country produced [in the peak of the second wave] has saved millions of people. It's difficult to put that into numbers, but we would have been in a very different place today.'[81]

Padma Shri awardee, Dr Devi Shetty said in an interview:

> I know a lot of people are criticizing the government, but I can tell you, the number of COVID patients we have, even if we present this to the US government, there is no way they can manage it ... forget any other country. These are astronomical numbers that no country in the world has the infrastructure to manage. In terms of oxygen, I can tell you, I have gone through the details. Our government has done a phenomenal job. They have moved Heaven and Earth to get the oxygen to the hospitals. Of course, a lot of people have suffered. But, then if the whole country is falling sick, there is no healthcare infrastructure in the world that can manage it.[82]

As we have seen earlier, the answers to some questions are better understood through counter-scenarios. It is no secret that for a number of days, the situation in the country was rather worrisome, despite a near ten-fold increase in oxygen supply and usage of all possible means of transportation for distribution. Could the GoI have done better? There always exists possibility of improvement. However, imagine a situation if all these efforts to augment production and distribution of oxygen were not taken in time. Each metric ton of oxygen saved innumerable lives. In retrospect, instant ramp up of oxygen by the GoI stood in stark contrast to Uttarakhand's tragic case where relief trucks did not leave for the destinations because top leaders of the Congress party could not find time to flag them off.

# 19

## MEDIA CAMPAIGN AND ROLE OF THE OPPOSITION

**1 MAY 2021**

INDIA | 33,49,564 ACTIVE CASES | 2,18,320 DEATHS | 12.63 CRORE VACCINE DOSES

WORLD | 1,47,01,140 ACTIVE CASES | 33,35,753 DEATHS | 60.62 CRORE VACCINE DOSES

In each of the last few days, India saw record after record shattered for the number of new cases logged, eclipsing everything at the worst of the outbreak. Today, on 1 May, India crossed a grave number of four lakh cases per day.[1] Many states had reinstituted curbs similar to those of last year's lockdown. People were once again placed under severe movement restrictions to control the spread of the contagion. The only difference being that introducing and lifting of restrictions remained each state's prerogative. This led to different states locking down at different times, with some allowing economic activities to function depending on the intensity of the caseload.

That being said, many cities and states were crumbling under the tsunami of the second wave. Their healthcare infrastructure had collapsed. Doctors from private hospitals were left to fend for themselves to arrange for drugs required for treatment. A doctor from a major private hospital in Mumbai, Dr J.P. attests that he and several other doctors from hospitals across the state had to repeatedly send out SOS messages to the opposition leader Devendra Fadnavis to make remdesivir and tocilizumab available for them because the state government was not able to cater to their supply. When Fadnavis did try to arrange from a manufacturer in Gujarat, the latter was booked by the police with heavy politics playing out. Such instances of dirty politicking over the miseries of the people became commonplace. People were angry and no state chief minister wanted to take the blame or accept any wrongdoing on their part.

While some states with decisive leadership managed to course correct pretty quickly, some failed at doing so for extended periods of time. The situation in the national capital had gotten very critical with the city clocking over 20,000 cases in a single day, for several weeks. Of course the health infrastructure of Delhi was so overwhelmed and the Government of National Capital Territory of Delhi was so inept at managing the crisis that the cases spilled over to the bordering states, which too fell to the same fate. Not only hospitals, even crematoriums began to be overwhelmed, with many of them conducting mass funerals. Pictures of these began to go viral all over the national and international media, causing emotional anxiety and distress to the people of the country. Photo journalists captured pictures of people in despair waiting outside hospitals, struggling to breathe. Some journalists like Barkha Dutt took to the road to investigate how mass funerals were taking place in smaller towns and villages and documented images of cremations done by immersing bodies in the Ganga, the holy river of the Hindus.[2] Dutt went so far as to sit on the roads outside crematoriums, hospitals and just about anywhere to demonstrate how she was the only 'chosen one' to reveal the Holy Grail. She'd interview men who'd be building pyres for the cremation of the Hindu individual; she'd interview rural folks in hamlets along the Ganga asking them questions about bodies being buried in the sand. She'd put up pictures of meals she's picking up off the streets during her travels with captions detailing the difficulty of her journey—it all seemed so rehearsed, so strategized. Sadly, she never saw fit to sit outside government offices where bureaucrats were working 24/7 or outside homes of folks who were recovering due to the incessant efforts of our healthcare workers, outside PDS ration shops to see how millions were being distributed food by the government so that they don't go hungry or even inside Muslim burial grounds for that matter. Did deaths of folks of other religions didn't warrant coverage? Or was the reward not as chunky as the reward for Hindu pyres? While haters of the establishment enjoyed the graveyard shift show that she put on, many eyes didn't fail to notice her blatant inclination to sell the emotion of Hindu pyres and deaths. Even when her own father unfortunately succumbed to COVID-19 during the second wave, there were those who saw her use the tragedy to get sympathetic coverage in the international media using the emotion of grief to further her agenda.[3] Multiple countries have seen a large number of deaths but the fascination of covering crematoriums in India among a section of Indian and international media has never been seen elsewhere. With the media flooded with pictures of floating bodies and overloaded crematoriums, several folks began to question if India was revealing the true figures of the COVID-19 death toll.

Typically, two out of three deaths in India occur at home and only about 86 per cent of all deaths are registered. In other words, 14 out of 100 deaths, even outside of a pandemic situation go entirely uncounted which is why researchers choose to use demographic surveys to confirm death rate.[4] Death rates in India are generally calculated from data extrapolated from the Civil Registration System (CRS) and the Sample Registration System (SRS). Now, it is also crucial to note that the government has increasingly invested in digitizing birth and death records which has had a positive impact on actual registration. In 2011, only 66 per cent of deaths were registered versus in 2019, when registrations increased to 92 per cent.[5]

The CRS is the body responsible for recording death data from local governments across states. It releases and corrects data after a considerable time lag. While data reporting highly varies across states, in rural areas deaths of women and children especially go unregistered. The SRS, on the other hand, is a large-scale demographic survey which is conducted annually by the Office of the Registrar General & Census Commissioner in India. Usually, the sample consists of 4,961 rural and 3,886 urban units covering a population of approximately 8.1 million people across states and UTs and is then adjusted relative to the entire population to calculate for total estimated deaths. However, the problem lies in the fact that death estimates from both systems vary significantly. Take the year 2019 for instance: according to the CRS, India had 1.1 million excess deaths as compared to average figures of 2015–18, but according to the SRS, death numbers from the same time period show that there was a marginal decline in deaths. In addition to these issues, for access to better medical facilities, folks from rural parts of the country travel to urban and semi-urban areas. If casualties occur in these urban areas where treatment centres are concentrated, that's where deaths would be registered, showing as a spike in death rates in urban areas versus rural ones. However, looking at this data on face value without factoring in the aforementioned considerations would lead to unreliable inferences—a rookie mistake most media sources were making when discussing India's death rate during the pandemic years. On similar lines, the problem with using the SRS is that it is only an estimate of deaths and not recorded deaths, making it less accurate for use in data collection, analysis and research.[6] For instance, if surveys were done in more high caseload areas, the generalization to total Indian population would not yield real numbers. Many health experts and data scientists such as Chinmay Tumbe[7], Abhishek Anand et al'[8] from the Center for Global Development, Bhramar Mukherjee[9] and many others came out with papers and opinion pieces analysing how India's death rates were anywhere between four to 10 times higher than official numbers. These studies used mostly SRS and Consumer Pyramids Household Surveys (CPHSs), which collected data from select households in the country and then generalized it to total population, basically working on estimates versus reality. In fact, CPHS mostly collected employment and income data, with mortality data as an add-on. Obviously, there was no way to ascertain if respondents answered to questions rather honestly or not. Oddly, the studies, despite using similar methodologies, contradicted themselves, with many saying that India's death rate was four times higher[10], while others pegging it at 10 times[11]. Such studies came to be quoted by several media organizations, pushing an already worried India population in the throes of sadness.

When the second wave of COVID-19 rampaged through the rural and semi-rural areas of the heartland states, several households didn't register deaths occurring. Driven into poverty after a year of the pandemic, many of them couldn't afford to purchase the wood for the pyre and other materials required for performing cremations. Instead, upholding the Hindu ritual of Jal Samadhi, many chose to immerse the dead in the Ganga or bury them in the sand along the banks of the holy river. Jal Samadhi, since generations, is especially common amongst select communities to cremate unmarried people.[12] In fact, every now and then as bodies float ashore, journalists put up pictures in the media questioning the ritual;

for instance, in 2015 when Gargi Rawat of NDTV tweeted, 'Shocker from Unnao in UP. Over 100 dead bodies floating in the #Ganga, many just lying in the shallow water #River'.[13] However, during the time of a pandemic, it drew heavy criticism, so much so that UP Chief Minister Yogi Adityanath hurriedly announced a proposal to construct crematoriums along the banks of the Ganga in an attempt to check unorganized cremation. The UP government also issued orders to provide up to ₹5,000 worth of financial assistance from the Namami Gange funds for each cremation.[14] Namami Gange is a flagship programme of the Modi government designed for arresting the pollution in the Ganga with the larger mission of Ganga conservation. Even Bihar announced that cremation of burial expenses of those dying due to COVID-19 would be borne by the government.[15] In addition, patrolling teams were set up along sites which saw an increase in cremations in the water or on the banks of the Ganga and its tributaries. Due to these measures, in a short period of time, there was a significant reduction in abandoned bodies in and along the river. However, despite that, the government found it difficult to maintain a balance between implementing awareness measures of stopping the jal samadhi ritual while also respecting religious sentiments.[16]

Yogi Adityanath and UP's response was singled out in attacks by the Opposition, perhaps due to the lingering sting of defeat for Rahul Gandhi, who lost his Lok Sabha seat from Amethi; a seat held by his family for decades. Even as the Tablighi episode was playing out in the media just at the onset of COVID-19 in India, *The Wire*, a left, anti-establishment online news platform, published an article about how Yogi Adityanath wanted to go ahead with a large Ram Navami celebration to take eyes off the Tablighis and wrongly attributed Acharya Paramhans's statement to the UP CM. Acharya Paramhans had quipped to the media that, 'Lord Ram would protect devotees from the coronavirus.'[17] Adityanath had issued no such statements and in fact Ayodhya's district magistrate and superintendent of police had issued a circular stating that devotees would not be allowed to gather for the event in view of the lockdown.[18] All through the pandemic, the opposition ecosystem's eyes remained trained on Adityanath. During the second wave, since there was a pouring in of cases from the NCR region into UP, Adityanath's response was particularly criticized by biased media channels frequently changing facts and digging out old photos to suit their narrative. However, in a report prepared by IIT

Kanpur, which took several indicators into consideration, concluded that UP had been able to do an exceptional job in not only swiftly bringing down the COVID-19 surge during the second wave but also to keep the economy of the state stable.[19] An important achievement for the Yogi government was that it was able to bring down unemployment rate in the state from about 10 per cent in March 2020 to about 4 per cent in June 2021 due to the extensive skill-mapping exercise it carried out for the returning migrants and further linking them to potential employers. The UP government provided about 39 metric tonnes of free ration during the second wave which works out to be about 100 kg per family, thus ensuring that the most populous state in India does not go hungry. Availability of COVID-19 beds was increased by 80,000 beds and healthcare manpower was significantly augmented to address the surge in cases. A COVID-19 monitoring committee was set up in every village equipped with a basic medical kit which could be given to anyone suspected to be infected. Timely restrictions on movement was key to UP's success in controlling the second wave. IIT's report shows that the lockdown was so timely that had it been done earlier, it wouldn't have contributed to reduction in caseload but would have significantly crippled the state's economy and any delay would have led to quick multiplication of cases. To keep an eagle's eye on the oxygen supply, the state had set up a 78-member team which constantly monitored the 15 oxygen plants which supplied oxygen to UP along with 133 oxygen tankers tagged with GPS and RFID which moved oxygen from them to various parts of the state.

◆

Coupled with the negative atmosphere countrywide, with no sight of emerging out of the wave and stories of despair and gloom plastered all over the media, the opposition began to blame the prime minister for the state of affairs. The fact that the former BJP chief minister of Uttarakhand Tirath Singh Rawat encouraged people to come to the Kumbha Mela in huge numbers only added to the resentment towards the prime minister. To top this, images of the prime minister addressing large rallies in West Bengal, fuelled the fire. After what they appreciated in the first wave, people expected the prime minister to get the house in order, even if it required a heavy hand. His decision to give autonomy to states began to be considered his weakness. His staunchest loyalists became disenchanted with his approach to handling the second wave and naturally his approval ratings dropped drastically.

The Opposition began to build on this mood. After all, why would they lose an opportunity to malign the leader responsible for their political defeat? The time was perfect. Attack the enemy when he's at his weakest.

◆

## 7 MAY 2021

INDIA | 37,25,991 ACTIVE CASES | 2,43,535 DEATHS | 13.22 CRORE VACCINE DOSES

WORLD | 1,76,45,313 ACTIVE CASES | 34,17,793 DEATHS | 64.79 CRORE VACCINE DOSES

The media narrative became ruthless towards the Centre and the prime minister. International media groups continuously ran stories projecting him as the chief villain responsible for India's crisis. Stories of efforts made by the government found no place in the narrative, perhaps because averting millions of deaths was simply not as sensational as pictures of mass funerals. While some reporting remained neutral, some was just outright biased and overtly exaggerated. On 28 April, *The Washington Post* published a front-page story which alleged that so many people were dying from the virus that Indians were burning bodies in their backyards.[20] This story was referenced in another story published in *Mail Online* on 25 April.[21] On 30 April, *The Straits Times* also reported that Indians were burning bodies on pavements, backyards, lawns and gardens.[22] All of these stories were inspired from a quote by Karnataka's former chief minister B.S. Yediyurappa, who had agreed to let families bury bodies in a decentralized manner to avoid crowding at cremation grounds in view of the raging second wave of infections.[23] Let me make a stronger case: the issue of overwhelmed cremation grounds was an urban one where the majority of the caseload was concentrated. Urban cities in Karnataka, the state whose chief minister's quote was lifted and where such guidelines were framed did not have homes with backyards and lawns. They were concrete jungles where people lived in compact apartments in buildings constructed very close to each other.

However, due to such unethical journalism, using striking headlines like 'Modi's pandemic choice: Protect his image or protect India. He chose himself'[24], 'India, the world's largest democracy, is now powered by a cult of personality' or Arundhati Roy's 'We are witnessing a crime against humanity' accompanied with a tag line 'it's hard to convey the full depth and range of the trauma, the chaos and the indignity that people are being subjected to; meanwhile, Modi and his allies are telling us not to complain'[25] became common reportage. Another serial critic, Ramachandra Guha wrote a piece titled 'Crisis-hit India needs a leader who listens, not one focused on building his brand'[26]. *The Australian* too published one titled, 'Modi leads India into viral apocalypse' with the tag line 'Arrogance, hyper-nationalism and bureaucratic incompetence have combined to create a crisis of epic proportions, critics say, as India's crowd-loving PM basks while citizens literally suffocate.'[27]

The aforementioned articles just scratch the surface of the scathing, offensive and predisposed narrative that the international media projected of India and the prime minister in a short span of time. The prejudice was so obvious that in a recent survey conducted of media professionals, 80 per cent noted that the coverage of COVID-19 in India by a section of the western media was biased and 71 per cent thought that the stories were not balanced. Sixty-nine per cent of the respondents stated that India's image took a beating by such negative coverage and about 56 per cent said that such reporting may have negatively influenced the opinion of Indians living abroad. The survey also posed questions to understand what media persons thought the possible reason for such biased reporting could be. As responses, 54 per cent thought that international politics was to blame and 47 per cent believed that internal politics in India could have played a major instigating role.[28] In fact, several distinguished international personalities noted the out-of-place, excessive criticism and made it appoint to call it out. For instance, bestselling author, former politician and international policy expert Bruno Maçães noted in a tweet, 'India really gets an odd treatment from global media. I think most people are only now discovering Delta is extraordinarily more contagious. A few months ago it was all about India's incapacities...'[29]

A fact which stood out was that the most derogatory pieces which the international media hosted were written by Indians as opinion pieces; however, that is no excuse to offer space to highly defamatory content for the head of a country. No other world leader in recent times has been subject to this kind of dire press coverage—one insulting opinion piece after the other. Regardless of this well-oiled machinery working in perfect tandem to constantly oppose, the prime minister, who is usually one to befittingly respond to critics with retaliations as sharp as a *kukri* knife, instead prioritized leading the country out of the devastating wave of infections. Possibly, this is the kind of wisdom which can be brought on only by decades of public service—choosing one's battles.

Barring some official objections raised by the Indian missions in the countries where these pieces were published, the GoI's machinery and the BJP's media cell failed to offer a sophisticated counter. In fact, some efforts to counter were counterproductive, i.e., a piece written and published by a party functionary in an Indian e-media outlet called *The Daily Guardian* titled in bold, capital letters, 'The prime minister has been "working hard", don't get trapped by the "opposition's barbs". This article was retweeted by multiple high-level functionaries of the party, starting with the head of the media cell Amit Malviya, followed by several ministers in the Union Cabinet.[30] Somehow, they didn't quite understand that media powerhouses like *The Washington Post* or *The Guardian* cannot be countered by a small, irrelevant Indian news portal which doesn't even have physical newspapers in circulation. Similarly, when *The Lancet* posted an editorial which held the administration fully responsible for India's COVID-19 emergency,[31] the then Union Health Minister Dr Harsh Vardhan, in response, shared a post from a blog named 'Pankaj Chaturvedi's Thoughts' with a note 'A fair rebuttal to the imbalanced editorial in *The Lancet* titled "India's COVID19 emergency" published on May 8th. While the COVID crisis did assume alarming proportions in India, it was indeed important to remain politically unbiased for a reputed journal.'[32] It was also shocking to see the former Union health minister responding to a giant in the world of scientific writing with a private individual's blog post which had an image of a cat as its thumbnail. It portrayed a lack of sophistication in responding to the international media community and understanding its nuances. The former health minister also engaged in several ill-timed activities which became opportune moments for the media to lambast him. For instance: when he graced along with Union Minister Nitin Gadkari, the launch of an Ayurvedic company's drug touted to be a cure for

COVID-19.[33] While Ayurveda, India's ancient medicine system, has a slew of products and concoctions which are proven to be immunity boosting, so much so that after the advent of the pandemic, turmeric-ginger cold-pressed shots became a rage, quickly flying off the grocery store shelves worldwide, the former health minister's choice of product to endorse and its timing was problematic.

◆

Through the month of May, several countries were sending various kinds of medical supplies in aid to India, including China, with whom we had just successfully concluded border disengagement talks. In our hour of crisis, many nations stood with us, as we did in theirs. Several sections of the media once again reported this as a dent on the prime minister's vision of a self-reliant India, completely undercutting the severity of the catastrophe. Little did they know that just a few months later, several other countries and their healthcare systems would be equally overwhelmed as ours as the Delta variant would rage in their countries. In fact, when Indonesia[34] and Bangladesh[35] became victims to intense surges of infections just months after our second wave, they too ran out of oxygen and we extended relief by sending them timely oxygen and concentrators.

As the authorities tried to steer the country out of the virus' grip, the mood in the PMO was also sombre. Every day brought with it several new challenges which needed to be resolved because millions of lives depended on the solution. At a later date, an advisor to the prime minister would recount, 'During the second wave, we were all coming to work, physically in the office. We could have worked from home, since we were holding all meetings virtually anyway. But none of us could go back home and get a full night's peaceful sleep because lives depended on us. We'd be in adjoining chambers, but we'd still hold virtual meetings, considering how bad the situation was in terms of the spread of the virus.'

◆

Enthused by the noise that the oxygen shortage episode created coupled with his ambitions to become a national political heavyweight, Kejriwal raked up several issues, many of them seeming headline-grabbing versus fact-based. Some of them hurt the country so severely that our Foreign

Service officers had to rush to control the damage. On 18 May, he had tweeted, 'The new variant of COVID-19 in Singapore is said to be very damaging for children. This can come to India in the form of a third wave. I appeal to the Centre to: Stop all flights to and from Singapore immediately, Start work on developing and vaccinating children on priority.'[36] Singapore's Health Ministry responded sharply calling him out for spreading misinformation, 'There is no truth whatsoever in the assertions found within the reports. There is no Singapore variant. The strain that is prevalent in many of the COVID-19 cases in recent weeks is the B.1.617.2 variant, which originated in India. Phylogenetic testing has shown this B.1.617.2 variant to be associated with several clusters in Singapore.'[37] Singapore's Foreign Minister also responded by saying, 'Politicians should stick to facts! There is no "Singapore variant".'[8] India's External Affairs Minister, S. Jaishankar had to intervene to sort out this diplomatic embarrassment and clearly convey that the Delhi chief minister does not speak for India. He tweeted, 'Singapore and India have been solid partners in the fight against Covid-19. Appreciate Singapore's role as a logistics hub and oxygen supplier. Their gesture of deploying military aircraft to help us speaks of our exceptional relationship. However, irresponsible comments from those who should know better can damage long-standing partnerships. So, let me clarify- Delhi CM does not speak for India.'[39] India's External Affairs Ministry also tweeted, 'Singapore Government called in our High Commissioner today to convey strong objection to Delhi CM's tweet on "Singapore variant". The Indian High Commissioner clarified that Delhi CM had no competence to pronounce on Covid variants or civil aviation policy.'[40] The whole episode turned out to be quite humiliating for Kejriwal, a man who clearly harbours national ambitions but falls desperately short of aptitude and skill.

However, Kejriwal didn't let one shameful incident deter him. He raised another issue with the Indian government's vaccination policy, hoping this time around it would stick. It did.

Other politicians dutifully followed. As the country braced itself for the tsunami of the virus, the opposition parties began to question several decisions made by the Union government on vaccine availability and its purchase, centralized distribution, eligibility criteria and price. Back in March, when the vaccine drive had opened up to immunize folks over 45 years of age with comorbidities and those over 60 years of age, Kejriwal had announced that if the Centre provided enough doses, he would put in place systems by which all of Delhi would be vaccinated in three months. With that, he also suggested, 'The Centre should make vaccines open for all those who are 18 years of age or above. India is producing enough COVID-19 vaccines now to get this done. Walk-in centres should be open for all. Our country is now doing good in terms of the production of vaccines. Rather than creating criteria on the eligibility, age groups with comorbidities, etc., we should create a category of ineligible people.'[41] This marked the beginning of vaccine politicization. His comments on the vaccine roll-out too came just a day after a video conference with the prime minister in which three other opposition parties' chief ministers had also requested for the expansion of the vaccine drive. Oddly, these states demanding for the opening up of the vaccination drive hadn't even completed vaccinating frontline workers and priority groups. The chief ministers were being informed in detail of the vaccine pipeline, how much stock they had and how much the Centre was expecting, on a regular basis by the health secretary and Dr V.K. Paul. Despite the knowledge, politicizing the vaccine roll-out took centre stage. In some states, shortages were deliberately made to appear so that this vaccine shortage narrative could be pushed forward. For instance, in Maharashtra, when a vaccine shortage situation was being politically created, the health minister Rajesh Tope was redirecting thousands of doses to his constituency Jalna, from the doses which were meant for high caseload areas, thus creating scarcity in other areas of the state.[42] Continued mud-slinging on the issue of vaccine shortage, pricing and the roll-out plan saw the Centre on the back foot with changing demands on-the-go from the Opposition-ruled states and parties.

By 1 May, the next phase of the vaccination drive which would include people over the age of 18 had opened up. The enthusiasm in the youth to get vaccinated was palpable, with over 1.2 crore individuals registering on CoWIN even before the slots to book vaccine appointments became available. Due to the limited amount of vaccines, not everyone who tried was able to make a booking. The situation remained like this for several weeks, until the time more vaccines became available, prompting the opposition parties to once again attack the government on vaccine shortages. Posters were put by various opposition parties in several cities calling out the Vaccine Maitri initiative, asking, 'Modiji, why did you send our kids' vaccines abroad?' The absurdity of the poster was that India hadn't approved any vaccines for children then, let alone fall short of them! The media was relentless in blaming the government about why enough pre-orders weren't placed with vaccine manufacturers and why certain foreign manufacturers were not given approvals. An article in BBC titled 'How India's vaccine drive went horribly wrong', written by two Indian freelance journalists, stated, 'India waited till January to place orders for its vaccines when it could have pre-ordered them much earlier. And it procured such paltry amounts.'[43]

These narratives were far from the truth. See, India operated with the awareness and knowledge that we had manufacturers working and producing vaccines in India. This meant that all production by them would be considered de facto an order for vaccines by the government, especially since it was ultimately the government's decision on when and how many vaccines could be exported and not totally the vaccine manufacturers' decision (apart from commitments from contractual obligations which were informed to NEGVAC in advance). Having incubated these companies, NEGVAC did not need to place formal 'orders' with any Indian vaccine manufacturers since their entire production was going to be for India.

Politicians from opposition parties and their lurid spokespersons took shots at the government shrieking on prime-time shows on news channels about how the Modi government had failed to protect the people by not having placed enough timely orders for the vaccines. As much as these stories made for great headlines, they didn't mean much. India was going to consume all vaccines made in the country; there was no doubt about that. As a matter of fact, countries which did need to place orders were those who didn't have in-house vaccine manufacturing capabilities; several of which despite placing orders in advance didn't receive the pre-ordered quantities. In fact, some opposition parties rather encouraged white supremacy alluding to the fact that when most major nations of the world were purchasing Pfizer and Moderna vaccines, why weren't we? They called out the Modi government of being 'callous' and 'cruel' for failing to do so. Their attitude of holding the international mRNA vaccines in superior light was quickly debunked when research surfaced showing Covaxin having similar levels of efficacy on variants.

On the contrary, the reality was that India was not only one of the five countries to manufacture its own indigenous vaccines but that we were on the cusp of becoming the largest manufacturer of vaccines in the world. Not only would India suffice its own people's needs but also the needs of a large chunk of the world's population. The opposition ecosystem's narrative operated from absolute ignorance about the fact that India did not need to place orders with companies which we had incubated.

Unfortunately, to take forward the plot, constant comparisons were made to link percentage of India's population vaccinated to percentages of other western nations running vaccination drives, despite the fact that India had administered more vaccine doses than all other countries by June 2020. But considering the vastness of our population, our percentage of population vaccinated would remain low as compared to nations with significantly lesser population. Running such conniving stories at the peak of a ghastly second wave was bringing the morale of the people down. The narrative in the media was so bitter that several world leaders stood up to defend India's vaccine policies. France's President Emmanuel Macron, in the presence of 26 EU nations at the India-EU virtual summit held during the peak of the wave, said, 'India does not need to be "lectured from anyone" on vaccine supplies. India has exported a lot for humanity to many countries. We know what situation India is in.'[44] The UN Secretary António Guterres was also prompted to tweet, 'I think the [vaccine] production capacity of India is the best asset that the world has today. I hope the world understands that it must be fully used.'[45]

Now, even as NEGVAC planned the vaccine drive, way back in the month of November, they were in full knowledge of the fact that the production of vaccines in India was going to be heavily back loaded. For the first seven months of the year, we would be seeing about 60 crore doses while over the remainder of the five months of 2021, we would have enough supplies to inoculate our entire population with both doses. However, 10 chief ministers of opposition-ruled states wrote to the prime minister several times, urging him to decentralize vaccine procurement. NEGVAC had been in talks with all vaccine manufacturers in India as well as over the world since mid-2020. By virtue of actual experience, they knew that opening up procurement would not yield any positive results. None of the vaccine manufacturers, who were coveted entities by several countries, would engage in procurement discussions on state levels. It wasn't going to happen. But owing to the constant pressure from the opposition parties, the government conceded and allowed state governments to procure vaccines. After a rough few weeks, where the tenders floated by states didn't attract any supplies, the same chief ministers who earlier forced the prime minister to open up procurement, made a U-turn asking the Centre to ensure that procurement and adequate supply of vaccines were made.

Finally, on 7 June, in an address to the nation, the prime minister announced that the Centre would take over the vaccination drive including vaccine procurement. The Centre, he announced, would also provide free vaccines to all those over the age of 18 in government-run vaccination centres. The Centre would buy 75 per cent of the vaccines, leaving 25 per cent for the private sector to purchase, which could then run paid vaccination drives at capped rates. Elaborating the sorry state of dependency and desperation which India faced in the past, the prime minister remarked, 'If you look at the history of vaccinations in India... you will see that India would have to wait decades for procuring vaccines from abroad. When vaccination programmes ended in other countries, it wouldn't have even begun in our country.'[46]

Vaccine nationalism is in the negative interest of the world and is entirely discreditable behaviour. However, this has been the norm for a long time. India, in the past, has been at the receiving end of the problem, having had to suffer for much longer periods of time and typically live with the diseases until vaccines would reach us, in some cases after over a decade. Taking a closer look, the rotavirus vaccines, while available to the world in 1998, reached India only in 2015. The Japanese encephalitis vaccine reached us in 2013 as compared to 1930, when it became available to wealthier countries. The Hepatitis B vaccine, which became available for the world in 1982, arrived in India for use only in 2002. While the world got the polio vaccine in 1955, it became available to India 22 years later, in 1978, after which we were able to become polio-free only in 2014. Even the tetanus vaccine took 54 years after the rest of the world to come to India for mass inoculation. The problem this time around was the behavioural pattern of the virus and its impact on entire countries due to high transmission rates because of which accessing enough doses for our population in the least possible time became absolutely crucial. Here is a shuddering thought: up until now, India used to be part of the developing world which wouldn't have access to vaccines for multiple years after the wealthier nations have inoculated their populations many times over and wasted millions of unused, over-ordered doses.

However, with the constant attacks back home, India was compelled to temporarily suspend the Vaccine Maitri initiative. Vaccine Maitri had not only brought India goodwill in the international community but also demonstrated the fact that as an important country in the vaccine supply chain, India was giving back as much as it was receiving. Let me explain. Vaccines are complex to manufacture and depend on a host of specifically engineered raw materials from around the world. For instance, the Pfizer COVID-19 vaccine reportedly depends on 280 ingredients and components sourced from 86 suppliers in 19 countries. Similarly, COVID-19 vaccines manufactured in India need about 360 ingredients sourced from over 10 countries. Over 200 of these ingredients are sourced from the US, about 100 from Germany and the rest from Singapore, Denmark, Poland and Japan. Supply chains of this entire ecosystem came to be disrupted when COVID-19 hit the world and the manufacturers of these ingredients had to significantly scale up to the sudden need—still falling short to meet demand. In such a scenario, where all manufacturers around the world were vying for the same ingredients, they were made available to India on priority mainly because India is an important link in the chain—both as a supplier of ingredients and the finished vaccines. The fact that India makes cost-effective vaccines for its own people as well as for countries across the globe makes us a tenable part of this global vaccine network. To ensure that India gets priority in the supply of ingredients, our diplomats worked aggressively with partner countries. To give you an example, the US had instituted an executive export embargo under the Defense Production Act (DPA) of 1950 across categories which would disallow raw materials from being exported. Adar Poonawalla even tweeted to that effect on 16 April, 'Respected @POTUS, if we are to truly unite in beating this virus, on behalf of the vaccine industry outside the U.S., I humbly request you to lift the embargo of raw material exports out of the U.S. so that vaccine production can ramp up. Your administration has the details.'[47] In order to ensure that our supplies were not disrupted, our diplomats worked closely with the US government behind the scenes to persuade it to lift the embargo. Given the excellent bilateral ties between the two countries, which have deepened considerably under Prime Minister Modi, the US suggested that India give them a specific list of ingredients which we would require the embargo to be lifted on. After working with the government, the Indian diplomats then went into individual manufacturers of the requisite raw materials, providing estimated quantities and a sound plan for them to be able to prioritize supplying to India. The prime minister, too, spoke with the US president, urging him to allow smooth supply chains, following which NSA Doval spoke with his counterpart in the US, Jake Sullivan, to discuss the finer points of the arrangement. The next day, Sullivan, in a statement, confirmed, '[The] United States has identified sources of specific raw material urgently required for Indian manufacture of Covishield vaccine that will immediately be made available for India.'[48] Due to relentless efforts from the very top of the government, supply chains remained open and Indian manufacturers were able to produce the large quantities required. However, when India suspended the Vaccine Maitri programme, from a security and market standpoint, we made way for the Chinese vaccine makers to access markets which were mostly dominated by Indian companies. A major Indian vaccine manufacturer would later vent, 'The people who created such a hue and cry about stopping the vaccine exports are such buffoons. They don't understand how much Modiji's vaccine export programme strengthened India's position in terms of bilateral and multilateral relations. Now that the Chinese and Koreans have taken over critical markets, due to our vaccine unavailability, how are we going to reclaim our positions of strength there?'

Case in point is SII's experience. Describing his frustrations, Mr Poonawalla said, 'Just when the pandemic began in March 2020, I was certain that SII would play a role in ensuring India's security. I first raised over 10,000 crores from the global community way back in March 2020, followed by another round of 6,000 crores. Most of this money came from countries which had placed advance orders with SII and some came from the COVAX program—under which SII was bound to supply a certain amount of doses to middle- and low-income countries within a certain time frame. In fact, with the export ban, SII was in such a tough spot that I had to offer to return this money we had raised.' The damage that the opposition network had done to India's credibility was immense. In fact, months later, when the prime minister spoke at the Global COVID-19 Summit, he had to commit to resuming vaccine exports in order to continue being a beneficiary of the global vaccine supply chain, assuring, 'We are leveraging India's manufacturing strength to produce vaccines for the Indo-Pacific region with the help of Quad partners. And as our production increases, we will be able to resume vaccine supplies to others too. For this, the supply chains of raw materials must be kept open.'[49]

◆

All through the second wave, there were media stories doing the rounds about an acute shortage of ventilators. All through 2020, the GoI along with private organizations had strived to meet the increased demand with funds allocated from PM CARES. Out of the total 60,000 units ordered, 49,960 ventilators had been sent to the states before the second wave and about 12,000 were dispatched during the second wave. Surprised to see stories of shortage, the prime minister ordered an immediate audit to look into reasons why the ventilators sent to the states were not put to use. Noticing that the states were crying foul about the quality of the ventilators, the MoHFW secretary had written to the states on 9 and 13 May,

> It has been found that there is a large gap between ventilators delivered and installed. It is understood that the non-installation is primarily on account of large number of them lying in warehouses, delay in allocation, preparing location for installation, absence of connectors with hospitals, lack of piped oxygen electrical fittings and trained manpower. In a number of hospitals the sites are not ready for ventilator installation. This includes lack of availability of piped oxygen supply system or lack of optimum oxygen pressure in the pipe system or even proper electrical fittings. It is again reiterated that the states may sensitize the consignee hospitals to ensure provisioning requisite number of ventilator connectors so that once the ventilators reach the hospitals their installation and commissioning does not get delayed.[50]

On the other side, the media was rife with stories about faulty ventilators provided to them by the Centre which had rendered the units useless. However, the audit brought to light several inadequacies on the part of states to use them appropriately. Let us consider the example below: Punjab and Rajasthan, both Congress-run states, first raised the issue of receiving faulty ventilators from the Centre. Punjab was first supplied about 100 ventilators in October 2020. The manufacturer of those ventilators, Jyoti CNC reached out to the Punjab government several times asking where they would want the units to be installed. During a video conference with the Punjab government officials, the latter apparently claimed that they didn't need the ventilators and that they should be taken back. By April 2021, about 809 ventilators had been supplied to the state, out of which a significant amount remained uninstalled.[51] After repeated reports of the state not even installing them, the secretary of the MoHFW wrote a letter to the chief secretary of Punjab asking the state to speed up installations, urging him that 'non-commissioning of the ventilators defeats the purpose of their use in the fight against Covid'. Finally, much after the second wave had reared its head, the Punjab government woke up to the need for ventilators and called the manufacturers to install them. When the team from the manufacturing company reached Punjab, they noticed that the hospitals where the ventilators needed to be installed hadn't even arranged for appropriate connectors (a specific part required to connect the hospitals' piped oxygen system). In addition to the lack of initiatives taken, the dispatched team also found that the oxygen pressure in hospitals was not adequate to operate several installed ventilators, which could easily lead to malfunction of the machines and eventually human casualties.[52]

When a second team of manufacturers from Bharat Electronics Limited (BEL) reached Punjab to investigate the causes for malfunctioning units produced by them, they found stunning revelations. According to M.V. Gowtham, Chief Managing Director of BEL, it was non-utilization of ventilators which was making them unfit for use. He further explained the Punjab government's irresponsibility,

> There are flow sensors connected with the patient's ICU and then there are oxygen sensors. When our team when to Faridkot, we saw that consumables were not replaced. It is mandatory to change the flow sensor each time a new patient comes to the ICU. Second, some ventilators were not calibrated along the latitude-longitude of Faridkot during installation. Whenever a ventilator changes location, oxygen pressure must be changed according to that location. Third, oxygen sensors have a shelf life. If you use it with a dozen patients

with 100% oxygen, it will deteriorate. It will not work. Oxygen sensors must be changed, which did not happen in Faridkot.[53]

Even more shocking was the revelation that the Centre supplied ventilators based on demand raised from states. After the first wave of COVID-19 ebbed in September 2020, and the first set of ventilators were dispatched, most states didn't even bother to order more quantities to prepare for future surges. They didn't pre-empt future surges and hence displayed this lacklustre attitude in installing them too. It was only during the time of the second wave when patients were stranded did they raise urgent requests for more units.

Now let us take Rajasthan's case as an example. The ventilators sent to Rajasthan from the PM CARES fund were further rented to private hospitals. The Centre had sent ventilators for every district in Rajasthan but the government of Rajasthan rented these out to private entities for ₹2,000 per day. Hence, the ventilator which was supposed to be used for free treatment for the common man was used to extract ₹50,000 per patient for treatment.[54] In another district—Churu in Rajasthan, the audit team dispatched by the Centre found that unopened boxes of ventilators were lying near the washroom area in a public hospital, eventually rendering them unusable. According to the management, they had no space to put them hence they chose to keep them near the toilets.[55] In Kotlipur, near Jaipur, ventilators remained unused due to the lack of adequate oxygen supply. What is unfortunate is that the chief minister of Rajasthan was quick to point fingers at the Centre for sending defective pieces before putting his own house in order![56]

Now let us also note that all of this narrative and media mud-slinging regarding ventilators took place in a limited time frame—the first three weeks of May. When the country was already struggling to control the second surge of the virus, it was generally easier for chief ministers to point fingers at the Centre versus being accountable and answering the public about their complacency and pandemic mismanagement.

◆

The Empowered Groups which had been condensed to six from the original 11, in view of the progression of the pandemic and the need to club some issued under certain groups were once again expanded to

10 groups. This time however, their ambit was expanded to specifically look into issues of oxygen availability, vaccination, emergency response and economic welfare measures. Dr Paul continued to remain the convener for Empowered Group 1, which oversaw vaccination, vaccine procurement, import and such other issues. This was the third specialty group after the VTF and NEGVAC which dealt with vaccination-related decisions. However, while the VTF initiated procurement conversations and the NEGVAC looked closely at the larger issues related to vaccine procurement, administration, import, export, priority groups and so on, the Empowered Group 1 dealt with day-to-day nitty-gritties of the vaccination drive. For instance, it would look at the status of the stock availability, accountability of manufacturers and amount of doses to import and export. Basically, VTF, NEGVAC and Empowered Group 1 operated simultaneously, overseeing interrelated arrangements to cover all issues related to India's vaccination journey.

◆

All through the second wave while the government struggled with optimizing resources, the high courts and the Supreme Court stayed heavily involved, forcing the central government as well as the state governments to allocate time from already stretched officers towards hearings. The fact that the courts became so involved in the government's pandemic management certainly warrants a discussion on the role of the judiciary as originally envisioned by the Indian Constitution. Many former Supreme Court justices have expressed opinions on the limitations and responsibilities of the Indian judiciary. Former Supreme Court Judge K.S. Radhakrishnan, in his comments to a media house during the COVID-19 hearing in Supreme Court, had explicitly noted, 'Administration is the job of the elected government. The Supreme Court cannot deal with highly sensitive and technical issues as it does not have the machinery for it.'[57] Considering that he spoke from experience, if the Supreme Court Bench led by Chief Justice S.A. Bobde including justices S. Ravindra Bhat and L. Nageswara Rao did not have the technical experience, was asking the Centre to submit a national COVID-19 management plan for review justified?[58] Or would that be considered judicial overreach into the executive and legislative branches of the Indian government? Now that we have the luxury to look back at past events in retrospect, let us take another example: during the hearing on the oxygen supply to Delhi, the Supreme Court ordered the Centre to provide 700 MT of oxygen on a daily basis. What became clear after the top Court ordered an oxygen audit on the Centre's insistence was that Delhi did not need that much oxygen. This episode let many journalists to conclude,

> Courts might have created more problems than they solved. Their decisions on fixing the quota that Chief Minister Kejriwal demanded for Delhi – 700 metric tonnes – resulted in states like Tamil Nadu and Karnataka also seeking judicial intervention for quotas. Clearly the messaging that went out was that the crying child gets the milk or rather oxygen![59]

This episode doesn't even scratch the surface of some of the ludicrous and unscientific statements that high courts have made through the pandemic. While hearing a case regarding COVID-19 management, the Allahabad High Court asked the UP government to 'consider producing COVID-19 vaccines themselves', in order to alleviate the state of affairs with regards to the pandemic. The Supreme Court had to intervene on 21 May 2021 by advising high courts across the country to avoid passing non-implementable orders regarding COVID-19 management.

So it is prudent to ask: was this excessive wading into the executive arm necessary? What was the norm regarding the role of the judiciary in other large democracies? In the US and the UK, very few cases were taken on regarding the government's COVID-19-management strategy and mostly the courts in those countries appeared supportive of the government's positions. Let us take for instance, the US Supreme Court's hearing regarding a plea challenging the COVID-19 vaccine mandate imposed by the employer of the petitioner. Justice Stephen G. Breyer, associate justice of the Supreme Court, didn't even consider the matter worthy to call for a response or refer the case to a full court. Only a week ago, he had rejected a challenge from the hospital workers of Massachusetts hospital system to block the US government's vaccine mandate.[60] On 30 October as well, the US Supreme Court had turned away healthcare workers who had been seeking a religious exemption to Maine's COVID-19 vaccine mandate.[61]

A similar pattern was observed in UK's top court. In a test case brought by the UK government's Financial Conduct Authority (FCA) regarding business interruption (BI) insurance policies providing insurance cover to policyholders in the COVID-19 context, the UK Supreme Court backed the FCA upholding that policyholders who were ordered to close business premises during the first national lockdown due to COVID-19 will be able to register valid claims with their insurers.[62]

A general opinion seems to be that since all three branches of the Indian government are envisioned to work together, is it responsible for one to overreach on matters exclusively allocated to the others by the Indian Constitution? Where should the fine line between interference and accountability be drawn? Due to the arms of the government not functioning in cohesion, the media, specifically the international media, gets an opportunity to comment on the country's credibility. Is that an outcome desirable in the best interest of the nation? Perhaps this is a matter better suited for debate in the Indian Parliament but certainly warrants discussions, deliberations and deep engagements by experts on the matter.

# 20

## INDIA'S ROLE IN SECURING THE WORLD

**24 JUNE 2021**

**INDIA | 6,15,055 ACTIVE CASES | 3,98,022 DEATHS | 24.76 CRORE VACCINE DOSES**

**WORLD | 1,13,06,942 ACTIVE CASES | 39,32,708 DEATHS | 176 CRORE VACCINE DOSES**

The second wave subsided as swiftly as it rose, making almost a vertical decline on the curve. All markers had begun to show that we were almost out of the grip of the second tsunami of cases. Many, many families had lost their loved ones this time around. In parts of India where the cases were unequally concentrated, everyone had closely experienced the struggle to procure beds, essential medicines or oxygen. Those horrifying memories weren't going to fade easily.

To be fair, in retrospect, no expert around the world had predicted this velocity and almost a vertical rise of a second surge of infections in India. As mentioned earlier, on the contrary, most of them had begun to release data in February 2021 indicating that the virus was on a subsiding trajectory in India.

It is rather unfortunate that India was so politically fractured during a time of a once-in-a-century global crisis and that people had to see such low-level politics play out. Political parties, their leaders, chief ministers, spokespersons, everyone had no qualms in unreservedly lying to the people about important issues which would impact the nation's state of mind during dealing with the pandemic. While we saw politics play out in other countries as well where governments have been under fire for their pandemic responses, it never got to a point where a leader of a nation was constantly shamed and ferociously attacked in the international press like India's prime minister was. Obviously this had an impact in the soft power India holds in the world order. For instance, in Japan's case, Japanese PM Yoshihide Suga had to resign owing to criticism of his COVID-19 handling.[1] But we didn't see brickbats flung at his dignity in the international media. Under the garb of free speech, these folks went too far, taking liberties which dented the very spirit of India. In October 2021, the prime minister finally let out what he may have thought about the excessive bias in the media against him driven by his opponents. In an interview to *Open* magazine, he reasoned why such a negative situation may have come to be,

> The problem here is not Modi…but when any person tries to see anything with a preconceived mindset, then either he is able to see only half of the view or is inspired to see wrong things. And if he is not able to see anything as per his preconceived notion, then he creates a perception to feed his preconceived mindset. We all know it is the nature of Man to not accept his mistakes easily. It takes courage to accept truth over your wrong notions. And it is because of this that one forms notions about a person even without meeting, knowing or understanding him. And even if they meet you in person and observe something different (as compared to their notion), they will still not accept it just to feed their ego. This is a natural tendency. However, it does not mean that Modi has no faults or there is no point on which Modi can be criticised. I feel, and this is my conviction, that for my own healthy development, I attach a big importance to criticism. I, with an honest mind, respect critics a lot. But, unfortunately, the number of critics is very few. Mostly, people only level allegations, the people who play games about perception are more in number. And the reason for this is that, for criticism, one has to do a lot of hard work, research and, in today's fast-paced world, maybe people don't have time. So sometimes, I miss critics.[2]

My view remains that the prime minister should have kept a heavy hand on the states, even if he came across as authoritarian. After the second wave shook the country, not one chief minister came forth to accept blame for their government's oversight. Not one chief minister admitted that they had been warned over and over by the prime minister—first in the second week of March 2021 all the way until May 2021—about how they need to be vigilant in controlling the surge and not let their guard down. Dispatches of advisories sent by the Ministry of Home Affairs and the MoHFW to the state leadership fell on deaf ears. Most chief ministers took for granted that if the surge was to come, it was going to be the Centre's problem and not theirs. Painfully, the prime minister repeatedly reiterated in his constant discourse with the chief ministers about the need to ramp up testing and contact tracing, the need to look out for mutations, the need to strengthen ambulance networks and many other vital issues.

I now understand that his intent was to entrust the state leadership and the elected chief ministers with more responsibility because he believed that they were equals in the exercise of keeping the nation safe. That in my opinion was a misjudgment of the abilities of various chief ministers. Several chief ministers hardly cared about the security of the nation and the safety of India, putting party politics above everything else.

◆

As of July, India's vaccination drive was yet to pick up the kind of speed that was needed to rapidly inoculate the country to meet the year-end target of vaccinating all 130 billion Indians. At this point, vaccination drives in other larger countries were achieving much more coverage than ours—a major reason being that the wealthy nations had invested large sums of money into vaccine manufactures, considering it to be risk funding, right from mid-2020. While India too had undertaken its own kind of risk funding by incubating companies with solid vaccine candidates, we obviously didn't have the risk appetite to put in billions of dollars into foreign companies whose candidates had not even begun Phase III vaccine trials, let alone demonstrate strong data. However, due to the pressure put on the government during the second wave to ramp up the pace of vaccinations, NEGVAC had started having advanced discussions with Pfizer and Moderna, despite their disagreeable terms. We changed our policy so that these candidates, which were now approved by the WHO or approved by regulatory authorities in Japan, Europe, the US or the UK and by now had immunized billions of people across the world would, not need to conduct bridge trials in India.

However, NEGVAC was clear in its approach, closely guided by the prime minister, that unless a fair deal was arrived at, India was not going to get strong-armed into any agreements detrimental to its sovereignty, even if that meant that the deal would fall through.

◆

## 5 JULY 2021

INDIA | 4,65,897 ACTIVE CASES | 4,08,211 DEATHS | 28.67 CRORE VACCINE DOSES

WORLD | 1,15,16,576 ACTIVE CASES | 40,15,824 DEATHS | 191 CRORE VACCINE DOSES

When we were in the midst of the crisis, over 40 countries sent us prompt aid which included 19 oxygen-generation plants, 11,058 oxygen generators, 13,496 oxygen cylinders, 7,365 ventilators, over 5.3 lakh vials of remdesivir and over 25,000 rapid antigen test kits. Many more who couldn't send help due to domestic requirements, sent us best wishes. This was a classic example of the *Vasudhaiva Kutumbakam* philosophy that India aspired to propagate. The world came together as a family as the second-most populous country was being attacked by our common enemy. When the time came, India would repay the generosity, surely.

Two months ago, when the CoWIN platform proved that it could hold its ground and truly become an asset, driving the largest vaccination drive in the world, the prime minister expressed to R.S. Sharma on 27 May that the platform should be open sourced and given to as many countries who wish to acquire and use it free of cost. To take this directive forward, on 5 July, a CoWIN conclave was organized since over 50 countries from Central Asia, Latin America and Africa had already expressed desire in using it. In his opening remarks, the prime minister reiterated his stand, 'The biggest lesson from the COVID-19 pandemic is that for humanity and the human cause, we have to work together and move ahead together. We have to learn from each other and guide each other about our best practices.'[3] At the conclave, where India demonstrated how the platform could be adapted to each country's requirements and used accordingly, health and technology experts from across the world were present. Sharma noted in his address that vaccinating 1.3 billion people was no trivial task, and now that we had used the platform to handle over 30 crore registrations, CoWIN had demonstrated that India had the capability to develop great scalable digital systems.

He noted that when we initially began to use the platform, several groups raised the issue of how the digital divide would be dealt with. The platform, he added, was fully capable of making on-the-spot registrations as well, for people who chose to walk into vaccination centres without prior appointments. By July, he said, over 80 per cent of Indians had been registered on the platform had gotten their vaccine doses without prior appointments. He proudly announced, 'I am proud to say the CoWIN is the fastest technology platform in the world.'[4]

In a later conversation, Sharma expressed how CoWIN could be repurposed post-pandemic to create a National Digital Health programme which could very quickly, within a couple of years, ensure that the entire country is connected through a grid that validates the identities of patients, healthcare providers, healthcare facilities and pharmacies. This would be an open and interoperable grid which would have the capability to leverage extensive internet connectivity and robust digital identities where Aadhaar would play a crucial part in plugging in gaps in the current healthcare delivery.

Eventually, CoWIN turned out to be a state-of-the art, top-class portal with sophisticated solutions which even several developed countries couldn't match. While countries like the UK and the US were issuing flimsy pieces of papers as vaccination records, we were issuing QR-coded vaccine certificates linked to Aadhaar numbers and available on WhatsApp and Digilocker on demand. The portal was also built in with some special features: people with disabilities didn't need to submit any documents at all apart from their unique disability registration number. If the vaccine certificate had errors, it could be corrected with just a click within 24 hours. To ensure that all vaccines administered came from legitimate, approved sources, a provision was added in the portal wherein slots at centres could be activated only once the vaccine manufacturer confirms supplies to that particular centre on the CoWIN portal. Also, doses would be auto calculated based on stock purchased versus used.

In September 2021, when the UK opened up travel to vaccinated Indians, it first announced that they would not recognize Covishield and

Covaxin and would need Indian passengers to finish their quarantine requirements. After pushback from the Indian government on the lines that Covisheild was the exact same formula which was used by them to inoculate their own citizens under AstraZeneca, they declared that they'd recognize Covishield but Indians would still need to quarantine since they didn't recognize CoWIN-issued digital certificates—a system manifold times more foolproof than their rickety cards issued in the name of vaccination records. The Indian government once again pushed back to diplomatically resolve this discriminatory policy. In fact, just a few days later, when the prime minister spoke at the Global COVID-19 Summit, he dealt with the matter head-on by stating that India was running the world's largest inoculation campaign and had recently vaccinated 25 million people in a single day and that this feat was achieved due to 'India's use of our innovative digital platform CoWIN'. He further expressed concern on the pandemic's economic impact, called for mutual recognition of COVID-19 vaccine certificates and urged countries to enable easier international travel.[5]

◆

## 1 SEPTEMBER 2021

INDIA | 3,96,207 ACTIVE CASES | 4,39,559 DEATHS | 67.10 CRORE VACCINE DOSES

WORLD | 1,89,40,415 ACTIVE CASES | 45,66,300 DEATHS | 317 CRORE VACCINE DOSES

India was geared up to vaccinate its entire, eligible adult population with both doses by the end of 2021. The systems put in place had ensured that the country could handle over a crore immunizations per day and had done so several times in the past month. Alongside, we came with the knowledge that all of the vaccine-manufacturing companies which we had painstakingly built over the last year were on the crux of delivering results. Zydus Cadila had already been granted emergency use authorization, becoming the fifth candidate to enter the market. Biological E and Genova Life Sciences were also on the verge of flooding the vaccine pool with their candidates. Soon, it would become a problem of plenty, where we would have more doses than our population. Oddly, Rahul Gandhi, Mamata Banerjee, Arvind Kejriwal and some other vocal opposition leaders went totally schtum on the subject of India's admirable vaccination drive. Mum. Silent. Not a word. A Congress spokesperson gave out just a by-the-way statement excusing Mr Gandhi's couple of missed days during the parliament session as a consequence of taking the jab.

India was not going to shy away from supplying cost-effective vaccines to the rest of the world, primarily to developing and underdeveloped nations. In the third week of September, the Union health minister announced that India was set to produce over 300 million doses by October. Since our security was ensured, we'd resume our Vaccine Maitri programme. The announcement was reiterated by the prime minister on his bilateral visit to the US for the Quad Summit, during his address to the 76th United Nations General Assembly and his remarks at the Global COVID-19 Summit later in the month.

The Indian economy markers were gaining solid footing showing that the economy was rapidly recovering from the COVID-19 impact, poised to grow at the world's fastest rate. The fact that we didn't lock down the country at the same time during the second wave, with states instituting lockdown measures only when required for very brief periods of time ensured that although economic recovery momentum had suffered, greater activity across sectors limited the economic damage. Experts believe that the rate of vaccinations picking up, rapid resumption in manufacturing activity and a milder hit on the services sector were some of the reasons that kept the economy afloat during the second wave. The RBI's low-interest regime and the GoI's bet on infrastructure investments had also helped to minimize the damage. In other words, the second wave did impact India's economy but many times lesser than the first wave.

India recorded a 20.1 per cent growth in GDP for the April–June 2021 quarter, bringing it on par with pre-pandemic levels and reaffirming its imminent V-shaped recovery forecast. For August 2021, ₹1,12,020 crore of gross GST revenue was collected, which was 30 per cent higher than GST revenues of the same month last year and 19 per cent higher than those collected in the same month in FY 2019–20.

These encouraging growth numbers reaffirmed the sound economic policies which India adopted from the start of the pandemic.

Ruchir Sharma, Morgan Stanley Investment Management's chief global strategist, wrote in the *Financial Times* that, 'Emerging economies that stimulated most aggressively (inspired by the US and other large developed countries "go-big" on economic stimulus) got no pay-off in a faster recovery. In fact, the big spenders like Greece, Hungary, Brazil and Phillipines who spent at least 16 percent of their GDP on stimulus, suffered higher inflation, higher interest rates and currency depreciation.' The reason he explains is that, 'Overspending often backfires, particularly in developing nations. They lack the financial credibility to ramp up spending without unbalancing the economy, and end up getting punished by global markets.'[6] Other noteworthy economists also shared similar views. R. Jagannathan published a piece titled 'Modi's socio-nomics starts to pay off' in the *Business Standard* on 2 November 2021 where he plainly predicted what could lie ahead for India. He predicted that a $10-trillion economy by 2030–32, a Sensex at 1,00,000 by 2025, monthly GST revenues at ₹2 trillion by 2024–25, 100 new unicorns by 2025 and poverty below 5 per cent by 2030 was well within reach.[7]

When India was crafting its economic response to the pandemic and very mindfully took the modified barbell approach, many people on the opposite side of the spectrum took a jaundiced view that India should have given large cash hand-outs like other countries. In May 2020, 20 opposition parties, led by the Congress, had demanded that ₹7,500 should be transferred to each family.[8] However, the prime minister took the explicit view that Indians by nature are not spenders, they are savers. He told his economic advisors that he was of the opinion that any cash hand-outs would not be used to purchase goods and services which was the purpose of the hand-outs in the first place—to influx cash into the markets. Instead, he believed that Indians will save the money for financial security, thus, making the policy goal of a cash hand-out counterproductive. He was aware through his decades of experience living among the people that the cash given out would not flow into the market, thus unable to stimulate it, as intended.

◆

In preparation for the imminent third wave, the Empowered Group 1, led by Dr Paul, had recommended in its July 2021 report, taking into account experiences from countries affected by the third wave, that a third surge of infections were likely to be as intense or slightly higher than the second wave, and that India should prepare for handling about four to five lakh cases per day. In terms of infrastructure preparedness, this would translate to having over 10 lakh COVID-19 isolation care beds, 7 lakh non-COVID hospital beds with 5 lakh enabled for oxygen delivery and 2 lakh ICU beds including 1.2 lakh ventilated beds. Five per cent of the ICU beds and 4 per cent of non-ICU beds were recommended to be earmarked for paediatric care. To enable this, India would need to further scale up around 80,000 ICU beds and over 1 lakh oxygen-enabled non-ICU beds as against the current status of availability. To enable judicious use of resources, the Group prepared a threadbare structure of a 'COVID saral ICU' which can be particularly erected as make-shift structures in rural and peri-urban areas, where populations are excessively vulnerable due to less exposure to the virus. The report also drew attention to realign preparedness to tackle a potential upsurge in disease in paediatric groups. However, if we are able to achieve wide vaccine coverage as planned and delay the surge by being vigilant, we may be able to escape a particularly fatal third wave.

♦

## 21 OCTOBER 2021

INDIA | 1,82,548 ACTIVE CASES | 4,53,076 DEATHS | 100 CRORE VACCINE DOSES

WORLD | 1,78,57,909 ACTIVE CASES | 49,45,246 DEATHS | 381 CRORE VACCINE DOSES

On 21 October, India crossed the mark of administering 1 billion vaccine doses to its people. A remarkable feat for the prime minister-led government machinery, the vaccine ecosystem and the healthcare workers of the country! In a televised address to the nation, the prime minister expressed his contentment and gratitude,

> 100 crore vaccinations are not just a figure, but a reflection of the strength of the country, it is the creation of a new chapter of history. This is a picture of a new India that sets difficult goals and knows how to achieve them. While people are comparing our vaccination

program to others around the world, the speed with which we have administered 1 billion doses is being appreciated. However, they often miss the point of where India began from. Developed countries had decades of expertise in researching and developing vaccines. India mostly depended on vaccines made by these countries. Thus, when the biggest pandemic of the century struck, various questions were raised about India's ability to fight it: From where will India get the money from to buy so many vaccines from other countries? When will India get the vaccine? Will the people of India even get the vaccine or not? Will India be able to vaccinate enough people to stop the pandemic from spreading? All these were answered by achieving this feat of administering 100 crore vaccinations that too free of cost to the people. India's vaccination drive has operated with a single mantra that if the disease does not discriminate, then there cannot be any discrimination in the vaccination, that's why it was ensured that the VIP culture of entitlement does not dominate the vaccination campaign. Regardless of class, money, access and privilege—every person was treated equally to get the vaccine.[9]

Speaking on vaccine hesitancy that is plaguing many nations, the prime minister said, 'Questions were raised whether most people in India would even go to the vaccination centre to get vaccinated. Vaccine hesitancy remains a major challenge even today in many major developed countries of the world. But the people of India have answered by taking 100 crore vaccine doses. The GoI made public participation the first line of defence in the country's fight against the pandemic.'[10]

He further expressed how the entire vaccination journey was a science-based one,

It is a matter of pride for all of us that the entire vaccination program of India has been science born, science driven and science-based. Before the vaccine was made and until the vaccine was administered, the entire campaign was based on a scientific approach. We encountered significant challenges in first scaling up production followed by distributing the vaccines to different states and timely delivery of vaccines to far-flung areas. But, with scientific methods and new innovations, the country has found solutions to these challenges. Resources were increased with extraordinary speed. The

CoWin platform, made in India, not only made it convenient for people to register for taking the vaccine but also made the work of our medical staff easier.[11]

In his op-ed, the prime minister revealed how difficult the challenge of running the largest and the fastest vaccination campaign in the world was. He wrote,

> It has been a truly Herculean, bhagirath effort involving multiple sections of society. For any effort to attain and sustain speed and scale, trust of all stakeholders is crucial. One reason for a successful campaign was the trust that people developed in the vaccine and the process followed, despite various efforts to create mistrust and panic. There are some who only trust foreign brands. However, when it came to something as crucial as the COVID-19 vaccine, Indians unanimously trusted 'Made in India' vaccines. This is a significant paradigm shift.[12]

Various experts on prime-time news channels concurred that it was only because of the pro-science approach that the prime minister had adopted from the beginning of the pandemic on various issues such as mask usage, lockdown, reopening the economy, oxygen supply and distribution that when it came to vaccines, Indians immediately trusted his word and chose to take the shots without blinking, despite the Opposition's efforts to shake their credibility.

In his piece, he also persuades one to think what if India had not developed its own vaccines. He writes,

> How would India have secured enough vaccines for such a large population? How many years would that have taken? It is here that credit should be given to Indian scientists and entrepreneurs for rising to the occasion. It is due to their talent and hard work that India is truly atmanirbhar when it comes to vaccines. Our vaccine manufacturers, by scaling up to meet the demands of such a large population, have shown that they are second to none. GoI has been an accelerator and enabler of progress. It partnered with vaccine-makers right from day one, and gave them support in the form of institutional assistance, scientific research, funding, as well as accelerated regulatory processes. All ministries came together to

facilitate and remove any bottlenecks as a result of the 'whole of government' approach. In a country of the scale of India, it is not enough to just produce. Focus has to be on last-mile delivery and seamless logistics. To understand the challenges involved, imagine the journey taken by one vial of vaccines. From a plant in Pune or Hyderabad, the vial is sent to a hub in any of the states, from where it is transported to the district hub. From there, it reaches a vaccination centre. This entails the deployment of thousands of trips taken by flights and trains. During this entire journey, the temperature has to be maintained in a particular range that is centrally monitored.[13]

To attest as to how much of a Himalayan a challenge this truly was, Mr Poonawalla confessed to me,

> When the government asked me to produce 250 million doses per month, I thought to myself, well... I can still pool resources, scale up production and achieve this number. But it is them who'd have to administer those shots. It would mean injecting 250 million times, the man-hours required from the healthcare workers and last-mile delivery pan-India would be enormous. To be honest, I was sceptical of them achieving this! But look at us now, I am pleasantly surprised.

Many world leaders congratulated India and the prime minister on crossing this crucial milestone. WHO Chief Tedros Ghebreyesus tweeted, 'Congratulations, Prime Minister Narendra Modi, the scientists, health workers and people of India, on your efforts to protect the vulnerable populations from COVID-19 and achieve #VaccinEquity targets.'[14] Bill Gates, in an opinion piece, highlighted five key ingredients because of which India was able to achieve this target: first, strong political will of the prime minister due to which state and local leaders responded with urgency; second, India's past experience with mass immunization campaigns lending experience, knowledge and infrastructure; third, harnessing of Indian expertise in vaccine and drug discovery and manufacturing; fourth, using its IT prowess to monitor the national vaccination drive and fifth, *jan bhagidari* or public participation.[15]

Most importantly, what achieving this milestone did for the country was that it made the citizens feel assured versus insecure, boosting confidence to continue our fight against the virus.

## 27 DECEMBER 2021

**INDIA | 81,906 ACTIVE CASES | 4,80,290 DEATHS | 141 CRORE VACCINE DOSES**

**WORLD | 23,84,131 ACTIVE CASES | 54,23,142 DEATHS | 450 CRORE VACCINE DOSES**

A few weeks before the year-end holidays, South Africa reported a sharp rise in COVID-19 cases owing to a new variant (B.1.1.29), which later came to known as Omicron, which showed significantly increased transmissibility as compared with other variants, including Delta.[16] In a matter of days, it was detected in several other countries in the world, leading to waves of infections around the holiday season. Very quickly, many countries closed borders for 'at-risk' nations, where the variant was believed to have spread rapidly. Scientists scrambled to figure out whether the new variant caused symptoms which were different from the previous variants, whether they were mild or severe and, most importantly, if the variant evaded the immunity generated by vaccines and previous infections. Early evidence suggested, providing much relief that Omicron resulted in only mild illness resembling that of a common cold in folks who were fully vaccinated. Cough, fatigue, tiredness and a runny nose seemed to be the most rampant symptoms generated. Vaccine manufacturers were quick to come out with supporting research on the effectiveness of their vaccines against Omicron and the need for booster doses to 'boost immunity' for better protection.[17] Even as countries in the developed world began to offer booster doses, many countries in the developing world remained without vaccines. The vaccine inequity was glaring. So disturbing was this hyper-nationalism of boosting its citizens and closing borders to at-risk nations including South Africa that the WHO chief announced that, 'Blanket booster programs are likely to prolong the pandemic, rather than ending it, by diverting supply to countries that already have high levels of vaccination coverage, giving the virus more opportunity to spread and mutate.' He added that, 'Vaccine inequality will allow the pandemic to continue. Countries with low access to initial doses of the vaccine will become breeding grounds for mutant variants of the virus.'[18]

Having been on the receiving end of low vaccine dose availability and discriminatory behaviour from nations such as blanket bans for our citizens during the Delta wave, India did not ban travel from at-risk nations. We escalated our testing and tracking strategy keeping a sharp focus on those arriving from these nations. We understood that blanket bans cannot stop the variant from spreading in our people and neither can it really buy us any significant amount of time. We also were more confident in the protection that our high-coverage vaccination drive provided to citizens in addition to the high rates of immunity due to previous infections as evidenced by our updated sero-surveillance, i.e., hybrid immunity.[19] Yet, sections of the media and the Opposition demanded that India begin to boost its people. The Lancet published a study[20] which suggested that protection offered by the Oxford AstraZeneca vaccine Covishield declines after three months. This stirred panic. The media and the Opposition amplified their demand for a blanket booster dose. However, after cautious analysis of the study, experts felt that the methodology used in the study was odd: one they had never seen before. President of the Indian Medical Association Dr J.A. Jayala went on to say,

> Unfortunately, this study has a strange methodology, which none of us, including my peers, had ever seen before... So my point is, without discrediting the study authors, methodologies are very important when we come to understanding conclusions. So my message is that one should never blindly jump to conclusions. This study is based on the author's conclusions. Most of the scientific data that is available says that vaccines provide antibodies and T cell immunity as well. It is based on certain facts. Most of the scientific data available from studies which have been conducted across the country and abroad have proved that antibody is not just stopping but it is continuing. We are concerned about the T cell immunity or/and cellular immunity which is long lasting by all chances and once you are getting infected with the virus or when you are getting the passive immunity by the Covishield, definitely you will have the effect of that sustaining for a longer time. It will be preventing you and helping you to come out of the severe infection you are getting.[21]

Another expert, chief of the Kerala State Indian Medical Association noted, 'Even till today, no decline has been observed as far as the protection offered by both vaccines, Covishield and Covaxin is concerned. No signal has come from anywhere in India that people are suddenly falling sick after taking these vaccines.'[22] After careful evidence-based consideration, on 25 December, the prime minister announced that in order to protect our most vulnerable groups, a pre-caution dose akin to a booster dose would be given to frontline workers, senior citizens and those over 45 years of age with comorbidities. He also announced that children between 15–18 years would be eligible to be vaccinated.[23] The prime minister also announced that a nasal vaccine would soon be available in India. A couple of days later, on 28 December, the DCGI approved two new vaccines, both manufactured in India: SII's Covovax and Biological E's Corbevax. The DCGI also approved molnupiravir, an antiviral drug which would be manufactured by 13 companies in India for restricted use under treatment of adult patients with COVID-19 who show a high risk of disease progression.[24] Covovax, a nanoparticle vaccine and Corbevax, India's first indigenously developed RBD protein (a critical component of the viral spike glycoprotein that is found in coronaviruses including SARS-CoV-2) subunit vaccine have both shown about 90 per cent efficacy in clinical trials. With these second-generation vaccines and drugs, India's arsenal has grown immensely to combat the virus with its variants.[25] Even as India worked on augmenting its resources, new research poured in about Omicron being some kind of an endemic-stage variant. A released pre-print paper showed that Omicron infection enhances neutralizing immunity against the Delta variant which essentially means that when an individual is infected with Omicron, the chances of him being reinfected with Delta goes down. The researchers also noted in their concluding remarks that, 'Along with emerging data indicating that Omicron, at this time of the pandemic, is less pathogenic than Delta, such an outcome may have positive implications in terms of decreasing the COVID-19 burden of severe disease.'[26]

While the debate is still on regarding the need to lock down cities as infection rates surge, many believe that with a less pathogenic variant like Omicron, perhaps a measure of damage must not be the number of registered cases anymore but rather the number of hospitalizations. Data coming in from various cities around the world have reported significantly lesser hospitalization rate as compared to previous variants.[27] The Indian response continues to be alert, cautious and watchful in order to fight the impending surge of cases which many cities have begun to experience.

◆

All in all, the pandemic has taught India several lessons from which we have emerged and grown. It may be premature to assume that more waves of the mutating virus will not hit us. However, we are far better prepared to deal with them. Combined with wide vaccine coverage and high immunity as revealed by sero-surveys, India believes that we may be able to face any upcoming waves of the virus, with much lower devastation. In a way, we have come to realize how protectionist and one-sided the world has come to be. Such a situation, compounded with the challenges during the pandemic years domestically, have compelled us to place much more emphasis on self-reliance by ushering in policies which are self-generating and self-sustaining.

Atmanirbharta by its very performance brings in greater innovation and creativity, while remaining an integral part of global networks. Atmanirbharta makes it clear that only when India's own production flourishes can it make an economic difference abroad. As the world revisits its supply chains, it is likely to see a greater deficit in the availability of global goods. Several countries are likely to reconsider rebuilding their supply chains and depending much lesser on countries which have maintained an opaque and territorial approach during the pandemic years. India, in such a situation, can be poised to take the place of a trustworthy ally, by vividly expressing its beliefs and traditions which speak volumes of our non-extremist attitude. Several countries, including major power nations, have come to realize that trade engagements based on economic outcomes are not sustainable, especially at the cost of running a risk of erosion of the social fabric. Due to this, moving forward, nations will also look to build stronger relations with countries who come from similar belief systems. India, over the past few years, has been forthcoming in asserting its role and thought processes in several global forums, giving the world an opportunity to get to know us better. We have demonstrated over and over that we aren't an expansionist regime. Instead, we call our motherland Bharat mata (mother), signifying our nurturing approach to multilateral and bilateral relations, a deeply maternal behaviour. In times of crisis, just like a mother would, we are fully capable of synchronizing our energies and displaying unimaginable strength to protect not just our own but all of humanity. For instance, during the pandemic, India stood firmly with partner countries by going the extra mile and delivering life-saving medicines, medical equipment and vaccines—much of which were given out as grants. In addition, we also sent out four medical missions to Kuwait, the Maldives, Mauritius and Comoros, establishing our credentials as not only a reliable pharmacy of the world but also as a premier health security responder for our allies. While it may be difficult to accurately say how the world will emerge on the other side of the pandemic, we can be sure that for a while, it will be in a period of uncertainty and transition. Who will emerge out of the pandemic with what extent of damage is impossible to predict. Also difficult to predict is which country will reinvent itself and which ones wouldn't be able to do so. It may take several years post the pandemic for all of these dynamics to emerge as a clear picture, after which forces in globalization and multilateral relations will likely shift like pieces of a Rubik's cube. In such a case, the best way forward for us would be to look inwards and work on clearly identifying our own preferences and hopes, set clear priorities and find workable solutions—become fully atmanirbhar. If we are able to overcome the needs and desires of 1.3 billion of us, it would only be a matter of time that the world begins to effectively utilize our worth and see clearly what we bring to the table. The prime minister often says that Indians have dared to dream, '*ekkeesvi sadi Bharat ki hi hogi*' (that the twenty-first century will belong to India). With the path we are on now, this dream may truly become a reality that forthcoming generations and perhaps even ours may be able to experience.

# ACKNOWLEDGEMENTS

All I started with at the beginning of this book was a clear intent to bring out India's efforts in fighting this once-in-a-century global pandemic. The anti-news and counter-propaganda to malign my country affected me deeply. However, as days passed during the journey of the book, unimaginable doors opened up and I received assistance from unexpected individuals. To all of you, a big, heartfelt thank you—without you the book wouldn't be anywhere near what it is. It is clear that the common thread that binds us all is incredible love for our nation.

Thank you to the fabulous team at Rupa Publications—in particular, Kapish Mehra, Dibakar Ghosh and Manali Das. You have been more than patient with me. The advice and assistance you have offered throughout the book has been top-class. I couldn't have asked for better partners.

And lastly, but more importantly, I want to express my most sincere gratitude to my family for their patience, advice, support and encouragement. You all make up the pieces of my heart.

# NOTES

## CHAPTER 1

1. All data sourced from: https://www.worldometers.info/coronavirus/country/india/. Accessed 6 December 2021.
2. https://worldpopulationreview.com/world-cities/wuhan-population. Accessed 6 December 2021.
3. Snehesh Alex Philip, 'Ajit Doval back as NSA, new Cabinet-rank status "reward" for first stint', *ThePrint*, 3 June 2019, https://theprint.in/india/governance/ajit-doval-back-as-nsa-new-cabinet-rank-status-reward-for-first-stint/244963/. Accessed 6 October 2021.
4. 'Half a million COVID-19 cases in India: How we got to where we are', *The Wire*, https://thewire.in/covid-19-india-timeline. Accessed 6 October 2021.
5. 'Seafood market closed after outbreak of "unidentified" pneumonia', *Global Times*, 1 January 2020, https://www.globaltimes.cn/content/1175369.shtml. Accessed 6 October 2021.
6. 'COVID-19–China', World Health Organization, https://www.who.int/emergencies/disease-outbreak-news/item/2020-DON229. Accessed 6 October 2021.
7. World Health Organization, https://twitter.com/who/status/1217043229427761152?lang=en. Accessed 6 October 2021. 'Exclusive WHO-led team expected in China in January to probe COVID-19 origins—experts', *Reuters*, 16 December 2020, https://www.reuters.com/business/healthcare-pharmaceuticals/exclusive-who-led-team-expected-china-january-probe-covid-19-origins-experts-2020-12-16/. Accessed 6 October 2021.
8. NITI Aayog is the Indian government's premier public policy think tank which replaced the Planning Commission of the United Progressive Alliance (UPA) era.
9. 'Seafood market closed after outbreak of "unidentified" pneumonia', *Global Times*, 1 January 2020, https://www.globaltimes.cn/content/1175369.shtml. Accessed 6 October 2021.
10. 'COVID-19 – China', World Health Organization, https://www.who.int/emergencies/disease-outbreak-news/item/2020-DON229. Accessed 6 October 2021.
11. Kate Kelland, 'China pneumonia outbreak may be linked to new virus – WHO', *Reuters*, 9 January 2020, https://www.reuters.com/article/uk-china-virus-who-idUKKBN1Z804X. Accessed 6 October 2021.
12. Bob Woodward, *Rage* (Simon & Schuster 2020), p. 217.
13. Stephanie Hegarty, 'The Chinese doctor who tried to warn others about

| | |
|---|---|
| | coronavirus,' *BBC News*, 6 February 2020, https://www.bbc.com/news/world-asia-china-51364382. Accessed 6 October 2021. |
| 14 | 'Health Ministry reviews preparedness for Novel Corona Virus (nCoV),' Press Release, Press Information Bureau (PIB), Government of India, 17 January 2020, https://pib.gov.in/PressReleseDetail.aspx?PRID=1599665. Accessed 6 October 2021. |
| 15 | Natasha Khan, 'New Virus Discovered by Chinese Scientists Investigating Pneumonia Outbreak,' *The Wall Street Journal*, 8 January 2020, https://www.wsj.com/articles/new-virus-discovered-by-chinese-scientists-investigating-pneumonia-outbreak-11578485668. Accessed 6 October 2021. |
| 16 | 'China releases genetic data on new coronavirus, now deadly,' Center for Infectious Disease Research and Policy (CIDRAP), 11 January 2020, https://www.cidrap.umn.edu/news-perspective/2020/01/china-releases-genetic-data-new-coronavirus-now-deadly. Accessed 6 October 2021. |
| 17 | Andrew Joseph, 'Woman with novel pneumonia virus hospitalized in Thailand—the first case outside China,' STAT, 13 January 2020, https://www.statnews.com/2020/01/13/woman-with-novel-pneumonia-virus-hospitalized-in-thailand-the-first-case-outside-china/. Accessed 6 October 2021. |
| 18 | 'Health Ministry reviews preparedness for Novel Corona Virus (nCoV),' Press Information Bureau (PIB), Government of India, 17 January 2020, https://pib.gov.in/PressReleseDetail.aspx?PRID=1599665. Accessed 6 October 2021. |
| 19 | 'Public Health Screening to Begin at 3 U.S. Airports for 2019 Novel Coronavirus ('2019-nCoV'),' Centers for Disease Control and Prevention, 17 January 2020, https://www.cdc.gov/media/releases/2020/p0117-coronavirus-screening.html. Accessed 6 October 2021. |
| 20 | Philip Ball, 'The lightning-fast quest for COVID vaccines—and what it means for other diseases,' *Nature*, 18 December 2020, https://www.nature.com/articles/d41586-020-03626-1. Accessed 6 October 2021. |
| 21 | Denis Mormile, 'Why airport screening won't stop the spread of coronavirus,' *Science*, 6 March 2020, https://www.science.org/news/2020/03/why-airport-screening-wont-stop-spread-coronavirus. Accessed 6 October 2021. |
| 22 | The Associated Press, 'China didn't warn public of likely pandemic for 6 key days,' *AP News*, 15 April 2020, https://apnews.com/68a9e1b91de4ffc166acd6012d82c2f9. Accessed 6 October 2021. |
| 23 | Shubhajit Roy, 'Explained: How India evacuated 654 individuals from Wuhan due to coronavirus outbreak,' *The Indian Express*, 5 February 2020, https://indianexpress.com/article/explained/coronavirus-outbreak-inside-the-wuhan-evacuation-indians-in-china-6251124/. Accessed 6 October 2021. |
| 24 | Press Trust of India, 'Indian embassy in Beijing cancels Republic Day ceremony due to coronavirus outbreak in China,' *India Today*, 24 January 2020, https://www.indiatoday.in/india/story/indian-embassy-beijing-cancels-republic-day-ceremony-due-to-coronavirus-outbreak-china-1639718-2020-01-24. Accessed 7 October 2021. |
| 25 | Special Correspondent, 'Indian embassy in Beijing starts hotline for coronavirus |

queries,' *The Hindu*, 24 January 2020, https://www.thehindu.com/news/national/indian-embassy-in-beijing-starts-hotline-for-coronavirus-queries/article30640708.ece. Accessed 7 October 2021.

26   'Principal Secretary to the Prime Minister chairs a high level meeting on Coronavirus outbreak,' Press Release, Press Information Bureau (PIB), Government of India, https://pib.gov.in/PressReleseDetail.aspx?PRID=1600552. Accessed 7 October 2021.

27   'Students should stay in Wuhan as Pakistan cannot treat coronavirus: Envoy,' *India Today*, 2 February 2020, https://www.indiatoday.in/world/story/pakistan-students-china-evacuation-coronavirus-treatment-envoy-1642527-2020-02-02. Accessed 24 January 2022.

28   Doan Loan, 'Vietnam stops flying to coronavirus-stricken areas in China,' *VNExpress International*, 30 January 2020, https://e.vnexpress.net/news/news/vietnam-stops-flying-to-coronavirus-stricken-areas-in-china-4047773.html. Accessed 7 October 2021.

29   https://twitter.com/ani/status/1222160667685179395. Accessed 7 October 2021.

30   'Xi Jinping meets with visiting World Health Organization (WHO) Director-General Tedros Adhanom Ghebreyesus,' Ministry of Foreign Affairs of the People's Republic of China, 29 January 2020, https://www.fmprc.gov.cn/mfa_eng/zxxx_662805/t1737014.shtml. Accessed 7 October 2021.

31   Nikkei staff writers, 'Three Japanese evacuees from Wuhan test positive for coronavirus,' *Nikkei Asia*, 30 January 2020, https://asia.nikkei.com/Spotlight/Coronavirus/Three-Japanese-evacuees-from-Wuhan-test-positive-for-coronavirus. Accessed 7 October 2021.

32   Bang Xiao, 'Australians in coronavirus epicentre of Wuhan could get evacuated by Australian Government,' *ABC News*, 26 January 2020, https://www.abc.net.au/news/2020-01-26/australians-in-coronavirus-epicentre-wuhan-trying-to-get-out/11902006. Accessed 7 October 2021.

33   'Coronavirus: Air New Zealand will charter flight to Wuhan,' *NewstalkZB*, 30 January 2020, https://www.newstalkzb.co.nz/news/coronavirus-health-minister-says-we-have-not-yet-had-a-case/. Accessed 7 October 2021.

34   Bill Chappell, 'Coronavirus: Americans Evacuated From Wuhan Will Remain At U.S. Air Base For 3 Days,' Npr, https://www.npr.org/sections/goatsandsoda/2020/01/29/800761987/coronavirus-americans-cheer-as-evacuation-flight-from-wuhan-reaches-u-s. Accessed 7 October 2021.

35   PTI, 'Will provide necessary assistance for evacuation of Indians, other nationals from Wuhan: China,' *The Hindu*, 29 January 2020, https://www.thehindu.com/news/national/coronavirus-outbreak-indians-in-china/article30684250.ece. Accessed 7 October 2021.

36   Vidya, 'Apocalypse: Air India pilot who planned Wuhan evacuation describes flying into coronavirus-hit city,' *India Today*, 15 February 2020, https://www.indiatoday.in/india/story/air-india-coronavirus-wuhan-evacuation-pilot-captain-amitabh-singh-experience-1646510-2020-02-14. Accessed 7 October 2021.

37  'Update on Novel Coronavirus: Quarantine centres are being established at Manesar and Chawla Camp,' Ministry of Health and Family Welfare, 31 January 2020, Press Information Bureau (PIB), New Delhi, https://pib.gov.in/PressReleaseIframePage.aspx?PRID=1601367. Accessed 7 October 2021.
38  Press Trust of India, 'PM Modi writes to Chinese President Xi, offers India's help to deal with coronavirus outbreak,' *India Today*, 9 February 2020, https://www.indiatoday.in/india/story/china-president-xi-pm-modi-offers-india-help-deal-coronavirus-outbreak-1644756-2020-02-09. Accessed 7 October 2021.
39  'Question No.3951 Medical Supply to China,' Ministry of External Affairs, 18 March 2020, https://mea.gov.in/lok-sabha.htm?dtl/32559/question+no3951+medical+supply+to+china. Accessed 7 October 2021.

# CHAPTER 2

1  P.S. Gopikrishnan Unnithan, 'Kerala reports first confirmed coronavirus case in India,' *India Today*, 30 January 2020, https://www.indiatoday.in/india/story/kerala-reports-first-confirmed-novel-coronavirus-case-in-india-1641593-2020-01-30. Accessed 7 October 2021.
2  M.A. Andrews, Binu Areekal, et al. 'First confirmed case of COVID-19 infection in India: A case report,' NCBI, May 2020, https://www.ncbi.nlm.nih.gov/pmc/articles/PMC7530459/. Accessed 7 October 2021.
3  Josephine Ma and Zhuang Pinghui, '5 million left Wuhan before lockdown, 1,000 new coronavirus cases expected in city,' *South China Morning Post*, 26 January 2020, https://www.scmp.com/news/china/society/article/3047720/chinese-premier-likeqiang-head-coronavirus-crisis-team-outbreak. Accessed 7 October 2021.
4  'China readies for world's biggest human migration,' https://www.bloomberg.com/news/articles/2020-01-20/china-readies-for-world-s-biggest-human-migration-quicktake. Accessed 10 November 2021.
5  Sandip Sen, 'How China locked down internally for COVID-19, but pushed foreign travel,' *The Economic Times*, 30 April 2020, https://economictimes.indiatimes.com/blogs/Whathappensif/how-china-locked-down-internally-for-covid-19-but-pushed-foreign-travel/. Accessed 7 October 2021.
6  'Transmission of 2019-nCoV infection from an asymptomatic contact in Germany,' *The New England Journal of Medicine*, 30 January 2020, https://www.nejm.org/doi/full/10.1056/NEJMc2001468. Accessed 7 October 2021.
7  Bethany Bell and Imogen Foulkes, 'Coronavirus: Defiant ski nations bid to save winter season,' *BBC News*, 5 December 2020, https://www.bbc.com/news/world-europe-55181518. Accessed 7 October 2021.
8  Vermeer Paul and Kreting Joris, *Religion and the Transmission of COVID-19 in The Netherlands* (Multidisciplinary Digital Publishing Institute, 2020).
9  Joshua Robinson, 'The soccer match that kicked off Italy's coronavirus disaster,' *The Wall Street Journal*, 1 April 2020, https://www.wsj.com/articles/the-soccer-match-that-kicked-off-italys-coronavirus-disaster-11585752012. Accessed 7 October 2021.

10  Smriti Mallapaty, 'What the cruise-ship outbreaks reveal about COVID-19,' *Nature*, 26 March 2020, https://www.nature.com/articles/d41586-020-00885-w. Accessed 7 October 2021.
11  Mizumoto Kenji and Chowell Gerardo, 'Transmission potential of the novel coronavirus (COVID-19) on board the Diamond Princess Cruises Ship,' *Infectious Disease Modelling*, 2020.
12  Rothe Camilla, Schunk Mirjam, Sothmann Peter, et al, 'Transmission of 2019-nCoV infection from an asymptomatic contact in Germany,' *The New England Journal of Medicine*, 30 January 2020.
13  'Report of the WHO-China Joint Mission on coronavirus disease 2019 (COVID-19),' https://www.who.int/docs/default-source/coronaviruse/who-china-joint-mission-on-covid-19-final-report.pdf. Accessed 7 October 2021.
14  'Cabinet Secretary reviews the preventive measures on "Novel Coronavirus" outbreak,' Press Release, Press Information Bureau (PIB), Government of India, 27 January 2020, https://pib.gov.in/PressReleaseIframePage.aspx?PRID=1600746. Accessed 7 October 2021.
15  'DGFT amends March 31 export policy to permit export of non-medical and non-surgical masks,' *Pharmabiz.com*, 18 May 2020, http://pharmabiz.com/NewsDetails.aspx?aid=124215&sid=2. Accessed 7 October 2021.
16  'High level Group of Ministers constituted on directions of PM, to review management of Novel Coronavirus; First meeting held today,' Press Release, Press Information Bureau (PIB), Government of India, 3 February 2020, https://pib.gov.in/PressReleseDetail.aspx?PRID=1601773. Accessed 7 October 2021.
17  'Mann Ki Baat: Prime Minister's Radio Programme on 23rd February 2020,' Government of India, https://www.mygov.in/talk/mann-ki-baat-prime-minister%E2%80%99s-radio-programme-23rd-february-2020/. Accessed 7 October 2021.
18  https://twitter.com/drharshvardhan/status/1239931131627098112?s=20 https://pib.gov.in/PressReleseDetail.aspx?PRID=1601773. Accessed 7 October 2021.
19  Tanvi Madan and Adrianna Pita, 'What did Trump's India trip accomplish?' *Brookings*, 27 February 2020, https://www.brookings.edu/podcast-episode/what-did-trumps-india-trip-accomplish/. Accessed 7 October 2021.
20  Bob Woodward, *Rage* (Simon & Schuster 2020), p. 250.
21  'Namaste Trump event to blame for over 800 coronavirus deaths in Gujarat: Congress,' *India Today*, 26 May 2020, https://www.indiatoday.in/india/story/namaste-trump-event-blame-coronavirus-deaths-gujarat-congress-1681848-2020-05-26. Accessed 6 January 2022.
22  'Report of the WHO-China Joint Mission on Coronavirus Disease 2019 (COVID-19),' https://www.who.int/docs/default-source/coronaviruse/who-china-joint-mission-on-covid-19-final-report.pdf. Accessed 7 October 2021.
23  'Report of the WHO-China Joint Mission on Coronavirus Disease 2019 (COVID-19),' https://www.who.int/docs/default-source/coronaviruse/who-china-joint-mission-on-covid-19-final-report.pdf. Accessed 7 October 2021.

## CHAPTER 3

1. Kamaljit Kaur Sandhu, '15 Italian tourists, 1 Indian driver test positive for coronavirus, says govt,' *India Today*, 4 March 2020, https://www.indiatoday.in/india/story/coronavirus-15-italian-tourists-test-positive-confirmed-cases-rise-to-21-in-india-1652237-2020-03-04. Accessed 7 October 2021.
2. Gulam Jeelani, 'Delhi coronavirus patient held birthday party at Hyatt hotel, confirm medical authorities,' *India Today*, 3 March 2020, https://www.indiatoday.in/india/story/delhi-coronavirus-patient-held-birthday-party-at-hyatt-hotel-confirm-medical-authorities-1652060-2020-03-03. Accessed 7 October 2021.
3. India Today Web Desk, 'No need to panic, says PM Modi after holding review meeting on coronavirus spread in India,' *India Today*, 3 March 2020, https://www.indiatoday.in/india/story/no-need-to-panic-over-coronavirus-says-pm-modi-1651969-2020-03-03. Accessed 7 October 2021.
4. https://twitter.com/narendramodi/status/1234762637361086465?ref_src=twsrc%5Etfw%7Ctwcamp%5Etweetembed%7Ctwterm%5E1234762662413660165%7Ctwgr%5E%7Ctwcon%5Es2_&ref_url=https%3A%2F%2Fwww.indiatoday.in%2Findia%2Fstory%2Fno-need-to-panic-over-coronavirus-says-pm-modi-1651969-2020-03-03. Accessed 7 October 2021.
5. https://twitter.com/narendramodi/status/1235083359501430789?ref_src=twsrc%5Etfw%7Ctwcamp%5Etweetembed%7Ctwterm%5E12350833595014307 89%7Ctwgr%5E%7Ctwcon%5Es1_&ref_url=https%3A%2F%2Fwww.indiatoday.in%2Findia%2Fstory%2Fpm-modi-says-no-to-holi-over-coronavirus-fears-1652281-2020-03-04. Accessed 7 October 2021.
6. PTI, 'PM, other top BJP leaders to stay away from Holi gatherings due to Coronavirus concerns,' *The Economic Times*, 4 March 2020, https://economictimes.indiatimes.com/news/politics-and-nation/coronavirus-pm-modi-cancels-holi-milan-events-to-avoid-mass-gatherings/articleshow/74471557.cms?from=mdr. Accessed 7 October 2021.
7. Rajiv Tikoo, 'India at 75 ranks below more than 100 countries on most development indices,' *The Times of India*, 16 August 2021, https://timesofindia.indiatimes.com/blogs/development-chaupal/india-at-75-ranks-below-more-than-100-countries-on-most-development-indices/. Accessed 7 October 2021.
8. 'Coronavirus: PMO holds high-level review meeting,' *The Times of India*, 4 March 2021, https://timesofindia.indiatimes.com/india/coronavirus-pmo-holds-high-level-review-meeting/articleshow/74478796.cms. Accessed 7 October 2021.
9. Scroll Staff, 'Coronavirus outbreak: Toll in China crosses 2,000, Hong Kong reports second death,' *Scroll.in*, 19 February 2020, https://scroll.in/latest/953606/coronavirus-outbreak-china-reports-136-more-deaths-toll-crosses-2000. Accessed 7 October 2021.
10. Tom Bower, *Boris Johnson: The Gambler* (Penguin Random House 2021), p. 443.
11. Yascha Mounk, 'The Extraordinary Decisions Facing Italian Doctors,' *The Atlantic*, 11 March 2020, https://www.theatlantic.com/ideas/archive/2020/03/who-gets-

hospital-bed/607807/. Accessed 7 October 2021.

12   AP, 'How Italy's Lombardy, home to Europe's "best medical system", became the epicentre of coronavirus crisis,' *The Hindu*, 27 April 2020, https://www.thehindu.com/news/international/why-italys-lombardy-was-the-hardest-hmany-failures-combined-to-unleash-death-on-italys-lombardy/article31441240.ece. Accessed 7 October 2021.

13   Tom Bower, *Boris Johnson: The Gambler* (Penguin Random House 2021), p. 453.

14   Ibid.

15   Ibid. 445–55.

16   Gregory Clary and Leah Asmelash, 'School closures of 8 weeks or more may better mitigate coronavirus spread, CDC says,' *CNN*, 14 March 2020, https://edition.cnn.com/2020/03/14/us/school-closures-cdc-long-term-trnd/index.html. Accessed 7 October 2021.

17   Fred Imbert, 'Dow drops nearly 3,000 points, as coronavirus collapse continues; worst day since '87,' *CNBC*, 15 March 2020, https://www.cnbc.com/2020/03/15/traders-await-futures-open-after-fed-cuts-rates-launches-easing-program.html. Accessed 7 October 2021.

18   Jason Horowitz, 'Italy announces restrictions over entire country in attempt to halt coronavirus,' *The New York Times*, 9 March 2020, https://www.nytimes.com/2020/03/09/world/europe/italy-lockdown-coronavirus.html. Accessed 7 October 2021.

19   Elisabeth Braw, 'The EU is abandoning Italy in its hour of need,' *Foreign Policy (FP)*, 14 March 2020, https://foreignpolicy.com/2020/03/14/coronavirus-eu-abandoning-italy-china-aid/. Accessed 7 October 2021.

20   *South Korea's Response to Covid-19*, U.S. Food & Drug Administration, 2020, p. 2.

21   Ibid. 3.

22   Tom Bower, *Boris Johnson: The Gambler* (Penguin Random House, 2021), p. 441.

## CHAPTER 4

1   PTI, 'Coronavirus: About 9,000 Tablighi Jamaat members, primary contacts quarantined in country, MHA says 2,' *The Times of India*, April 2020, https://timesofindia.indiatimes.com/india/coronavirus-about-9000-tablighi-jamaat-members-primary-contacts-quarantined-in-country-mha-says/articleshow/74948832.cms. Accessed 7 October 2021.

2   Hannah Beech, '"None of us have a fear of corona": The faithful at an outbreak's center,' *The New York Times*, 20 March 2020, https://www.nytimes.com/2020/03/20/world/asia/coronavirus-malaysia-muslims-outbreak.html. Accessed 7 October 2021.

3   Sruthi Radhakrishnan, 'Tablighi Jamaat and COVID-19: The story so far,' *The Hindu*, 2 April 2020, https://www.thehindu.com/news/national/tablighi-jamaat-and-covid-

4   Pankaj Jain, 'Delhi govt declares coronavirus an epidemic, cinema halls, schools and colleges shut till March 31,' *India Today*, 13 March 2020, https://www.indiatoday.in/india/story/coronavirus-delhi-cinema-halls-schools-colleges-shut-kejriwal-1654856-2020-03-12. Accessed 7 October 2021.

5   Tanseem Haider, 'Timeline of how Nizamuddin Markaz defied lockdown with 3,400 people at Tablighi Jamaat event,' *India Today*, 31 March 2020, https://www.indiatoday.in/india/story/timeline-of-nizamuddin-markaz-event-of-tablighi-jamaat-in-delhi-1661726-2020-03-31. Accessed 7 October 2021.

6   Jyotika Sood, 'No model good enough to predict Covid wave,' *Outlook*, 25 May 2021, https://www.outlookindia.com/website/story/india-news-no-model-good-enough-to-predict-covid-wave-before-2-4-weeks-johns-hopkins-expert-david-peters/383571. Accessed 7 October 2021.

7   Tom Bower, *Boris Johnson: The Gambler* (Penguin Random House, 2021), p. 434.

8   'Special report: The simulations driving the world's response to COVID-19,' *Nature*, 3 April 2020, https://www.nature.com/articles/d41586-020-01003-6. Accessed 7 October 2021.

9   'Coronavirus: the first three months as it happened,' *Nature*, 22 April 2020, https://www.nature.com/articles/d41586-020-00154-w. Accessed 7 October 2021.

10  'High level Group of Ministers reviews current status, and actions for prevention and management of COVID-19,' Press Release, Press Information Bureau (PIB), Government of India, 11 March 2020, https://pib.gov.in/PressReleseDetail.aspx?PRID=1606056. Accessed 7 October 2021.

11  'WHO announces COVID-19 outbreak a pandemic,' World Health Organization, 12 March 2020, https://www.euro.who.int/en/health-topics/health-emergencies/coronavirus-covid-19/news/news/2020/3/who-announces-covid-19-outbreak-a-pandemic. Accessed 7 October 2021.

12  Amit Mudgill, 'Phew!!! Sensex crashed over 1,000 points 14 times in 2020,' *The Economic Times*, 31 December 2020, https://economictimes.indiatimes.com/markets/stocks/news/phew-sensex-crashed-over-1000-points-14-times-in-2020/articleshow/80040882.cms. Accessed 7 October 2021.

13  Gaurav Laghate, 'BCCI suspends IPL till April 15 due to coronavirus,' *The Economic Times*, 13 March 2020, https://economictimes.indiatimes.com/news/sports/ipl-postponed-till-april-15-due-to-coronavirus/articleshow/74594836.cms?from=mdr. Accessed 7 October 2021.

14  Jyoti Shelar, '82 from Hinduja hospital under observation,' *The Hindu*, 14 March 2020, https://www.thehindu.com/news/cities/mumbai/82-from-hinduja-hospital-under-observation/article31064905.ece. Accessed 7 October 2021.

15  'First COVID-19 death in Maharashtra: 63-year-old passes away in Mumbai,' *Mumbai Mirror*, 17 March 2020, https://mumbaimirror.indiatimes.com/coronavirus/news/first-covid-19-death-in-maharashtra-64-year-old-passes-away-in-mumbai/articleshow/74668738.cms. Accessed 7 October 2021.

16   'Adding cruelty to coronavirus: Ghatkopar housing society faces social boycott,' *Mumbai Mirror*, 15 March 2020, https://mumbaimirror.indiatimes.com/coronavirus/news/adding-cruelty-to-coronavirus/articleshow/74633061.cms. Accessed 7 October 2021.

## CHAPTER 5

1   'Lock down completely now: To learn from other countries' tragedies and fight Covid-19, here's what we must do,' *The Times of India*, 22 March 2020, https://timesofindia.indiatimes.com/blogs/toi-edit-page/lock-down-completely-now-to-learn-from-other-countries-tragedies-and-fight-covid-19-heres-what-we-must-do/. Accessed 8 October 2021.

2   Shashank R. Joshi, 'Smart-locking India: India has political will, resources to shut down country intelligently to counter coronavirus spread,' *The Indian Express*, 16 March 2020, https://indianexpress.com/article/opinion/columns/coronavirus-covid-19-outbreak-india-world-cases-deaths-vaccine-6315850/. Accessed 6 December 2021.

3   Sangeeta Barooah Pisharoty, 'Revisiting Partition: Gandhi's Role in Integrating the Northeast with Independent India,' *The Wire*, 9 August 2017, https://thewire.in/history/partition-gandhi-northeast-independence. Accessed 28 December 2021.

4   https://twitter.com/narendramodi/status/1238371182094639104?lang=en. Accessed 8 October 2021.

5   'SAARC summit to be cancelled,' *The Hindu*, 3 November 2016, https://www.thehindu.com/news/international/SAARC-summit-to-be-cancelled/article15004093.ece. Accessed 8 October 2021.

6   Nayanima Basu, 'Modi makes surprise call to SAARC nations to "fight coronavirus"—after 4 yrs of stalemate,' *ThePrint*, 13 March 2020, https://theprint.in/diplomacy/modi-makes-surprise-call-to-saarc-nations-to-fight-coronavirus-after-4-years-of-stalemate/380689/. Accessed 8 October 2021.

7   https://twitter.com/PMBhutan/status/1238395565571883009?ref_src=twsrc%5Etfw%7Ctwcamp%5Etweetembed%7Ctwterm%5E1238395565571883009%7Ctwgr%5Ehb_2_7%7Ctwcon%5Es1_&ref_url=https%3A%2F%2Ftheprint.in%2Fdiplomacy%2Fmodi-makes-surprise-call-to-saarc-nations-to-fight-coronavirus-after-4-years-of-stalemate%2F380689%2F. Accessed 23 December 2021.

8.  Scroll Staff, 'Coronavirus: Narendra Modi calls on SAARC leaders to together chalk out strategy to fight pandemic,' *Scroll.in*, 13 March 2020, https://scroll.in/latest/956069/coronavirus-narendra-modi-calls-on-saarc-leaders-to-together-chalk-out-strategy-to-fight-pandemic. Accessed 29 December 2021.

9.  Ibid.

10  https://twitter.com/narendramodi/status/1239225502495158272?lang=en. Accessed 8 October 2021.

11  'PM Modi's opening remarks at video conference of SAARC nations on fighting Coronavirus,' YouTube, 15 March 2020, https://youtu.be/MbJ8vzpRRN8. Accessed 23 December 2021.

12. 'PM Modi's remarks on way forward at video conference of SAARC leaders on combating COVID-19,' 16 March 2020, *YouTube*, https://youtu.be/CZQUoUbURlg. Accessed 8 October 2021.
13. 'PM Modi's closing remarks at video conference of SAARC nations on fighting Coronavirus,' 16 March 2020, YouTube, https://youtu.be/HMc283uoc9E. Accessed 8 October 2021.
14. 'As Nizamuddin meet comes under spotlight, restrictions continue in Telangana's Karimnagar,' *The News Minute*, 31 March 2020, https://www.thenewsminute.com/article/nizamuddin-meet-comes-under-spotlight-restrictions-continue-telangana-s-karimnagar-121555. Accessed 8 October 2021.
15. Sruthisagar Yamunan, 'Tablighi Jamaat: How did the government fail to detect a coronavirus infection hotspot?' *Scroll.in*, 1 April 2020, https://scroll.in/article/957891/tablighi-jamaat-how-did-the-government-fail-to-detect-a-coronavirus-infection-hotspot. Accessed 8 October 2021.
16. '2100 foreigners visited India for Tablighi activities this year: MHA,' *The Economic Times*, 31 March 2020.
17. 'Venture capitalists, start-ups appeal PM Modi to impose strict lock-downs amid Coronavirus scare,' *New Delhi Times*, 18 March 2020, https://www.newdelhitimes.com/venture-capitalists-start-ups-appeal-pm-modi-to-impose-strict-lock-downs-amid-coronavirus-scare/. Accessed 8 October 2021.
18. 'P. Chidambaram wants Modi govt to partially lockdown towns, cities to check coronavirus,' *The Economic Times*, 16 March 2020, https://economictimes.indiatimes.com/news/politics-and-nation/p-chidambaram-wants-modi-govt-to-partially-lockdown-towns-cities-to-check-coronavirus/articleshow/74647312.cms?from=mdr. Accessed 8 October 2021.
19. '"A tsunami is coming": Rahul Gandhi warns Centre over coronavirus, economy,' *The Hindustan Times*, 17 March 2020, https://www.hindustantimes.com/india-news/a-tsunami-is-coming-rahul-gandhi-warns-centre-over-coronavirus-economy/story-yAJxx0xsfiNAvEOZYn7xSM.html. Accessed 8 October 2021.
20. PIB Delhi, 'Text of Prime Minister's address to the nation on combating COVID-19,' Prime Minister's Office, 19 March 2020, https://pib.gov.in/PressReleasePage.aspx?PRID=1607254. Accessed 6 December 2021.
21. Ibid.
22. PM Modi addresses nation on Coronavirus outbreak | March 19, 2020, YouTube, https://www.youtube.com/watch?v=XPTyktyBj5k. Accessed 23 December 2021.

## CHAPTER 6

1. Wright Lawrence, *The Plague Year: America in the time of Covid* (Penguin Random House, 2020), p. 92.

# CHAPTER 7

1. Pranjal Baruah, 'Janata Curfew unites Northeast', *The Telegraph*, 7 December 2021, https://www.telegraphindia.com/north-east/janata-curfew-unites-northeast/cid/1756873. Accessed 7 December 2021.
2. PIB Delhi, 'Text of PM's address to the nation on Vital aspects relating to the menace of COVID-19', Prime Minister's Office, 24 March 2020, https://pib.gov.in/PressReleseDetailm.aspx?PRID=1607995. Accessed 7 December 2021.
3. 'PM Modi addresses the Nation on vital aspects relating to the menace of COVID-19', YouTube, Streamed live on 24 March 2020, https://youtu.be/iSdXynpQkUA. Accessed 7 December 2021.
4. *Economic Times*, https://mobile.twitter.com/economictimes/status/1243085045188800512. Accessed 7 December 2021.
5. Rajeev Kumar, 'Rs 50 Lakh cover! Who will benefit from Modi govt's Special Insurance Scheme for Covid-19?' *Financial Express*, 26 March 2020, https://www.financialexpress.com/money/insurance/modi-govt-special-insurance-scheme-for-covid-19-who-will-get-rs-50-lakh-cover/1910295/. Accessed 7 December 2021.
6. Kanika Verma, 'India's finance minister announces giant economic stimulus to fight Covid-19', *Invest India*, 26 March 2020, https://www.investindia.gov.in/team-india-blogs/indias-finance-minister-announces-giant-economic-stimulus-fight-covid-19. Accessed 7 December 2021.
7. Lev Facher, 'Trump says his belief in one potential coronavirus drug is "just a feeling,"' Statnews, 20 March 2020, https://www.statnews.com/2020/03/20/trump-coronavirus-drug-just-a-feeling/. Accessed 7 December 2021.
8. Michael M. Grynbaum 'Fox News Stars Trumpeted a Malaria Drug, Until They Didn't', *The New York Times*, 23 April 2020, https://www.nytimes.com/2020/04/22/business/media/virus-fox-news-hydroxychloroquine.html. Accessed 7 December 2021.
9. Himani Chandana, 'India bans export of Hydroxychloroquine but Trump is counting on Modi for urgent supply', *ThePrint*, 5 April 2020, https://theprint.in/india/governance/india-bans-export-of-hydroxychloroquine-as-coronavirus-cases-jump-to-over-3000/395766/. Accessed 29 December 2021.
10. 'A moment when India can save lives, we can't let it go: PM Modi', *The Times of India*, 12 April 2020, https://timesofindia.indiatimes.com/india/a-moment-when-india-can-save-lives-we-cant-let-it-go-pm/articleshow/75102677.cms. Accessed 7 December 2021.
11. Suhasini Haidar, 'India revokes ban on export of hydroxychloroquine, drug used in treatment for COVID-19', *The Hindu*, 8 April 2020, https://www.thehindu.com/news/national/india-revokes-ban-on-export-of-malaria-drug-hydroxychloroquine/article31277664.ece. Accessed 7 December 2021.
12. 'Will not be forgotten: Donald Trump thanks India, PM Modi for supplying hydroxychloroquine to US', *India Today*, 9 April 2020, https://www.indiatoday.in/india/story/donald-trump-thanks-india-pm-modi-for-supplying-

hydroxychloroquine-to-us-1664892-2020-04-09. Accessed 7 December 2021.

13. 'Brazil receives vaccine from India, PM Bolsonaro tweets thanks to India with picture of Lord Hanuman,' *Deccan Herald*, 23 January 2021, https://www.deccanherald.com/international/world-news-politics/brazil-receives-vaccine-from-india-pm-bolsonaro-tweets-thanks-to-india-with-picture-of-lord-hanuman-942306.html. Accessed 7 December 2021.

14. Stacy Chen, 'Taiwan to donate 10 million masks to countries hit hardest by coronavirus,' abcnews, 2 April 2020, https://abcnews.go.com/Health/taiwan-donate-10-million-masks-countries-hit-hardest/story?id=69918187. Accessed 7 December 2021.

15. Alex Ward, 'How masks helped Hong Kong control the coronavirus,' Vox, 18 May 2020, https://www.vox.com/2020/5/18/21262273/coronavirus-hong-kong-masks-deaths-new-york. Accessed 7 December 2021.

16. Lawrence Wright, *The Plague Year: America in the Time of Covid* (Penguin Random House, 2020), p. 148.

17. Tom Bowler, *Boris Johnson: The Gambler* (Penguin Random House, 2020), p. 437.

18. Xiaopeng Liu and Sisen Zhang, 'COVID-19: Face masks and human-to-human transmission,' Wiley Online Library, 29 March 2020, https://onlinelibrary.wiley.com/doi/10.1111/irv.12740. Accessed 7 December 2021.

19. 'Respiratory virus shedding in exhaled breath and efficacy of face masks,' *naturemedicine*, https://www.nature.com/articles/s41591-020-0843-2?fbclid=IwAR3Wsl4YU3D7Q_1non7ZG88H-sYzBZI9fYSErhv7hYs_HASwpaOmOff0d9c. Accessed 7 December 2021.

20. Jeremy Howard et al., 'An evidence review of face masks against COVID-19,' PNAS, 26 January 2021, https://www.pnas.org/content/118/4/e2014564118. Accessed 7 December 2021.

21. Kevin Breuninger, Jessica Bursztynsky and Kif Leswing, 'Trump says new mask guidelines will be out in coming days, global coronavirus cases top 1 million,' CNBC, 2 April 2020, https://www.cnbc.com/2020/04/02/coronavirus-latest-updates.html. Accessed 7 December 2021.

22. Our World in Data, https://ourworldindata.org/grapher/covid-19-testing-policy. Accessed 7 December 2021.

23. 'India, several other nations receive faulty coronavirus test kits from China,' WION, 16 April 2020, https://www.wionews.com/india-news/india-several-other-nations-receive-faulty-coronavirus-test-kits-from-china-292974. Accessed 7 December 2021.

24. Ashley Yeager, 'Inside the effort to make India's first COVID-19 test,' *The Scientist*, 6 July 2020, https://www.the-scientist.com/notebook/inside-the-effort-to-make-indias-first-covid-19-test-67686. Accessed 7 December 2021.

25. Aparna Banerjea, 'Pune woman makes India's 1st Covid-19 testing kit hours before delivering her baby,' *LiveMint*, 29 March 2020, https://www.livemint.com/news/india/pune-woman-makes-india-s-1st-covid-19-testing-kit-hours-before-delivering-her-baby-11585476163000.html. Accessed 7 December 2021.

26. Press Trust of India, 'Delhi Police video shows cops urged Nizamuddin markaz members to vacate area,' *Hindustan Times*, 1 April 2020, https://www.hindustantimes.com/india-news/coronavirus-update-delhi-police-video-shows-cops-urged-nizamuddin-markaz-members-to-vacate-area/story-zKNftKgzfJluFm85BZItwO.html. Accessed 7 December 2021.

27. Sruthisagar Yamunan, 'Tablighi Jamaat: How did the government fail to detect a coronavirus infection hotspot?' *Scroll.in*, 1 April 2020, https://scroll.in/article/957891/tablighi-jamaat-how-did-the-government-fail-to-detect-a-coronavirus-infection-hotspot. Accessed 7 December 2021.

28. 'Tablighi Jamaat: How Maulana Saad Set Off Covid-19 Clusters, Newstrack with Rahul Kanwal,' YouTube, https://www.youtube.com/watch?v=wrV9xWAtS68. Accessed 7 December 2021.

29. 'Delhi violence: Deadly protests rock the national capital,' *The Economic Times*, 26 February 2020, https://economictimes.indiatimes.com/news/politics-and-nation/delhi-violence-deadly-protests-rock-the-national-capital/articleshow/74311186.cms. Accessed 7 December 2021.

30. Akash Bisht and Sadiq Naqvi, 'How Tablighi Jamaat event became India's worst coronavirus vector,' *Aljazeera*, 7 April 2020, https://www.aljazeera.com/news/2020/4/7/how-tablighi-jamaat-event-became-indias-worst-coronavirus-vector. Accessed 7 December 2021.

31. 'Markaz leadership resisted, then NSA Ajit Doval dropped by at 2 am,' *Hindustan Times*, 2 April 2020, https://www.hindustantimes.com/india-news/markaz-leadership-resisted-then-nsa-ajit-doval-dropped-by-at-2-am/story-RhL243HMbRgTGBbriNIVzL.html. Accessed 7 December 2021.

32. Cheena Kapoor, India: Government acts against Tablighi Jamaat,' *World Asia-Pacific*, 3 April 2020, 'https://www.aa.com.tr/en/asia-pacific/india-government-acts-against-tablighi-jamaat-/1791305. Accessed 7 December 2021.

33. Tanseem Haider, 'Tablighi Jamaat leader asks followers to follow govt orders, says he's in isolation,' *India Today*, 2 April 2020, https://www.indiatoday.in/india/story/tablighi-jamaat-maulana-saad-audio-message-coronavirus-case-cluster-1662405-2020-04-02. Accessed 7 December 2021.

34. 'Maulana Saad Makes First Public Appearance, Visits Mosque in Delhi With 20 People: Sources,' YouTube, 12 June 2020, https://www.youtube.com/watch?v=7NwlOJm06q4. Accessed 7 December 2021.

35. 25 March 2020, https://www.youtube.com/watch?v=T23oNAN38iI. Accessed 7 December 2021.

36. 'Muskurayega India | An initiative by Jjust Music and Cape of Good Films,' YouTube, 6 April 2020, https://www.youtube.com/watch?v=wh-sRmTWGTw. Accessed 7 December 2021.

37. 'Akshay Kumar Hosts Concert With Asha Bhosle, Other Veterans To Raise Funds, PM Modi Reacts,' RepublicWorld.com, 11 April, 2020, https://www.republicworld.com/entertainment-news/bollywood-news/akshay-kumar-pm-cares-concert-sangeet-setu-singers-asha-alka-songs-hit.html. Accessed 7 December 2021.

38    'For want of buyers, sections of farmers dump produce,' *The Hindu*, 5 April 2020, https://www.thehindu.com/news/national/tamil-nadu/for-want-of-buyers-sections-of-farmers-dump-produce/article31264981.ece. Accessed 7 December 2021.

39    'Home delivery of essential items allowed in Noida hotspots: DM,' *Outlook*, 11 April 2020, https://www.outlookindia.com/newsscroll/home-delivery-of-essential-items-allowed-in-noida-hotspots-dm/1798807. Accessed 7 December 2021.

40    Gaurav Noronha, 'Finance Ministry issues guidelines for relaxation of procurement, expenditure and transportation norms of medical and other essential supplies,' *The Economic Times*, 30 March 2020, https://economictimes.indiatimes.com/news/economy/policy/finance-ministry-issues-guidelines-for-relaxation-of-procurement-expenditure-and-transportation-norms-of-medical-and-other-essential-supplies/articleshow/74898998.cms?from=mdr. Accessed 7 December 2021.

# CHAPTER 8

1    Rukmini S., 'Why India's "migrants" went back home,' *LiveMint*, 28 May 2020, https://www.livemint.com/news/india/why-india-migrants-walked-back-home-11590564390171.html. Accessed 9 December 2021.

2    Sanjay Singh, 'Migrant workers crowd Anand Vihar bus terminus to return to their villages,' 28 March 2020, *The Economic Times*, https://economictimes.indiatimes.com/news/politics-and-nation/migrant-workers-crowd-anand-vihar-bus-terminus-to-return-to-their-villages/articleshow/74863940.cms. Accessed 9 November 2021.

3    'MHA issues advisory to all States/UTs to make adequate arrangements for migrant workers, students etc from outside the States to facilitate Social Distancing for COVID-19,' Press Information Bureau, Government of India, 27 March 2020, https://www.mha.gov.in/sites/default/files/PressRelease%20MHAAdvisory_27032020.pdf. Accessed 9 December 2021.

4    'Leaving the City Behind: A Rapid Assessment with Migrant Workers in Maharashtra,' Terwilliger Center for Innovation in Shelter, August 2020, https://www.habitat.org/sites/default/files/documents/Leaving-the-City-Behind_Rapid-assessment-with-migrant-workers-Maharashtra.pdf. Accessed 9 December 2021.

5    Anulekha Ray, '"One Nation, One Ration card" to be a reality soon, says PM Narendra Modi. How it will benefit,' *LiveMint*, 30 June 2020, https://www.livemint.com/news/india/-one-nation-one-ration-card-to-be-a-reality-soon-says-pm-modi-11593518071166.html. Accessed 9 December 2021.

6    'Leaving the City Behind: A Rapid Assessment with Migrant Workers in Maharashtra,' Terwilliger Center for Innovation in Shelter, August 2020, https://www.habitat.org/sites/default/files/documents/Leaving-the-City-Behind_Rapid-assessment-with-migrant-workers-Maharashtra.pdf. Accessed 9 December 2021.

7    'Coronavirus Lockdown: Rahul Gandhi tweets video of migrant exodus, slams govt,' *Hindustan Times*, 28 March 2020, https://www.hindustantimes.com/india-news/coronavirus-lockdown-rahul-gandhi-tweets-video-of-migrant-exodus-slams-govt/story-guwAzFzsuwvLPBqlG7zXcP.html. Accessed 9 December 2021.

8 PTI, '"Please Don't Go To Your Villages," Arvind Kejriwal Urges Migrants,' NDTV, 29 March 2020, https://www.ndtv.com/india-news/coronavirus-updates-delhi-chief-minister-arvind-kejriwal-appeals-to-migrant-workers-do-not-go-to-nat-2202477. Accessed 9 December 2021.

9 'Uddhav Thackeray appeals to migrant workers in Maharashtra to stay put,' *The Hindu BusinessLine*, 28 March 2020, https://www.thehindubusinessline.com/news/uddhav-thackeray-appeals-to-migrant-workers-in-maharashtra-to-stay-put/article31189724.ece. Accessed 9 December 2021.

10 Ranabir Samaddar, 'Not Just the Media, Organised Politics Too Failed India's Migrant Workers,' *The Wire*, 1 July 2020, https://thewire.in/politics/migrant-workers-political-parties-failure. Accessed 9 December 2021.

11 Manu Sebastian, 'SC Says Fake News Triggered Migration of Labourers; Asks Media to Publish Official Version on COVID-19,' LiveLawin, 31 March 2020, https://www.livelaw.in/top-stories/migration-of-labourers-triggered-by-fake-news-observes-sc-calls-for-responsible-media-coverage-on-covid-19-154607.

12 Dyani Lewis, 'Why many countries failed at COVID contact-tracing—but some got it right,' *Nature*, https://www.nature.com/articles/d41586-020-03518-4. Accessed 9 December 2021.

13 Robin Dubey, 'Privacy in a Pandemic: Is the Aarogya Setu App legal?' *Bar and Bench*, 12 May 2020, https://www.barandbench.com/columns/privacy-in-a-pandemic-is-the-aarogya-setu-app-legal. Accessed 9 December 2021.

14 Karishma Mehrotra, 'Behind Aarogya Setu app push: "At least 50% people must download for impact",' *The Indian Express*, 11 April 2020, https://indianexpress.com/article/coronavirus/behind-aarogya-setu-app-push-at-least-50-people-must-download-for-impact-6357121/. Accessed 9 December 2021.

15 Shubham Verma, 'Aarogya Setu now world's most downloaded covid-19 tracking app,' *India Today*, 16 July 2020, https://www.indiatoday.in/technology/news/story/aarogya-setu-now-world-s-most-downloaded-covid-19-tracking-app-1701273-2020-07-16. Accessed 9 December 2021.

## CHAPTER 9

1 'Text of PM's Address to the Nation,' *The Free Press Journal*, 3 April 2020, https://www.freepressjournal.in/india/full-text-of-pm-narendra-modis-9-am-speech-on-april-3-2020. Accessed 9 December 2021.

2 https://twitter.com/shashitharoor/status/1246306192596652033. Accessed 23 December 2021.

3 https://twitter.com/sardesairajdeep/status/1246346841970466816. Accessed 23 December 2021.

4 'Power Ministry issues clarification on rumours of massive Power Grid failure,' DD News, 4 April 2020, https://www.ddnews.gov.in/national/power-ministry-issues-clarification-rumours-massive-power-grid-failure-due-turning-lights-9. Accessed 23 December 2021.

5. https://twitter.com/rautsanjay61/status/1372534457467465731. Accessed 23 December 2021.
6. https://twitter.com/sardesairajdeep/status/1246838817518235650. Accessed 23 December 2021.
7. https://twitter.com/awhadspeaks/status/1246847990846742528. Accessed 23 December 2021.
8. 'FAKE ALERT: Two month old visuals of fire at Solapur Airport tweeted after 9 pm candlelight vigil,' *The Times of India*, https://timesofindia.indiatimes.com/times-fact-check/news/fake-alert-two-month-old-visuals-of-fire-at-solapur-airport-tweeted-after-9-pm-candlelight-vigil/articleshow_comments/75014965.cms?from=mdr. Accessed 23 December 2021.
9. https://twitter.com/sardesairajdeep/status/1247224703820783621. Accessed 23 December 2021.
10. https://twitter.com/sjhdelhi/status/1246395553077800960. Accessed 23 December 2021.
11. 'India Today takes Sardesai off-air, docks salary over wrong tweet,' *The Indian Express*, 29 January 2021, https://indianexpress.com/article/india/india-today-takes-sardesai-off-air-docks-salary-over-wrong-tweet-7165951/#:~:text=The%20India%20Today%20Group%20Thursday,Delhi%20on%20January%2026%20had
12. '400 positive cases linked to Tablighi Jamaat event, about 9,000 people quarantined: Govt,' *India Today*, 2 April 2020, https://www.indiatoday.in/india/story/400-positive-cases-linked-to-tablighi-jamaat-event-about-9-000-people-quarantined-govt-1662576-2020-04-02. Accessed 9 December 2021.
13. Vijaita Singh, 'Coronavirus: MHA tells States to track foreign Tablighi members,' *The Hindu*, 1 April 2020, https://www.thehindu.com/news/national/2100-foreigners-visited-india-for-tablighi-activities-this-year-says-mha/article31219576.ece. Accessed 9 December 2021.
14. Vijaita Singh, 'Home Ministry asked States to identify 824 foreign Tablighi members,' *The Hindu*, 13 April 2020, https://www.thehindu.com/news/national/home-ministry-to-blacklist-800-tablighi-preachers-from-indonesia-for-violation-of-visa-rules/article31214048.ece. Accessed 9 December 2021.
15. 'Here are 20 incidents where members of Tablighi Jamaat engaged in unlawful behaviour with doctors, police and government officials,' *OpIndia*, 27 April 2020, https://www.opindia.com/2020/04/tablighi-jamaat-crimes-coronavirus-doctors-police-government-officials/. Accessed 9 December 2021.
16. 'Tabligh Jamaat members harass nurses, Uttar Pradesh government to invoke NSA,' *The Economic Times*, 3 April 2020, https://economictimes.indiatimes.com/news/politics-and-nation/tabligh-jamaat-members-harass-nurses-uttar-pradesh-government-to-invoke-nsa/articleshow/74968361.cms?from=mdr. Accessed 10 December 2021.
17. 'Family of man who died due to COVID-19 attack doctors at Hyderabad hospital,' *The News Minute*, 1 April 2020, https://www.thenewsminute.com/article/family-man-who-died-due-covid-19-attack-doctors-hyderabad-hospital-121646. Accessed

10 December 2021.

18 'Bullets in Bihar, stone-pelting in Gujarat: Police face challenges in locating Tablighi Jamaatis,' *OpIndia*, 1 April 2020, https://www.opindia.com/2020/04/bihar-muslim-mob-attack-stone-pelting-police-mass-namaz-coronavirus-lockdown-gujarat/. Accessed 10 December 2021.

19 'Govt says legal action against housing societies, home owners asking doctors, nurses to vacate,' *The Indian Express*, 26 March 2020, https://indianexpress.com/article/cities/mumbai/govt-housing-societies-home-owners-who-ask-doctors-nurses-to-vacate-rental-properties-to-face-legal-action-6333157/. Accessed 10 December 2021.

20 'Yogi Adityanath orders NSA against Jamaat members for alleged misbehaviour,' *Hindustan Times*, 3 April 2020, https://www.hindustantimes.com/india-news/yogi-adityanath-orders-nsa-against-misbehaving-jamaat-members/story-YYsjhu56cz7NHrmCCxJlrL.html. Accessed 10 December 2021.

21 'Promulgation of an Ordinance to amend the Epidemic Diseases Act, 1897 in the light of the pandemic situation of COVID-19,' Ministry of Health and Family Welfare, 22 April 2020, Press Information Bureau, Government of India, https://pib.gov.in/PressReleseDetail.aspx?PRID=1617327. Accessed 11 December 2021.

22 'On directions of the Prime Minister, Home Ministry approves release of Rs 11,092 crores under State Disaster Risk Management Fund to All States,' 3 April 2020, Ministry of Home Affairs, Press Information Bureau, Government of India, https://www.pib.gov.in/PressReleasePage.aspx?PRID=1610756. Accessed 11 December 2021.

23 Aditya Kalra and Alexandra Ulmer, 'Donations pour in but India's 'PM CARES' coronavirus fund faces criticism,' *Reuters*, 8 April 2020, https://www.reuters.com/article/us-health-coronavirus-india-fund-idUSKBN21Q19B. Accessed 11 December 2021.

24 Priscilla Jebaraj, 'PM CARES Fund collected over ₹3,000 crore in 2019-20,' *The Hindu*, 18 August 2020, https://www.thehindu.com/news/national/pm-cares-fund-collected-over-3000-crore-in-2019-20/article32380967.ece. Accessed 11 December 2021.

25 Shishir Sinha, 'Contributions to PM CARES Fund will be considered as CSR: Centre,' *The Hindu BusinessLine*, 27 May 2020, https://www.thehindubusinessline.com/economy/policy/contributions-to-pm-cares-fund-will-be-considered-as-csr-centre/article31684769.ece. Accessed 11 December 2021.

26 'PM CARES Fund is black hole of lies, corruption: Congress,' DevDiscourse, 8 August 2021, https://www.devdiscourse.com/article/headlines/1684983-pm-cares-fund-is-black-hole-of-lies-corruption-congress. Accessed 11 December 2021.

27 Scroll staff, 'Stop media ads, transfer PM CARES fund for Covid-19, Sonia Gandhi tells Modi,' *Scroll.in*, 7 April 2020, https://scroll.in/latest/958465/stop-media-ads-transfer-pm-cares-fund-for-covid-19-sonia-gandhi-tells-modi. Accessed 11 December 2021.

28 'Now, PMO says Prime Minister's National Relief Fund not a "public

|    | |
|----|---|
| | authority" under RTI Act,' *National Herald*, 23 October 2020, https://www.nationalheraldindia.com/india/now-pmo-says-prime-ministers-national-relief-fund-not-a-public-authority-under-rti-act. Accessed 11 December 2021. |
| 29 | OpIndia Staff, 'Did you know that the Prime Minister's National Relief Fund had the President of Congress party in its managing committee,' *OpIndia*, 3 April 2020, https://www.opindia.com/2020/04/pmnrf-managing-committee-congress-president-all-you-need-to-know/. Accessed 11 December 2021. |
| 30 | Special correspondent, 'Rajiv Gandhi Foundation got funds from PMNRF during UPA regime, says BJP chief Nadda,' *The Hindu*, 26 June 2020, https://www.thehindu.com/news/national/rajiv-gandhi-foundation-got-funds-from-pmnrf-during-upa-regime-says-bjp-chief-nadda/article31921071.ece. Accessed 11 December 2021. |
| 31 | Samanwaya Rautray, 'Supreme Court refuses to direct Modi government on PM CARES Fund,' *The Economic Times*, 19 August 2020, https://economictimes.indiatimes.com/news/politics-and-nation/sc-refuses-plea-to-transfer-pm-cares-fund-to-ndrf/articleshow/77606706.cms?from=mdr. Accessed 11 December 2021. |
| 32 | 'Mumbai: Amid corruption allegations, probe ordered into BMC covid-related expenditure,' *The Indian Express*, 24 December 2020, https://indianexpress.com/article/cities/mumbai/mumbai-amid-corruption-allegations-probe-ordered-into-bmc-covid-related-expenditure-7117682/. Accessed 11 December 2021. |
| 33 | Krishna Kumar, 'BMC chief Praveen Pardeshi transferred as Mumbai struggles...' *The Economic Times*, 9 May 2020, https://economictimes.indiatimes.com/news/politics-and-nation/bmc-chief-pardeshi-transferred-as-mumbai-struggles-/articleshow/75635885.cms. Accessed 11 December 2021. |
| 34 | 'Kolkata: West Bengal government to probe alleged corruption in COVID-19 equipment procurement matter,' *Times Now Digital*, 20 August 2020, https://www.timesnownews.com/kolkata/article/kolkata-west-bengal-government-to-probe-alleged-corruption-in-covid-19-equipment-procurement-matter/640193. Accessed 11 December 2021. |
| 35 | 'Centre tells West Bengal Chief Secretary to report to Delhi after Mamata Banerjee skips meeting with Narendra Modi,' *The Hindu*, 28 May 2021, https://www.thehindu.com/news/cities/kolkata/west-bengal-chief-secretary-attached-to-centre-after-mamata-skips-meeting-with-pm/article34671108.ece. Accessed 11 December 2021. |
| 36 | Bhanu P. Lohumi, 'PPE kits scam: Close aide of ex-Himachal BJP chief held,' *Tribune India*, 7 June, https://www.tribuneindia.com/news/himachal/ppe-kits-scam-close-aide-of-ex-himachal-bjp-chief-held-95816. Accessed 11 December 2021. |
| 37 | Howard Jeremy, Huang Austin, Li Zhiyuan, et al, *An evidence review of face masks against Covid-19*, PNAS (January, 2020). |
| 38 | 'PM addresses the nation for 4th time in 4 Weeks in India's fight against COVID-19,' *Narendra Modi*, 14 April 2020, https://www.narendramodi.in/prime-minister-narendra-modi-s-address-to-the-nation-on-covid-19-14-04-2020-549256. Accessed 11 December 2021. |

# CHAPTER 10

1. 'Coronavirus (COVID-19) Update: FDA Authorizes First Antigen Test to Help in the Rapid Detection of the Virus that Causes COVID-19 in Patients,' US Food & Drug Administration, 9 May 2020, https://www.fda.gov/news-events/press-announcements/coronavirus-covid-19-update-fda-authorizes-first-antigen-test-help-rapid-detection-virus-causes. Accessed 23 December 2021
2. 'Coronavirus in Context: Eric Topol Explains the Emerging Research,' *MedScape*, 25 March 2020, https://www.medscape.com/viewarticle/927357#vp_1. Accessed 23 December 2021.
3. Geeta Mohan, 'After failing across countries, faulty Chinese testing kits now hamper India's fight against COVID-19,' *The Hindu*, 22 April 2020, https://www.indiatoday.in/india/story/chinese-testing-kits-now-hamper-india-fight-against-covid-19-1669786-2020-04-22. Accessed 11 December 2021.
4. 'Coronavirus: India cancels order for "faulty" China rapid test kits,' BBC News, 20 April 2020, https://www.bbc.com/news/world-asia-india-52451455. Accessed 11 December 2021.
5. Elizabeth Roche, 'SD Biosensor starts manufacturing COVID-19 kits for India at Manesar Plant,' *LiveMint*, 19 April 2020, https://www.livemint.com/companies/news/sd-biosensor-starts-manufacturing-covid-19-test-kits-for-india-at-manesar-plant-11587302011626.html. Accessed 11 December 2021.
6. ET Online, 'How India, which did not manufacture personal protective equipment, became a PPE giant,' *The Economic Times*, 28 February 2021, https://economictimes.indiatimes.com/industry/miscellaneous/how-india-which-did-not-manufacture-personal-protective-equipment-became-a-ppe-giant/operation-ppe-coverall/slideshow/81257264.cms. Accessed 23 December 2021.
7. 'India produced 60 mn PPEs, 150 mn N-95 masks till Oct from zero in March, says Irani,' *LiveMint*, 11 December 2020, https://www.livemint.com/news/india/india-produced-60-mn-ppes-150-mn-n-95-masks-till-oct-from-zero-in-march-says-irani-11607701181407.html. Accessed 11 December 2021.
8. Ananya Varma, 'Massive feat: India Scales Up Ventilator Production to 50K in a Year; Produces Them at 10% Cost,' Republic World, 16 May 2021, https://www.republicworld.com/india-news/general-news/india-scales-up-ventilator-production-to-50k-in-a-year-produces-them-at-10-percent-cost.html. Accessed 11 December 2021.
9. 'Ready to help India to procure ventilators, but scaling-up production a challenge: China,' *The Economic Times*, 1 April 2020, https://economictimes.indiatimes.com/news/politics-and-nation/ready-to-help-india-to-procure-ventilators-but-scaling-up-production-a-challenge-china/articleshow/74933098.cms?from=mdr. Accessed 11 December 2021.
10. John Miller, 'UK faces "massive shortage" of ventilators - Swiss manufacturer,' *Reuters*, 19 March 2020, https://www.reuters.com/article/us-health-coronavirus-ventilators-idUSKBN2153JV. Accessed 23 December 2021.

11. 'There Aren't Enough Ventilators to Cope with the Coronavirus,' *The New York Times*, 18 March 2020, https://www.nytimes.com/2020/03/18/business/coronavirus-ventilator-shortage.html. Accessed 11 December 2021.
12. 'COVID-19 Update: Availability of PPE kits, N95 masks and ventilators,' Ministry of Health and Family, 30 March 2020, Welfare, https://pib.gov.in/PressReleaseIframePage.aspx?PRID=1609263. Accessed 11 December 2021.
13. https://twitter.com/anandmahindra/status/1241622109752676352?lang=en. Accessed 11 December 2021.
14. 'Maruti Suzuki ties up with AgVa Healthcare for production of ventilators, aims to make 10,000/month,' *Express Drives*, 29 March 2020, https://www.financialexpress.com/auto/industry/maruti-suzuki-agva-healthcare-ventilators-face-masks-coronavirus-pandemic-lockdown-covid19/1912676/. Accessed 11 December 2021.
15. Ankita Sharma, Kanika Verma and Aarushi Aggarwal, 'Helping India Breathe: Ventilator Manufacturing During Covid-19,' Strategic Investment Research Unit, https://www.investindia.gov.in/siru/helping-india-breathe-ventilator-manufacturing-during-covid-19. Accessed 11 December 2021.
16. 'Coronavirus: PM CARES Fund allotted ₹2,000 crore to supply 50,000 Made-in-India ventilators, says Centre,' *The Hindu*, 23 June 2020, https://www.thehindu.com/news/national/coronavirus-pm-cares-fund-allotted-2000-crore-to-supply-50000-made-in-india-ventilators-says-centre/article31897228.ece. Accessed 11 December 2021.
17. 'Indian ventilators will be geo-tagged to prevent misuse: Health ministry,' *Hindustan Times*, 6 August 2020, https://www.hindustantimes.com/india-news/indian-ventilators-will-be-geo-tagged-to-prevent-misuse-health-ministry/story-YelSyGN6mv8W56qCXlyJ4L.html. Accessed 11 December 2021.
18. '"Made in India" Ventilators have strengthened Infrastructure of Hospitals for Effective COVID management', Ministry of Health and Family Welfare, https://pib.gov.in/PressReleseDetail.aspx?PRID=1718183. Accessed 11 December 2021.
19. 'Over 36,000 'Make in India' ventilators delivered to govt hospitals amid COVID: Govt,' *The New Indian Express*, 31 December 2020, https://www.newindianexpress.com/nation/2020/dec/31/over-36000-make-in-india-ventilators-delivered-to-govt-hospitals-amid-covid-govt-2243631.html. Accessed 11 December 2021.
20. Wright Lawrence, *The Plague Year: America in the Time of Covid* (Penguin Random House, 2020), p. 141.
21. 'BoE warns UK set to enter worst recession for 300 years,' *Financial Times*, 7 May 2020, https://www.ft.com/content/734e604b-93d9-43a6-a6ec-19e8b22dad3c. Accessed 11 December 2021.
22. Wright Lawrence, *The Plague Year: America in the time of Covid* (Penguin Random House, 2020), p. 91.
23. 'World Renowned Columbia Economists Review Impact of COVID-19,' Columbia Global Centers, 27 March 2020, https://globalcenters.columbia.edu/news/world-renowned-columbia-economists-review-impact-covid-19. Accessed 11 December 2021.

24 'How to break the COVID doom loop,' *Open Democracy*, 16 October 2020, https://www.opendemocracy.net/en/oureconomy/how-break-covid-doom-loop/. Accessed 11 December 2021.

25 Economic Sutra: Decoding Economic Policies with Sanjeev Sanyal, Ep-01, YouTube, https://www.youtube.com/watch?v=WcWRp67rt68. Accessed 11 December 2021.

26 Karishma Mehrotra, 'Explained: India enforced one of the strongest lockdowns, here's how it stacks up against other countries,' *The Indian Express*, 8 May 2020, https://indianexpress.com/article/explained/coronavirus-india-lockdown-vs-global-lockdown-covid-19-deaths-cases-cure-6399181/. Accessed 30 December 2021.

27 Economic Sutra: Decoding Economic Policies with Sanjeev Sanyal, Ep-01, YouTube, https://www.youtube.com/watch?v=WcWRp67rt68. Accessed 11 December 2021.

28 'UK Government announces employee "furlough" scheme,' *Mayer Brown*, 23 March 2020, https://www.mayerbrown.com/en/perspectives-events/blogs/2020/03/uk-government-announces-employee-furlough-scheme#:~:text=On%2020%20March%2C%20the%20UK,see%20the%20Chancellor's%20speech%20here). Accessed 11 December 2021.

29 'President Trump Signs CARES Act into Law,' *Steptoe*, 25 March 2020, https://www.steptoe.com/en/news-publications/president-trump-signs-cares-act-into-law.html. Accessed 11 December 2021.

30 Bertrand Benoit and Tom Fairless, 'Germany Boosts Already Hefty Coronavirus Stimulus,' *The Wall Street Journal*, 26 August 2020, https://www.wsj.com/articles/germany-boosts-already-hefty-coronavirus-stimulus-11598440184

31 Sopel Jon, *UnPresidented: Politics, pandemics and the race that Trumped all others* (BBC Books, 2021), p. 106.

32 https://twitter.com/pib_india/status/1336274769478443008?lang=en. Accessed 11 December 2021

33 'Meeting schedule of the PMO constituted vaccine task force (VTF),' https://static.psa.gov.in/psa-prod/psa_custom_files/Meeting%20schedule%20of%20the%20PMO%20Constituted%20VTF.pdf. Accessed 11 December 2021.

## CHAPTER 11

1 '588 flights operated under Lifeline Udan: Hardeep Singh Puri,' ANI, 20 June 2020, https://www.aninews.in/news/national/general-news/588-flights-operated-under-lifeline-udan-hardeep-singh-puri20200620153503/. Accessed 11 December 2021.

2 PM's address to the Nation on 12.5.2020, 12 May 2020, https://www.pmindia.gov.in/en/news_updates/pms-address-to-the-nation-on-12-5-2020/. Accessed 11 December 2021.

3 https://www.pmindia.gov.in/en/news_updates/pms-address-to-the-nation-on-12-5-2020/. Accessed 11 December 2021.

4 'Economic stimulus package | Details of ₹20-lakh-crore package announced by

Union Finance Minister Nirmala Sitharaman in five tranches,' *The Hindu*, 17 May 2020, https://www.thehindu.com/news/resources/economic-stimulus-package-details-of-20-lakh-crore-package-announced-by-union-finance-minister-nirmala-sitharaman-in-five-tranches/article31606806.ece. Accessed 11 December 2021.

5    'Migrants, in Thousands, Gather Outside Bandra Station Yet Again; Only 1,000 Allowed to Board Trains,' *India.com*, 19 May 2020, https://www.india.com/news/india/migrants-in-thousands-gather-outside-bandra-station-yet-again-only-1000-allowed-to-board-trains-4033612/. Accessed 11 December 2021.

6    Ibid.

7    'Maharashtra: War of words between govt, Railways over Shramik trains,' *The Indian Express*, 25 May 2020, https://indianexpress.com/article/cities/mumbai/maharashtra-war-of-words-between-govt-railways-over-shramik-trains-6425651/. Accessed 11 December 2021.

8    'Piyush Goyal's 2 am tweet: "Where is list for 125 trains from Maharashtra?"' *The Indian Express*, 25 May 2020, https://indianexpress.com/article/india/piyush-goyal-uddhav-thackeray-maharashtra-migrants-train-list-6426554/. Accessed 30 December 2021.

9    Central Railway press release dated 24.5.2020, https://cr.indianrailways.gov.in/view_detail.jsp?lang=0&id=0,4,268&dcd=5414&did=1590396037417926D55289CB17F2FA5830D1F46D0AE87. Accessed 11 December 2021.

10    https://twitter.com/piyushgoyal/status/1264657825705259008?lang=en. Accessed 11 December 2021.

11    'Shramik Specials: railways say "sending States" will have to pay ticket costs,' *The Hindu*, 4 May 2020, https://www.thehindu.com/news/national/shramik-special-now-railways-says-sending-states-will-have-to-pay-ticket-costs/article31499523.ece. Accessed 11 December 2021.

12    'Congress will pay for rail travel of migrant workers, says Sonia Gandhi,' *The Hindu*, 4 May 2020, https://www.thehindu.com/news/national/congress-will-pay-for-rail-travel-of-migrant-workers-says-sonia-gandhi/article31497707.ece. Accessed 11 December 2021.

13    'Standoff ends, Congress buses for migrants turn back from Rajasthan-UP border,' *The Times of India*, 20 May 2020, https://timesofindia.indiatimes.com/india/congress-arranged-buses-for-migrants-return-from-rajasthan-up-border/articleshow/75848877.cms. Accessed 11 December 2021.

14    '"This Is Hell." Prime Minister Modi's Failure to Lead Is Deepening India's COVID-19 Crisis,' *TIME*, https://time.com/5957118/india-covid-19-modi/. Accessed 11 December 2021.

15    Simrin Sirur, 'Only way to give back is to tell a powerful story: Inside Barkha Dutt's 84-day Covid journey,' *ThePrint*, 9 June 2020, https://theprint.in/india/only-way-to-give-back-is-to-tell-a-powerful-story-inside-barkha-dutts-84-day-covid-journey/437847/. Accessed 11 December 2021.

16    https://twitter.com/BDUTT/status/1381534299124600834. Accessed 11 December 2021.

17  Discovery Plus to stream a documentary, "Covid-19: India's war against the virus", Best Media Info, 7 July 2020, https://bestmediainfo.com/2020/07/discovery-plus-to-stream-a-documentary-covid-19-india-s-war-against-the-virus/. Accessed 11 December 2021.
18  Mudit Kapoor and Shamika Ravi, 'Poverty, Pandemic and Elections: Analysis of Bihar Assembly Elections' (*Indian Journal of Human Development*, 4 April 2020).

## CHAPTER 12

1  Geeta Mohan, 'Can't rely solely on China, India needs to become part of global supply chain: Denmark PM to India Today,' *India Today*, 11 October 2021, https://www.indiatoday.in/india/story/india-denmark-pm-mette-frederikson-china-supply-chain-climate-change-1863517-2021-10-11. Accessed 11 December 2021.
2  'Galwan Valley: China and India clash on freezing and inhospitable battlefield,' BBC News, 17 June 2020, https://www.bbc.com/news/world-asia-india-53076781. Accessed 11 December 2021.
3  'China suffered 43 casualties during face-off with India in Ladakh: Report,' *India Today*, 16 June 2020, https://www.indiatoday.in/india/story/india-china-face-off-ladakh-lac-chinese-casualties-pla-1689714-2020-06-16. Accessed 11 December 2021.
4  'Rahul Gandhi lacks "either aptitude or passion to master subject", says Obama in new memoir,' *ThePrint*, 13 November 2020, https://theprint.in/world/rahul-gandhi-lacks-either-aptitude-or-passion-to-master-subject-says-obama-in-new-memoir/543228/. Accessed 11 December 2021.
5  https://twitter.com/rahulgandhi/status/1293887589930344448?lang=en. Accessed 11 December 2021.
6  'PM Modi's statement on India-China clashes at Galwan valley in Ladakh,' YouTube, 17 June 2020, https://www.youtube.com/watch?v=pdzSrwh6FPM. Accessed 23 December 2021.
7  'PM visits Nimu in Ladakh to interact with Indian troops,' PMIndia, 3 July 2020, https://www.pmindia.gov.in/en/news_updates/pm-visits-nimu-in-ladakh-to-interact-with-indian-troops/. Accessed 11 December 2021.
8  'PM Modi visit to Odisha HIGHLIGHTS: PM takes aerial survey of cyclone Amphan-hit areas, announces Rs 500 cr for Odisha,' *Financial Express*, 22 May 2020, https://www.financialexpress.com/india-news/cyclone-amphan-pm-modi-west-bengal-kolkata-odisha-visit-mamata-banerjee-naveen-patnaik-latest-updates/1967038/. Accessed 11 December 2021.
9  Ananth Krishnan and Suhasini Haidar, 'Jaishankar, Wang differ on way forward for India-China ties,' *The Hindu*, 15 July 2021, https://www.thehindu.com/news/international/jaishankar-wang-differ-on-way-forward-for-india-china-ties/article35335065.ece. Accessed 11 December 2021.
10  https://www.theaustralian.com.au/commentary/india-the-sensible-substitute-for-belligerent-beijing/news-story/2d7940c990e38bb4c4574c38c2c45e79.

## CHAPTER 13

1. 'AstraZeneca takes next steps towards broad and equitable access to Oxford University's potential COVID-19 vaccine,' *AstraZeneca*, 4 June 2020, https://www.astrazeneca.com/media-centre/articles/2020/astrazeneca-takes-next-steps-towards-broad-and-equitable-access-to-oxford-universitys-potential-covid-19-vaccine.html. Accessed 11 December 2021.
2. 'Gave some aid for clinical trials of Covaxin and Covishield, not R&D: Centre to SC,' *The Times of India*, 10 May 2021, https://timesofindia.indiatimes.com/india/gave-some-aid-for-clinical-trials-of-covaxin-and-covishield-not-rd-centre-to-sc/articleshow/82524449.cms. Accessed 11 December 2021.
3. 'Gave some aid for clinical trials of Covaxin and Covishield, not R&D: Centre to SC,' *The Times of India*, 10 May 2021, https://timesofindia.indiatimes.com/india/gave-some-aid-for-clinical-trials-of-covaxin-and-covishield-not-rd-centre-to-sc/articleshow/82524449.cms. Accessed 11 December 2021.
4. 'The unequal scramble for coronavirus vaccines—by the numbers,' *nature*, 24 August 2020, https://www.nature.com/articles/d41586-020-02450-x. Accessed 11 December 2021.
5. https://cmie.com/kommon/bin/sr.php?kall=warticle&dt=2020-12-15%2010:21:21&msec=266. Accessed 11 December 2021.
6. Atul Thakur, 'When India locked down, this Bihar district started up,' *The Times of India*, 16 August 2021, https://timesofindia.indiatimes.com/india/when-india-locked-down-this-bihar-district-started-up/articleshow/85237952.cms. Accessed 11 December 2021.
7. Indivjal Dhasmana, 'GST collections cross Rs 1 trillion in October for first time in 8 months,' *Business Standard*, 2 November 2020, https://www.business-standard.com/article/economy-policy/gst-collections-cross-rs-1-trillion-in-october-for-first-time-in-8-months-120110100248_1.html. Accessed 11 December 2021.
8. 'Indian Economy Heading For A "V- Shaped" Recovery, Says Finance Ministry,' AbpNews, 4 December 2020, https://news.abplive.com/news/finance-ministry-says-indian-economy-heading-for-a-v-shaped-recovery-1403566. Accessed 11 December 2021.
9. PTI, 'Nearly 40 lakh people in Bihar watched Shah's virtual rally: state BJP chief,' *Outlook*, 7 June 2020, https://www.outlookindia.com/newsscroll/nearly-40-lakh-people-in-bihar-watched-shah-s-virtual-rally-state-bjp-chief/1859068. Accessed 12 December 2021.
10. Dipak Mishra, 'Can't match BJP's e-rallies, so Bihar opposition now wants EC to allow traditional rallies,' *ThePrint*, 27 June 2020, https://theprint.in/politics/cant-match-bjps-e-rallies-so-bihar-opposition-now-wants-ec-to-allow-traditional-rallies/449835/. Accessed 12 December 2021.
11. Ibid.
12. Rohit Kumar Singh, 'Thousands thronged poll rallies but Bihar miraculously managed to keep Covid cases under control,' *India Today*, 13 November 2020,

https://www.indiatoday.in/india/story/bihar-covid19-coronavirus-cases-under-controll-assembly-election-poll-1740778-2020-11-13. Accessed 12 December 2021.
13. 'Global overview of Covid-19 impact on elections,' IDEA, 10 December 2021, https://www.idea.int/news-media/multimedia-reports/global-overview-covid-19-impact-elections. Accessed 12 December 2021.

## CHAPTER 14

1. Nikita Prasad, 'Atmanirbhar Bharat 3.0: Key Takeaways From Finance Minister's Stimulus Package,' NDTV, 12 November 2020, https://www.ndtv.com/business/atmanirbhar-3-0-12-key-takeaways-from-fm-sitharamans-economic-stimulus-package-2324335. Accessed 12 December 2021.
2. 'Pfizer ready to supply 5 crore Covid-19 doses to India this year: Report,' *LiveMint*, 25 May 2021, https://www.livemint.com/news/india/pfizer-ready-to-supply-5-crore-covid-19-doses-to-india-this-year-report-11621954927656.html. Accessed 12 December 2021.
3. Sriram Iyer, 'India may consider indemnity for Pfizer and Moderna vaccines on one condition,' *Business Insider*, 3 August 2021, https://www.businessinsider.in/india/news/pfizer-and-moderna-covid-19-vaccines-can-get-indemnity-on-one-condition-as-per-dr-nk-arora/articleshow/84996625.cms. Accessed 12 December 2021.
4. 'BioNTech signs Covid-19 vaccine deals with Pfizer and Fosun,' *Pharmaceutical Techonology*, 17 March 2021, https://www.pharmaceutical-technology.com/news/biontech-pfizer-fosun-covid-19-vaccine/. Accessed 12 December 2021..
5. Pfizerleak: Exposing the Pfizer manufacturing and supply agreement, https://threadreaderapp.com/thread/1419653002818990085.html. Accessed 12 December 2021.
6. 'Investigation: Drugmaker "bullied" Latin American nations,' *Aljazeera*, 11 March 2021, https://www.aljazeera.com/news/2021/3/11/investigation-pfizer-bullied-latin-american-nations. Accessed 12 December 2021.
7. Milan Sharma, 'Inside Modi government's Covid-19 vaccine rollout plan,' *India Today*, 21 October 2020, https://www.indiatoday.in/india/story/inside-modi-government-s-covid-19-vaccine-rollout-plan-1733886-2020-10-21. Accessed 12 December 2021.
8. https://twitter.com/pmoindia/status/1332263149483900936. Accessed 12 December 2021.
9. PTI, 'Modi lands in Hyderabad, to visit Bharat Biotech manufacturing facility,' *The Hindu BusinessLine*, 28 November 2020, https://www.thehindubusinessline.com/news/national/coronavirus-vaccine-development-in-india-pm-narendra-modis-three-city-tour/article33198502.ece. Accessed 12 December 2021.
10. 'PM Modi concludes 3-city visit to review Covid vaccine development,' *LiveMint*, 28 November 2020, https://www.livemint.com/news/india/pm-modi-concludes-3-city-visit-to-review-covid-vaccine-development-11606568584737.html. Accessed 12 December 2021.

## CHAPTER 15

1. 'President Kovind gives his assent for 3 farm bills passed by Parliament,' *LiveMint*, 27 September 2020, https://www.livemint.com/news/india/president-kovind-gives-his-assent-for-three-farm-bills-passed-by-parliament-11601210482225.html. Accessed 12 December 2021.
2. Karan Bhasin and Rashi Sharma, 'Towards a new deal for Indian farmers,' ORF, 9 October 2020, https://www.orfonline.org/research/towards-a-new-deal-for-indian-farmers/. Accessed 12 December 2021.
3. Bobins Abraham, 'With Ration Stocked For 6 Months, Protesting Farmers Continue March To Delhi In Chilly Weather,' *IndiaTimes*, 28 November 2020, https://www.indiatimes.com/news/india/farmer-protests-delhi-chalo-haryana-updates-ration-stocked-528513.html. Accessed 12 December 2021.
4. Saurabh Shukla, 'Farmers Brave Tear Gas, Water Cannons, Push Into Haryana For Delhi March,' NDTV, 26 November 2020, https://www.ndtv.com/india-news/delhi-borders-sealed-metro-services-affected-as-farmers-gather-for-march-10-points-2330331. Accessed 12 December 2021.
5. 'Farmers protest: Two lakh more set to reach Delhi in 40km-long cavalcade,' *Business Standard*, 28 November 2020, https://www.business-standard.com/article/current-affairs/farmers-protest-two-lakh-more-set-to-reach-delhi-in-40km-long-cavalcade-120112800158_1.html. Accessed 12 December 2021.
6. '"Ready for talks, shift to Burari ground": Shah reaches out to protesting farmers, they say "it's not good",' Times Now Digital, 28 November 2020, https://www.timesnownews.com/india/article/shift-to-burari-ground-will-provide-drinking-water-ambulance-amit-shah-reaches-out-to-protesting-farmers/687994. Accessed 12 December 2021.
7. Scroll Staff, 'Farmers' unions reject Amit Shah's offer for early talks, want to go to Jantar Mantar to protest,' *Scroll.in*, 29 November 2020, https://scroll.in/latest/979777/farmers-unions-reject-amit-shahs-offer-for-early-talks-want-to-go-to-jantar-mantar-to-protest. Accessed 12 December 2021.
8. FP Staff, 'Farmers' Protests: Negotiations deadlocked as farmers blame govt's "ego", Centre says takes two to tango,' *Firstpost*, 4 January 2021, https://www.firstpost.com/india/farmers-protests-negotiations-deadlocked-as-farmers-blame-govts-ego-centre-says-takes-two-to-tango-9170501.html. Accessed 12 December 2021.
9. Aparna Banerjea, 'No changes will be made in MSP: Agriculture minister assures farmer leaders, next meeting on 5 Dec,' *LiveMint*, 3 December 2020, https://www.livemint.com/news/india/no-changes-will-be-made-in-msp-agriculture-minister-responds-to-farmer-leaders-during-meeting-at-vigyaan-bhawan-11607002782440.html. Accessed 12 December 2021.
10. Sumeda, 'SC sets up committee to resolve farm law impasse, farmers raise fingers over its neutrality | Recap,' *India Today*, 13 January 2021, https://www.indiatoday.in/india/story/supreme-court-hold-farm-laws-committee-resolve-impasse-developments-updates-1758326-2021-01-12. Accessed 12 December 2021.

11. 'First Biryani, Now Pizza: Farmers Having 'Lavish' Meals at Protests Outrages Netizens,' News18, 12 December 2020, https://www.news18.com/news/buzz/first-biryani-now-pizza-farmers-having-lavish-meals-at-protests-outrage-netizens-3171158.html. Accessed 12 December 2021.

12. '"Why protest when matter is in court", Supreme Court asks farmers,' *The Tribune*, 5 October 2021, http://www.tribuneindia.com/news/nation/why-protest-when-matter-is-in-court-supreme-court-asks-farmers-320013. Accessed 12 December 2021.

13. Mayank Bhardwaj, Indian opposition demands repeal of farm laws after protests,' *Reuters*, 24 December 2020, https://www.reuters.com/article/us-india-farms-protests-idUSKBN28Y17H. Accessed 12 December 2021.

14. Sahil Joshi, 'Farmers' protest: Where does Sharad Pawar exactly stand on new farm laws?' *India Today*, 7 December 2020, https://www.indiatoday.in/india/story/farmers-protest-where-sharad-pawar-exactly-stand-bjp-new-farm-laws-1747491-2020-12-07. Accessed 12 December 2021.

15. 'Sharad Pawar's U-turn on farm laws? Advocated same changes in past, wrote to these CMs,' DNA, https://www.dnaindia.com/india/news-farmers-protest-sharad-pawar-s-u-turn-on-farm-laws-advocated-same-changes-in-past-wrote-to-cms-2860392. Accessed 12 December 2021.

16. 'Prime Minister Dr Manmohan Singh's interview with Wall Street Journal Editorial Board,' 22 September 2004, https://www.mea.gov.in/interviews.htm?dtl/4562/Prime+Minister+Dr+Manmohan+Singhs+interview+with+Wall+Street+Journal+Editorial+Board. Accessed 6 January 2022.

17. 'PM Modi Quotes Manmohan Singh in "Congress U-Turn" Charge over Farm Laws,' YouTube, https://www.youtube.com/watch?v=565UHUHIE8A. Accessed 12 December 2021.

18. 'Second wave: The link between Covid-19 variants and the spike—Explained,' *Financial Express*, 8 May 2021, https://www.financialexpress.com/lifestyle/health/second-wave-the-link-between-covid-19-variants-and-the-spike-explained/2248390/. Accessed 12 December 2021.

19. Venu Gopal Narayanan, 'Data Story: Did the "Farmers' Protest" Cause the Second Wave of Covid-19 in India?' *Swarajya*, 11 May 2021, https://swarajyamag.com/politics/data-story-did-the-farmers-protest-cause-the-second-wave-of-covid-19-in-india. Accessed 12 December 2021.

20. Sanjay Singh, 'The day Narendra Modi finally acknowledged BJP's biggest asset: Rahul Gandhi,' *Firstpost*, 22 December 2016, https://www.firstpost.com/politics/the-day-narendra-modi-finally-acknowledged-bjps-biggest-asset-rahul-gandhi-3169184.html. Accessed 12 December 2021.

21. Recommendations of the SEC meeting to examine COVID-19 related proposal under accelerated approval process made in its 130th meeting held on 09.12.2020 at CDSCO, HQ New Delhi, https://cdsco.gov.in/opencms/opencms/system/modules/CDSCO.WEB/elements/common_download.jsp?num_id_pk=MTI3NQ==. Accessed 12 December 2021.

22  Ibid.
23  'Boris Johnson announces new restrictions in UK amid second wave of coronavirus infections,' 22 September 2020, https://www.abc.net.au/news/2020-09-22/boris-johnson-new-restrictions-uk-second-wave-covid19/12690804. Accessed 12 December 2021.
24  'Second wave: The link between Covid-19 variants and the spike—Explained,' *Financial Express*, 8 May 2021, https://www.financialexpress.com/lifestyle/health/second-wave-the-link-between-covid-19-variants-and-the-spike-explained/2248390/. Accessed 12 December 2021.

## CHAPTER 16

1  'AZD1222 Oxford Phase III trials interim analysis results published in The Lancet,' *AstaZeneca*, 8 December 2020, https://www.astrazeneca.com/media-centre/press-releases/2020/azd1222-oxford-phase-iii-trials-interim-analysis-results-published-in-the-lancet.html. Accesses 12 December 2021.
2  James Gallagher and Nick Triggle, 'Covid-19: Oxford-AstraZeneca vaccine approved for use in UK,' BBC News, 30 December 2020, https://www.bbc.com/news/health-55280671. Accessed 12 December 2021.
3  'Credibility crisis: How effective are Chinese Covid vaccines?' WOIN, 18 July 2021, https://www.wionews.com/world/credibility-crisis-how-effective-are-chinese-covid-vaccines-398874. Accessed 12 December 2021.
4  'Oxford Covid-19 vaccine, Bharat Biotech's Covaxin get DCGI approval for emergency use,' *The Indian Express*, 3 January 2021, https://indianexpress.com/article/india/covid-19-vaccine-announcement-dcgi-presser-covishield-oxford-covaxin-7130635/. Accessed 12 December 2021.
5  'Congress leaders question "modification" of protocols to approve Covaxin,' *The Hindu*, 3 January 2020, https://www.thehindu.com/news/national/congress-leaders-raise-concern-over-grant-of-permission-for-restricted-use-of-covid-19-vaccine/article33485769.ece. Accessed 12 December 2021.
6  '"Premature approval": Shashi Tharoor questions authorisation for Covaxin vaccine,' *The Week*, 3 January 2021, https://www.theweek.in/news/india/2021/01/03/premature-approval-mp-shashi-tharoor-questions-authorisation-for-covaxin-vaccine.html. Accessed 12 December 2021.
7  Asad Rehman, 'Won't take "BJP vaccine",' says Akhilesh Yadav; attracts flak,' *The Indian Express*, 3 January 2021, https://indianexpress.com/article/india/akhilesh-yadav-coronavirus-vaccine-bjp-7130434/. Accessed 2021.
8  100 cr Covid doses : Why India's economic recovery is linked to mass vaccination : Shamika Ravi, YouTube, https://www.youtube.com/watch?v=9WIbxxTRZnI. Accessed 12 December 2021.
9  https://www.google.com/search?q=akhilesh+yadav+says+bjp+vaccine&rlz=1C1SQJL_enIN776IN776&oq=akhilesh+yadav+says+bjp+vaccine&aqs=chrome..69i57j69i60.7182j0j9&sourceid=chrome&ie=UTF-8

10. https://www.google.com/search?rlz=1C1SQJL_enIN776IN776&tbm=vid&sxsrf=AOaemvJM2-SIKk1h094bD0bu6IJCEjls9w:1637339357918&q=akhilesh+yadav+campaign+without+vaccine&spell=1&sa=X&ved=2ahUKEwiEnLi27KT0AhUUE4gKHeYdAW8QBSgAegQIARBI&biw=1462&bih=762&dpr=1.25

11. https://twitter.com/jpnadda/status/1345685960743399425. Accessed 31 December 2021.

12. Dr Krishna Ella CMD, Bharat Biotech shares his journey to Covaxin approval | Times Now Summit 2021', https://www.timesnownews.com/videos/times-now/india/dr-krishna-ella-cmd-bharat-biotech-shares-his-journey-to-covaxin-approval-times-now-summit/113499. Accessed 23 December 2021.

13. 'COVID-19 vaccination drive to kick off in India on Jan 16', *Telegana Today*, 9 January 2021, https://telanganatoday.com/covid-19-vaccination-drive-to-kick-off-in-india-on-jan-16. Accessed 23 Deecember 2021.

14. Govindraj Ethiraj, 'Is CoWin data safe? – and other queries answered by the CEO of the agency that runs the vaccine app', *Scroll.in*, https://scroll.in/article/996155/is-cowin-data-safe-and-other-questions-answered-by-the-ceo-of-the-agency-that-runs-the-vaccine-app. Accessed 13 December 2021.

15. Author's notes with Dr Ram Sewak Sharma.

16. Rupsa Chakraborty, 'Mumbai: Some domestic passengers use fake Covid-19 reports to fly', *Hindustan Times*, 16 March 2021, https://www.hindustantimes.com/cities/mumbai-news/mumbai-some-domestic-passengers-use-fake-covid-19-reports-to-fly-101615834372383.html. Accessed 13 December 2021.

17. 'India opposes vaccine passport at G7 meet', *The Hindu BusinessLine*, 6 June 2021, https://www.thehindubusinessline.com/news/india-opposes-vaccine-passport-at-g7-meet/article34740274.ece. Accessed 13 December 2021.

18. 'COVID-19 vaccine patent waiver talks get massive backing at G7 summit: MEA', *BusinessToday.in*, https://www.businesstoday.in/latest/economy-politics/story/covid-19-vaccine-patent-waiver-talks-get-massive-backing-at-g7-summit-mea-298592-2021-06-14

19. Vijayta Lalwani, 'The new laws will kill us': Three small farmers explain agricultural economics for city dwellers', *Scroll.in*, 9 December 2020, https://scroll.in/article/980669/the-new-laws-will-kill-us-three-small-farmers-explain-agricultural-economics-for-city-dwellers. Accessed 13 December 2021.

20. Ananya Varma, 'Route for 'Kisan Tractor Rally' on Republic Day Finalized, No Entry into Delhi: Sources', RepublicWorld.com, 24 January 2021, https://www.republicworld.com/india-news/general-news/route-for-kisan-tractor-rally-on-republic-day-finalized-no-entry-into-delhi-sources.html. Accessed 13 December 2021.

21. Raakhi Jagga, Liz Mathew and Jignasa Sinha, 'Farmers draw hard line, reject Centre's offer to stay farm laws', *The Indian Express*, 22 January 2021, https://indianexpress.com/article/india/farmers-draw-hard-line-reject-centres-offer-to-stay-laws-7156526/. Accessed 13 December 2021.

22. Revathi Krishnan, 'Breaking barriers to Red Fort march—timeline of how farmer

|    | |
|----|---|
|    | protest turned ugly within hours,' *ThePrint*, 26 January 2021, https://theprint.in/india/breaking-barriers-to-red-fort-march-timeline-of-how-farmer-protest-turned-ugly-within-hours/592514/. Accessed 13 December 2021. |
| 23 | 'Indian farmers ramp up their protest by riding tractors into the capital,' *Saudi Gazette*, 26 January 2021, https://saudigazette.com.sa/article/602911. Accessed 13 December 2021. |
| 24 | Raj Sekhar, 'Delhi: Khalistan flags at Red Fort? Probe launched,' *The Times of India*, 27 January 2021, https://timesofindia.indiatimes.com/city/delhi/khalistan-flags-at-red-fort-probe-launched/articleshow/80471652.cms. Accessed 13 December 2021. |
| 25 | https://twitter.com/rihanna/status/1356625889602199552?lang=en. Accessed 13 December 2021. |
| 26 | 'After Thunberg and Rihana, Kamala Harris' niece tweets in support of farmers protest in India,' *The Times of India*, 3 February 2021, https://timesofindia.indiatimes.com/india/after-thunberg-and-rihana-kamala-harris-niece-tweets-in-support-of-farmers-protest/articleshow/80662175.cms. Accessed 13 December 2021. |
| 27 | Mallica Joshi, 'Explained: Why is Delhi Police probing a farmers' protest "toolkit" tweeted by Greta Thunberg?' *The Indian Express*, 22 February 2021, https://indianexpress.com/article/explained/greta-thunberg-toolkit-farmers-protest-fir-delhi-police-7176187/. Accessed 13 December 2021. |
| 28 | 'Mia Khalifa tweets in support of farmers' protest after Rihanna and Greta Thunberg,' *India Today*, https://www.indiatoday.in/trending-news/story/mia-khalifa-tweets-in-support-of-farmers-protest-after-rihanna-and-greta-thunberg-1765411-2021-02-03. Accessed 13 December 2021. |
| 29 | 'A conversation with Rupi Kaur and Rana Ayyub,' https://www.facebook.com/watch/?v=206718647749421. Accessed 13 December 2021. |
| 30 | https://twitter.com/rupikaur_/status/1360882070873112579. Accessed 13 December 2021. |
| 31 | 'Canadian Khalistani outfit behind toolkit on farmers protests shared by Greta, says Delhi Police,' *BusinessToday*, 3 February 2021, https://www.businesstoday.in/latest/economy-politics/story/canadian-khalistani-outfit-behind-toolkit-on-farmers-protests-shared-by-greta-says-delhi-police-286792-2021-02-05. Accessed 13 December 2021. |
| 32 | 'Rihanna Paid $2.5 million by PR Firm with Khalistani Links to Tweet in Support of Farmers: Report,' News 19, 7 February 2021. https://www.news18.com/news/india/rihanna-was-paid-2-5-million-by-pr-firm-with-khalistani-links-to-tweet-in-support-of-farmers-report-3394502.html. Accessed 13 January 2022. |
| 33 | Anand Patel, 'Congress to recruit 5 lakh 'social media warriors' to counter BJP IT cell,' *India Today*, 6 February 2021, https://www.indiatoday.in/india/story/congress-to-recruit-5-lakh-social-media-warriors-to-counter-bjp-it-cell-1766687-2021-02-06. Accessed 13 December 2021. |
| 34 | Anonna Dutt, 'Alpha to Delta switch behind city's 4th wave,' *Hindustan Times*, 5 June 2021, https://www.hindustantimes.com/india-news/alpha-to-delta-switch-behind- |

city-s-4th-wave-101622838952997.html. Accessed 13 December 2021.
35. https://www.indiatoday.in/india/story/govt-will-repeal-three-farm-laws-farmers-pm-modi-1878436-2021-11-19

# CHAPTER 17

1. Press Trust of India, 'Two new COVID-19 mutations found in samples from Maharashtra's Amravati and Yavatmal, say researchers,' *Firstpost*, 19 February 2021, https://www.firstpost.com/health/two-new-covid-19-mutations-found-in-samples-from-maharashtras-amravati-and-yavatmal-say-researchers-9321281.html. Accessed 13 December 2021.
2. Rupsa Chakraborty, 'Maharashtra: Rigorous testing brings down positivity rate in Amravati and Yavatmal,' *Hindustan Times*, 19 March 2021, https://www.hindustantimes.com/cities/mumbai-news/maharashtrarigorous-testing-brings-down-positivity-rate-in-amravati-and-yavatmal-101616093056992.html Accessed 13 December 2021.
3. Sushmi Dey, 'Surge in Maharashtra & Kerala not linked to new strains, says ICMR DG,' *The Times of India*, 23 February 2021, https://timesofindia.indiatimes.com/india/surge-in-maharashtra-kerala-not-linked-to-new-strains-says-icmr-dg/articleshow/81177312.cms. Accessed 13 December 2021.
4. '6 cases of new Covid-19 strain detected in Kerala,' *Hindustan Times*, 4 January 2021, https://www.hindustantimes.com/kerala/6-cases-of-new-covid-19-strain-detected-in-kerala/story-24jLfOc7aTi1XUmFKpDuYM.html. Accessed 13 December 2021.
5. Anonna Dutt, 'Delhi's April Covid surge was driven by Delta replacing Alpha variant: Paper,' *Hindustan Times*, 4 January 2021, https://www.hindustantimes.com/cities/delhi-news/delhis-april-covid-surge-was-driven-by-delta-replacing-alpha-variantpaper-101622791336090.html. Accessed 13 December 2021.
6. https://mobile.twitter.com/economictimes/status/1362049160753594370
7. 'Experts say India's Covid-19 "human barricade" to keep cases under control,' *Hindustan Times*, 17 February 2021, https://www.hindustantimes.com/india-news/experts-say-india-s-covid-19-human-barricade-to-keep-cases-under-control-101613567028418.html. Accessed 13 December 2021.
8. Prashasti Awasthi, 'Second wave of Covid-19 pandemic in India will not be as severe: Experts,' The Hindubusinessline, 27 February 2020, https://www.thehindubusinessline.com/news/second-wave-of-covid-19-pandemic-in-india-will-not-be-as-severe-experts/article33947310.ece. Accessed 23 December 2021.
9. Tariq Hashmat, 'The worst may be over but we are certainly not out of the woods,' *Health Analytics Asia*, 15 January 2021, https://www.ha-asia.com/the-worse-may-be-over-but-we-are-certainly-not-out-of-the-woods/. Accessed 23 December 2021.
10. Pankaj Upadhyay, 'How close are we to the end of Covid-19 pandemic? Here's what experts say,' *India Today*, 25 January 2021, https://www.indiatoday.in/india/story/how-close-are-we-to-the-end-of-covid-19-pandemic-here-s-what-experts-

say-1762426-2021-01-25. Accessed 23 December 2021.
11. P. Chidambaram, 'Pandemic, vaccine and controversy,' *The Indian Express*, 10 January 2021, https://indianexpress.com/article/opinion/columns/covid-19-pandemic-vaccine-controversy-p-chidambaram-7140020/. Accessed 13 December 2021.
12. 'Opinion: Is Kumbh a soft target?' News18, 20 May 2021, https://www.news18.com/news/opinion/is-the-kumbh-a-soft-target-3757106.html. Accessed 13 December 2021.
13. Ibid.
14. 'Covid Rules Tossed Aside at UP Cleric's Funeral, Thousands Attend,' NDTV, 10 May 2021, https://www.ndtv.com/india-news/uttar-pradesh-badaun-covid-rules-tossed-aside-at-up-clerics-funeral-thousands-attend-2439023. Accessed 13 December 2021.
15. Manisha Mondal, 'Thousands gather for Hola Mohalla festival in Punjab, give masks & social distancing a miss,' *ThePrint*, 29 March 2021, https://theprint.in/in-pictures/thousands-gather-for-hola-mohalla-festival-in-punjab-give-masks-social-distancing-a-miss/630597/. Accessed 13 December 2021.
16. 'Amid Covid-19 surge in Punjab, a tussle over restrictions on religious festivals,' *The Indian Express*, 24 March 2021, https://indianexpress.com/article/explained/punjab-religious-festivals-covid-19-restrictions-7242413/. Accessed 13 December 2021.
17. 'PM interacts with the Chief Ministers on Covid-19 situation,' Press Information Bureau, 17 March 2021, https://pib.gov.in/PressReleseDetail.aspx?PRID=1705457. Accessed 23 December 2021.
18. MHA Guidelines for effective control of COVID-19, Ministry of Home Affairs, PIB Delhi, 23 March 2021, https://pib.gov.in/PressReleasePage.aspx?PRID=1706966. Accessed 23 December 2021.

# CHAPTER 18

1. PM interacts with the Chief Ministers on Covid-19 situation, https://pib.gov.in/PressReleseDetail.aspx?PMO=3&PRID=1705457. Accessed 13 December 2021.
2. 'Maharashtra: High-flow tube is guzzler of oxygen, avoid it, says task force,' *The Times of India*, 16 April 2021, https://timesofindia.indiatimes.com/city/mumbai/maharashtra-high-flow-tube-is-guzzler-of-oxygen-avoid-it-says-task-force/articleshow/82091980.cms. Accessed 13 December 2021.
3. Johnson TA, 'To breathe easy, use NIV instead of HFNO to conserve Oxygen stock, Karnataka Govt urges hospitals,' *The Indian Express*, 17 May 2021, https://indianexpress.com/article/cities/bangalore/to-breathe-easy-use-niv-instead-of-hfno-to-conserve-oxygen-stock-urges-karnataka-govt-to-hospitals-7317281/. Accessed 13 December 2021.
4. 'Oxygen audit panels set up in all hospitals,' *The Hindu*, Thiruvananthapuram, 15 May 2021.

5   Joshua Cohen, 'The Grimmest Days of the Covid-19 Pandemic Coincide with the Most Severe Forms of Rationing', *Forbes*, 8 January 2021, https://www.forbes.com/sites/joshuacohen/2021/01/08/the-grimmest-days-of-the-covid-19-pandemic-coincide-with-the-most-severe-forms-of-rationing/?sh=5a8358e0211d. Accessed 13 December 2021.

6   '"1 In 30 Now Has Covid": London Mayor Declares "Major Incident"', NDTV, 8 January 2021, https://www.ndtv.com/world-news/one-in-30-now-has-covid-london-mayor-sadiq-khan-declares-major-incident-2349777. Accessed 23 December 2021.

7   Ibid.

8   Charlotte Peet, '"Brazil is suffocating": COVID surge creates severe oxygen crisis', *Aljazeera*, 24 March 2021, https://www.aljazeera.com/news/2021/3/24/brazil-is-suffocating-covid-surge-creates-severe-oxygen-crisis. Accessed 13 December 2021.

9   'Patients should use as much oxygen as they need, says Piyush Goyal amid criticism', *The Week*, 19 April 2021, https://www.theweek.in/news/india/2021/04/19/patients-should-use-as-much-oxygen-as-they-need-says-piyush-goyal-amid-criticism.html. Accessed 13 December 2021.

10  'States should control oxygen demand, says minister Piyush Goyal; "how stupid", says Digvijaya', *India Today*, 19 April 2021, https://www.indiatoday.in/coronavirus-outbreak/story/states-should-control-oxygen-demand-says-piyush-goyal-1792437-2021-04-19. Accessed 13 December 2021.

11  'PM reviews COVID-19 Pandemic situation and Vaccination Program in India', Prime Minister's Office, 4 April 2021, https://pib.gov.in/PressReleseDetail.aspx?PMO=3&PRID=1709503. Accessed 13 December 2021.

12  'English rendering of PM's remarks at meeting with CMs of all states and UTs to take stock of the COVID-19 situation', Prime Minister's Office, 8 April 2021, https://pib.gov.in/PressReleasePage.aspx?PRID=1710541. Accessed 13 December 2021.

13  https://mobile.twitter.com/ShekharGupta/status/1331631583430787072. Accessed 13 December 2021.

14  '"At 6 p.m, life stops": Europe uses night curfews to fight COVID-19 crisis', *New Indian Express*, 15 January 2021, https://www.newindianexpress.com/world/2021/jan/15/at-6-pm-life-stops-europe-uses-night-curfews-to-fight-covid-19-crisis-2250437.html. Accessed 13 December 2021.

15  'California's Covid curfew to begin, as US cases hit 12-million mark', BBC News, 20 November 2020, https://www.bbc.com/news/world-us-canada-55030611. Accessed 13 December 2021.

16  'Sri Lanka lifts lockdown, retains curfew at night', *The Hindu*, 1 October 2021, https://www.thehindu.com/news/international/sri-lanka-lifts-lockdown-retains-curfew-at-night/article36783784.ece. Accessed 13 December 2021.

17  https://mobile.twitter.com/kiranshaw/status/1331639985443725317. Accessed 13 December 2021.

18  Karan Thapar, 'Coronavirus Lockdown: "Food Riots Are a Very Real Possibility," Says Pronob Sen', *The Wire*, 27 March 2020, https://thewire.in/food/pronob-sen-

karan-thapar-coronavirus-food-riots. Accessed 23 December 2021.
19. 'English rendering of PM's remarks at meeting with CMs of all states and UTs to take stock of the COVID-19 situation,' Prime Minister's Office, 8 April 2021, https://pib.gov.in/PressReleseDetail.aspx?PMO=3&PRID=1710541
20. 'English rendering of PM's remarks at meeting with CMs of all states and UTs to take stock of the COVID-19 situation,' Prime Minister's Office, 8 April 2021, https://pib.gov.in/PressReleseDetail.aspx?PMO=3&PRID=1710541. Accessed 13 December 2021.
21. Ibid.
22. Biman Mukherji, 'India has always had enough oxygen,' *Fortune*, 18 May 2021, https://fortune.com/2021/05/18/india-covid-cases-crisis-oxygen-shortage-supply/. Accessed 13 December 2021.
23. 'Medical oxygen requirement increased 7 times; met 60% demand: Inox Air,' *Business Standard*, 20 April 2021, https://www.business-standard.com/article/companies/medical-oxygen-requirement-increased-7-times-met-60-demand-inox-air-121042000030_1.html. Accessed 13 December 2021.
24. 'PM reviews status of oxygen availability to ensure adequate supply,' Prime Minister's Office, 16 April 2021, https://pib.gov.in/PressReleseDetail.aspx?PMO=3&PRID=1712222. Accessed 13 December 2021.
25. 'Gujarat cadre IAS officer Guruprasad Mohapatra dies of Covid-related complications,' *The Indian Express*, 20 June 2021, https://indianexpress.com/article/cities/ahmedabad/dpiit-secretary-guruprasad-mohapatra-dies-of-covid-7366007/. Accessed 13 December 2021.
26. 'India clocks over 2 lakh fresh cases in new record: How nation's daily COVID-19 tally doubled in just 10 days,' *Times Now Digital*, 15 April 2021, https://www.timesnownews.com/india/article/india-clocks-over-2-lakh-fresh-cases-in-new-record-how-nations-daily-covid-19-tally-doubled-in-just-10-days/745381. Accessed 13 December 2021.
27. Parimal Kumar, 'With 3.14 Lakh Covid Cases, India Records World's Biggest Daily Spike,' NDTV, 22 April 2021, https://www.ndtv.com/india-news/coronavirus-over-3-lakh-fresh-covid-19-cases-reported-in-india-for-the-first-time-2-104-deaths-highest-in-24-hours-2419238. Accessed 13 December 2021.
28. Biman Mukherji, 'India has always had enough oxygen,' *Fortune*, 18 May 2021, https://fortune.com/2021/05/18/india-covid-cases-crisis-oxygen-shortage-supply/. Accessed 13 Dcember 2021.
29. 'Maharashtra requests for Air Force help for supply of oxygen,' *LiveMint*, 13 April 2021, https://www.livemint.com/news/india/maharashtra-requests-for-air-force-help-for-supply-of-oxygen-11618327831840.html. Accessed 13 December 2021.
30. Arun Kumar Das, 'Indian Railways Ready To Roll Out Wagons With Oxygen Tankers,' *Swarajya*, 19 April 2021, https://swarajyamag.com/news-brief/indian-railways-ready-to-roll-out-wagons-with-oxygen-tankers. Accessed 13 December 2021.
31. 'Covid crisis: Govt to set up 10,000 beds in temporary hospitals near oxygen plants,'

32. *The Tribune*, 3 May 2021, https://www.tribuneindia.com/news/nation/covid-crisis-govt-to-set-up-10-000-beds-in-temporary-hospitals-near-oxygen-plants-247283. Accessed 13 December 2021.
33. Ibid.
34. Union Home Secretary writes to Chief Secretaries of States and Administrators of Union Territories to take necessary measures to prohibit supply of oxygen for Industrial Purposes in view of rising cases of Covid-19, 18 April 2021, https://pib.gov.in/PressReleasePage.aspx?PRID=1712589. Accessed 23 December 2021.
35. Snehesh Alex Philip, 'DRDO reopens makeshift Covid hospital in Delhi, 5 other facilities to come up across India,' *ThePrint*, 19 April 2021, https://theprint.in/defence/drdo-reopens-makeshift-covid-hospital-in-delhi-5-other-facilities-to-come-up-across-india/642341/. Accessed 13 December 2021.
36. "'Don't blame Centre, poor data by states caused oxygen crisis'": Iqbal Singh Chahal, YouTube, 7 May 2021, https://www.youtube.com/watch?v=ckkGYuA4NkU. Accessed 23 December 2021.
37. 'Iqbal Singh Chahal: If Mumbai has 6-7% positivity rate, why should we suffer a national lockdown? Decision should be left to states,' *The Indian Express*, 10 May 2021, https://indianexpress.com/article/india/iqbal-singh-chahal-maharashtra-covid-cases-bmc-oxygen-vaccine-shortage-second-wave-7308663/
38. 'Uddhav Thackeray dials PM Modi for remdesivir, told he's campaigning in Bengal,' *India Today*, 17 April 2021, https://www.indiatoday.in/coronavirus-outbreak/video/uddhav-thackeray-dials-pm-modi-for-remdesivir-told-he-s-campaigning-in-bengal-1792047-2021-04-17. Accessed 13 December 2021.
39. 'PM Modi interacts with vaccine manufacturers from across the country,' Prime Minister's Office, 20 April 2021, https://pib.gov.in/PressReleseDetail.aspx?PMO=3&PRID=1713044. Accessed 13 December 2021.
40. Ibid.
41. 'English rendering of PM's address to the nation on the COVID-19 situation,' Prime Minister's Office, 20 April 2021, https://pib.gov.in/PressReleseDetail.aspx?PMO=3&PRID=1713117. Accessed 13 December 2021.
42. 'PM interacts with leaders of pharma industry,' Prime Minister's Office, 19 April 2021, https://pib.gov.in/PressReleseDetail.aspx?PMO=3&PRID=1712726. Accessed 13 December 2021.
43. 'PM Modi holds meeting with oxygen manufacturers,' *The Times of India*, 23 April 2021, https://timesofindia.indiatimes.com/videos/news/pm-modi-holds-meeting-with-oxygen-manufacturers/videoshow/82218156.cms. Accessed 13 December 2021.
44. Outlook Web Bureau, 'Beg, Borrow, Steal, It's Your Job to Get Oxygen: HC Tells Centre,' *Outlook*, 22 April 2021, https://www.outlookindia.com/website/story/india-news-beg-borrow-steal-its-your-job-to-get-oxygen-hc-tells-centre/380949. Accessed 14 December 2021.
45. https://twitter.com/barandbench/status/1388067067459375106. Accessed 13 December 2021.

45  https://twitter.com/barandbench/status/1388067325102882824. Accessed 13 December 2021.

46  ANI, 'Haryana, UP govt officials hindering Delhi's oxygen supply, says Delhi deputy CM Manish Sisodia,' *The Times of India*, 22 April 2021, https://timesofindia.indiatimes.com/city/delhi/haryana-up-govt-officials-hindering-delhis-oxygen-supply-says-delhi-deputy-cm-manish-sisodia/articleshow/82197002.cms. Accessed 14 December 2021.

47  https://www.newslaundry.com/2021/04/21/did-haryana-block-oxygen-supply-to-delhis-hospitalsAccessed 13 December 2021.

48  https://twitter.com/PTI_News/status/1384844986336874496?ref_src=twsrc%5Etfw%7Ctwcamp%5Etweetembed%7Ctwterm%5E1384844986336874496%7Ctwgr%5E%7Ctwcon%5Es1_&ref_url=https%3A%2F%2Fwww.newslaundry.com%2F2021%2F04%2F21%2Fdid-haryana-block-oxygen-supply-to-delhis-hospitals. Accessed 23 December 2021.

49  Nikhil M. Babu, 'As oxygen supply dips, 25 die in Delhi's Ganga Ram hospital,' *The Hindu*, 23 April 2021, https://www.thehindu.com/news/cities/Delhi/as-oxygen-supply-dips-25-die-in-delhis-ganga-ram-hospital/article34390060.ece. Accessed 13 December 2021.

50  '25 Sickest Patients Have Died": After Ganga Ram Hospital SOS, 2 Versions,' NDTV, 23 April 2021, https://www.ndtv.com/india-news/25-sickest-patients-have-died-in-last-24-hours-oxygen-will-last-another-2-hours-delhis-ganga-ram-hospital-2419999. Accessed 13 December 2021.

51  Richa Banka, '21 at Jaipur Golden hospital succumbed to comorbidities, not O2 shortage: Delhi govt to High Court,' *Hindustan Times*, 4 May 2021, https://www.hindustantimes.com/cities/delhi-news/21-at-jaipur-golden-hospital-succumbed-to-comorbidities-not-o2-shortage-delhi-govt-to-high-court-101620067639441.html. Accessed 14 December 2021.

52  '21 patients died of 'respiratory failure' and not due to lack of medical oxygen, Delhi govt tells HC,' *The Indian Express*, https://indianexpress.com/article/cities/delhi/delhi-jaipur-golden-hospital-deaths-oxygen-govt-hc-7301714/. Accessed 13 December 2021.

53  https://twitter.com/MeghaSPrasad/status/1386605709702230016. Accessed 23 December 2021.

54  Sourav Roy Barman, 'Kejriwal writes to Piyush Goyal over oxygen diversion and availability,' *The Indian Express*, 18 April 2021, https://indianexpress.com/article/india/kejriwal-writes-to-piyush-goyal-over-oxygen-diversion-and-availability-delhi-covid-7279210/. Accessed 14 December 2021.

55  'AAP supported farmer protests hampering war against Covid-19, oxygen supplier writes to GOI saying tankers delayed due to roadblocks by protestors,' *OpIndia*, 20 April 2021, https://www.opindia.com/2021/04/oxygen-supplier-says-its-trucks-are-delayed-due-to-farmer-protests-in-delhi/. Accessed on 15 January 2022.

56  https://twitter.com/barandbench/status/1386581458580434944. Accessed 14 December 2021.

57. "Delhi's govt was just complaining, not trying to handle logistics of oxygen supply": Director of INOX,' *OpIndia*, 14 May 2021, https://www.opindia.com/2021/05/delhi-wasnt-organising-the-logistics-and-was-just-complaining-siddharth-jain-director-of-inox-air-products/. Accessed 13 January 2022.
58. PTI, 'HC takes strong note of black marketing of oxygen cylinders in Delhi, asks govt to take action,' *The Economic Times*, 26 April 2021, https://economictimes.indiatimes.com/news/india/hc-takes-strong-note-of-black-marketing-of-oxygen-cylinders-in-delhi-asks-govt-to-take-action/articleshow/82259530.cms?from=mdr. Accessed 14 December 2021.
59. Sofi Ahsan, 'HC slams Delhi Govt for oxygen mess: If you can't manage, will ask Centre to step in,' *The Indian Express*, 28 April 2021. https://indianexpress.com/article/cities/delhi/delhi-high-court-government-oxygen-shortage-covid-19-7291390/. Accessed 3 January 2021
60. Ibid.
61. Ibid.
62. Aamir Khan, 'Set your house in order, we can't let people die, HC tells Delhi govt,' *The Times of India*, 28 April 2021, https://timesofindia.indiatimes.com/city/delhi/set-your-house-in-order-we-cant-let-people-die-hc-tells-delhi-govt/articleshow/82283730.cms. Accessed 14 December 2021.
63. 'PM Modi reviews public health response to Covid-19,' Prime Minister's Office, 6 May 2021, https://pib.gov.in/PressReleseDetail.aspx?PMO=3&PRID=1716474. Accessed 14 December 2021.
64. 'PM Modi pulls up Arvind Kejriwal for live telecast of Covid-19 review meeting,' *India Today*, 23 April 2021, https://www.indiatoday.in/india/story/pm-modi-pulls-up-arvind-kejriwal-live-telecast-covid-meeting-protocol-1794293-2021-04-23. Accessed 23 December 2021.
65. 'Kejriwal Draws Flak for Starting Live Telecast of his Address during Meeting with PM,' News18, 23 April 2021, https://www.news18.com/news/india/kejriwal-draws-flak-for-starting-live-telecast-of-his-address-during-meeting-with-pm-3669446.html. Accessed 14 December 2021.
66. Staff Reporter, 'Face contempt proceedings if oxygen supply is not met: Delhi HC warns Centre,' *The Hindu*, 1 May 2021, https://www.thehindu.com/news/cities/Delhi/supply-490-mt-oxygen-to-delhi-today-or-face-contempt-hc-to-centre/article34457413.ece. Accessed 14 December 2021.
67. PTI, 'Delhi government to import 18 oxygen tankers from Bangkok: Kejriwal,' *The Economic Times*, 27 April 2021, https://economictimes.indiatimes.com/news/india/delhi-government-to-import-18-oxygen-tankers-from-bangkok-kejriwal/articleshow/82272644.cms. Accessed 14 December 2021.
68. Susmita Pakrasi, 'Centre moves SC challenging Delhi HC's show cause notice of contempt over deficit in oxygen supply to Capital,' *Hindustan Times*, 5 May 2021, https://www.hindustantimes.com/india-news/centre-moves-supreme-court-challenging-delhi-hc-s-show-cause-notice-of-contempt-against-them-over-deficit-in-oxygen-supply-to-capital-101620194469063.html. Accessed 14 December 2021.

69. 'Coronavirus | Centre owes a "special responsibility" to Delhi, says Supreme Court,' *The Hindu*, 30 April 2021, https://www.thehindu.com/news/national/centre-owes-a-special-responsibility-to-delhi-says-supreme-court/article34451726.ece. Accessed 23 December.
70. Krishnadas Rajagopal, 'Supreme Court forms National Task Force for transparent oxygen allocation,' *The Hindu*, 8 May 2021, https://www.thehindu.com/news/national/supreme-court-sets-up-national-task-force-for-transparent-oxygen-allocation/article34515284.ece. Accessed 23 December 2021.
71. 'Don't blame Centre, poor data by states caused oxygen crisis': Iqbal Singh Chahal, YouTube, https://www.youtube.com/watch?v=ckkGYuA4NkU. Accessed 14 December 2021.
72. Report of Oxygen Audit in NCT of Delhi, Submitted by Subgroup Constituted by Supreme Court of India, July 2021.
73. OpIndia Staff, 'While Delhi govt was alleging inadequate oxygen supply, data show it was returning oxygen to suppliers, asked them to store the excess,' *OpIndia*, 13 May 2021, https://www.opindia.com/2021/05/delhi-was-returning-oxygen-to-suppliers-asked-them-to-store-the-excess/. Accessed 14 December 2021.
74. Rahul Shrivastava, 'Mumbai vs Delhi: Why the capital is facing an oxygen crisis?' *India Today*, 7 May 2021, https://www.indiatoday.in/coronavirus-outbreak/story/mumbai-delhi-oxygen-crisis-covid-cases-deaths-1799979-2021-05-07. Accessed 14 December 2021.
75. Sanjay Sharma, 'Delhi govt sought 4 times more oxygen than it needed during 2nd wave, says SC audit panel,' *India Today*, 25 June 2021, https://www.indiatoday.in/coronavirus-outbreak/story/oxygen-audit-panel-says-delhi-govt-sought-far-more-oxygen-1819103-2021-06-25. Accessed 14 December 2021.
76. Report of Oxygen Audit in NCT of Delhi, Submitted by Subgroup Constituted by Supreme Court of India, July 2021.
77. Sanjay Sharma, 'Delhi govt sought 4 times more oxygen than it needed during 2nd wave, says SC audit panel,' *India Today*, 25 June 2021, https://www.indiatoday.in/coronavirus-outbreak/story/oxygen-audit-panel-says-delhi-govt-sought-far-more-oxygen-1819103-2021-06-25. Accessed 14 December 2021.
78. India Today Web Desk, '"My fault was...": Kejriwal after SC panel says Delhi inflated oxygen need: Top points,' *India Today*, 25 June 2021, https://www.indiatoday.in/coronavirus-outbreak/story/my-fault-was-arvind-kejriwal-sc-panel-delhi-inflated-oxygen-need-top-points-1819334-2021-06-25. Accessed 14 December 2021.
79. ANI, 'COVID-19: Odisha supplies surplus oxygen to different states,' *LiveMint*, 25 April 2021, https://www.livemint.com/news/india/covid19-odisha-supplies-surplus-oxygen-to-different-states-11619357599158.html. Accessed 14 December 2021.
80. 'How states are using triage centres to manage the Covid-19 situation,' *Deccan Herald*, 27 April 2021, https://www.deccanherald.com/national/how-states-are-using-triage-centres-to-manage-the-covid-19-situation-979435.html. Accessed 14 December 2021.

81. '"Hope we never have to see it again": INOX Air Products chief on oxygen crisis,' *The News Minute*, 10 June 2021, https://www.thenewsminute.com/article/hope-we-never-have-see-it-again-inox-air-products-chief-oxygen-crisis-150413. Accessed 14 December 2021.
82. Dr Devi Shetty's Mantra To Fight The Pandemic: 3 Point Vaccine Plan & Double The Medical Workforce, https://www.youtube.com/watch?v=7aYUs9TpPTQ. Accessed 6 January 2022.

## CHAPTER 19

1. 'India crosses a grim milestone of 4 lakh cases daily with over 3500 deaths in the last 24 hours,' *Business Insider*, 1 May 2021, https://www.businessinsider.in/india/news/india-crosses-a-grim-milestone-of-4-lakh-cases-daily-with-over-3500-deaths-in-the-last-24-hours/articleshow/82331604.cms. Accessed 14 December 2021.
2. Manisha Inamdar, 'Besides COVID-19, India is also fighting with vulture journalists, who are spreading more panic and despair than pandemic,' *The Hindu*, 29 May 2021, https://www.theaustraliatoday.com.au/besides-covid-19-india-is-also-fighting-with-vulture-journalists-who-are-spreading-more-panic-and-despair-than-pandemic/
3. Manisha Inamdar, 'Besides COVID-19, India is also fighting with vulture journalists, who are spreading more panic and despair than pandemic,' *Opinion*, 29 May 2021, https://www.theaustraliatoday.com.au/besides-covid-19-india-is-also-fighting-with-vulture-journalists-who-are-spreading-more-panic-and-despair-than-pandemic/. Accessed 14 December 2021.
4. 'Indian Population Clock,' https://www.medindia.net/patients/calculators/pop_clock.asp. Accessed 14 December 2021.
5. 'In conversation with Shamika Ravi on reporting of COVID deaths in India,' YouTube, 31 July 2021, https://www.youtube.com/watch?v=oOjiafNOX78. Accessed 14 December 2021.
6. Shamika Ravi, 'Counting deaths in India is difficult,' *Hindustan Times*, 14 July 2021, https://www.hindustantimes.com/opinion/counting-deaths-in-india-is-difficult-101626273326958.html. Accessed 14 December 2021.
7. 'Why "excess mortality" figures for Covid must be calculated,' *The Indian Express*, 26 May 2021, https://indianexpress.com/article/opinion/columns/why-excess-mortality-figures-for-covid-must-be-calculated-7330348/. Accessed 14 December 2021.
8. Abhishek Anand, Justin Sandefur and Arvind Subramanian, 'Three New Estimates of India's All-Cause Excess Mortality during the COVID-19 Pandemic,' Center for Global Development, 20 July 2021, https://cgdev.org/publication/three-new-estimates-indias-all-cause-excess-mortality-during-covid-19-pandemic. Accessed 14 December 2021.
9. Soumik Purkayastha, Ritoban Kundu, Ritwik Bhaduri, Daniel Barker, Michael Kleinsasser, Debashree Ray and Bhramar Mukherjee, 'Estimating the wave 1 and

wave 2 infection fatality rates from SARS-CoV-2 in India,' Medrxiv, https://www.medrxiv.org/content/10.1101/2021.05.25.21257823v1

10   Kalyan Ray, 'India's Covid-19 death toll may be 4-11 times higher, economic cost is 30% of GDP: Study,' *Deccan Herald*, 16 September 2021, https://www.deccanherald.com/national/india-s-covid-19-death-toll-may-be-4-11-times-higher-economic-cost-is-30-of-gdp-study-1030812.html. Accessed 14 December 2021.

11   'India's Covid-19 deaths 10 times higher than reported: Study,' *LiveMint*, 20 July 2021, https://www.livemint.com/news/india/indias-covid-19-deaths-10-times-higher-than-reported-study-11626767976960.html. Accessed 14 December 2021.

12   '"Jal samadhi" ritual sinks clean Ganga drive in Haridwar's Neel Dhara,' *Hindustan Times*, https://www.hindustantimes.com/dehradun/jal-samadhi-ritual-sinks-clean-ganga-drive-in-haridwar-s-neel-dhara/story-MtqB4mWq7an7xZZe2vLCuI.html. Accessed 14 December 2021.

13   https://twitter.com/gargirawat/status/555162281093251072?lang=en. Accessed 14 December 2021.

14   'Fresh orders issued for payment to kin for cremation of Covid victims,' *Daily Pioneer*, 17 May 2021, https://www.dailypioneer.com/2021/state-editions/fresh-orders-issued-for-payment-to-kin-for----cremation-of-covid-victims.html. Accessed 14 December 2021.

15   Faryal Rumi, 'Covid victims to be cremated for free: Patna Municipal Corporation,' *The Times of India*, 16 April 2021, https://timesofindia.indiatimes.com/city/patna/covid-victims-to-be-cremated-for-free-pmc/articleshow/82089643.cms. Accessed 14 December 2021.

16   'Jal samadhi ritual in Uttarakhand gives tough time to police,' *Hindustan Times*, 11 September 2018, https://www.hindustantimes.com/dehradun/jal-samadhi-ritual-in-uttarakhand-gives-tough-time-to-police/story-F6P6btm0Pud0NPwadV9WFJ.html. Accessed 14 December 2021.

17   Omar Rashid, 'Uttar Pradesh police lodge FIR against the editor of The Wire for "objectionable article" against Yogi Adityanath,' *The Hindu*, 2 April 2020, https://www.thehindu.com/news/national/other-states/uttar-pradesh-police-lodge-fir-against-the-editor-of-the-wire-siddharth-varadarajan/article31231478.ece. Accessed 23 December 2021.

18   'UP Police Serve Notice on The Wire, Summon Founding Editor to Ayodhya Despite Lockdown,' *The Wire*, 11 April 2020, https://thewire.in/media/up-police-serve-notice-on-the-wire-summon-founding-editor-to-ayodhya-despite-lockdown. Accessed 23 December 2021.

19   https://drive.google.com/file/d/12Hp6LPYBXmrguADWVbc8fwYO4pGTkkvA/view.

20   Sumit Ganguly, 'Modi's pandemic choice: Protect his image or protect India. He chose himself,' *The Washington Post*, 28 April 2021, https://www.washingtonpost.com/outlook/modis-pandemic-choice-protect-his-image-or-protect-india-he-chose-himself/2021/04/28/44cc0d22-a79e-11eb-bca5-048b2759a489_story.html. Accessed 14 December 2021.

21. Jack Newman and Faith Ridler, 'Indian families are told to bury their dead in their back gardens as crematoriums buckle under strain of record Covid surge that saw 350,000 cases in one day', *Mail Online*, 27 April 2021, https://www.dailymail.co.uk/news/article-9509181/Indian-families-told-bury-dead-gardens-crematoriums-buckle-Covid-strain.html?ito=facebook_share_article-top&fbclid=IwAR1MldVNmtaiNDIyKzZcPJHbH0gTx_M0_Fbb8PICg62CfOInA6NbaX8uyZA, Accessed 14 December 2021.

22. Debarshi Dasgupta and Rohini Mohan, 'Families allowed to bury dead in backyards as India's Covid-19 surge overwhelms crematoriums', *The Straits Times*, 30 April 2021, https://www.straitstimes.com/asia/south-asia/families-allowed-to-bury-dead-in-their-backyard-with-crematoriums-overwhelmed-by?utm_source=fark&utm_medium=website&utm_content=link&ICID=ref_fark. Accessed 14 December 2021.

23. 'Covid deaths: Karnataka govt allows cremation, burial of dead bodies at pvt lands, farmhouses', *The Indian Express*, 22 April 2021, https://indianexpress.com/article/coronavirus/covid-deaths-karnataka-govt-allows-cremation-burial-of-dead-bodies-at-pvt-lands-farmhouses-7283651/. Accesssed 14 December 2021.

24. 'Modi's pandemic choice: Protect his image or protect India. He chose himself.' *The Washington Post*, https://www.washingtonpost.com/outlook/modis-pandemic-choice-protect-his-image-or-protect-india-he-chose-himself/2021/04/28/44cc0d22-a79e-11eb-bca5-048b2759a489_story.html. Accessed 14 December 2021.

25. Arundhati Roy, '"We are witnessing a crime against humanity": Arundhati Roy on India's Covid catastrophe', *The Guardian*, 28 April 2021,303https://www.theguardian.com/news/2021/apr/28/crime-against-humanity-arundhati-roy-india-covid-catastrophe. Accessed 14 December 2021.

26. Ramachandra Guha, 'Ramachandra Guha: Crisis-hit India needs a leader who listens, not one focused on building his brand', *Scroll.in*, 25 April 2021, https://scroll.in/article/993177/ramachandra-guha-crisis-hit-india-needs-a-government-that-listens-not-one-dedicated-to-a-brand. Accessed 14 December 2021.

27. 'Modi leads India into viral apocalypse', *The Australia*, https://www.google.com/search?q=%E2%80%9CModi+leads+India+into+viral+apocalypse%E2%80%9D&rlz=1C1SQJL_enIN776IN776&oq=%E2%80%9CModi+leads+India+into+viral+apocalypse%E2%80%9D&aqs=chrome..69i57j0i10i22i30.717j0j4&sourceid=chrome&ie=UTF-8. Accessed 14 December 2021.

28. '82% media persons reveal 'Western Media' is biased in COVID-19 pandemic coverage of India', *Organiser*, 18 July 2021, https://www.organiser.org/media-3432.html. Accessed 14 December 2021.

29. https://twitter.com/macaesbruno/status/1412127833426640897?lang=en. Accessed 14 December 2021.

30. 'Several Ministers Share Article by BJP Member Praising Modi's "Hard Work" to Tackle COVID', *The Wire*, 11 May 2021, https://thewire.in/politics/narendra-modi-covid-19-crisis-daily-guardian-bjp-ministers-sudesh-varma. Accessed 14 December 2021.

31  'India's COVID-19 emergency,' *The Lancet*, Volume 397, Issue 10286, p. 1683, 8 May 2021, https://www.thelancet.com/journals/lancet/article/PIIS0140-6736(21)01052-7/fulltext. Accessed 14 December 2021.

32  '"A masterly academic response": Twitter stunned as Health Minister rebuts Lancet editorial by sharing blog post,' *Free Press Journal*, 18 May 2021, https://www.freepressjournal.in/viral/a-masterly-academic-response-twitter-stunned-as-health-minister-rebuts-lancet-editorial-by-sharing-blog-post. Accessed 14 December 2021.

33  'Watch: Ramdev launches Covid-19 medicine Coronil, Harsh Vardhan attends event,' *Hindustan Times*, 19 February 2021, https://www.hindustantimes.com/videos/news/watch-ramdev-launches-covid-19-medicine-coronil-harsh-vardhan-attends-event-101613737807861.html. Accessed 14 December 2021.

34  Abhishek Bhalla, 'India sends 100 MT oxygen, 300 concentrators to Indonesia as Covid relief material,' *India Today*, 24 July 2021, https://www.indiatoday.in/india/story/india-sends-100-mt-oxygen-300-concentrators-to-indonesia-as-covid-relief-material-1832139-2021-07-24. Accessed 14 December 2021.

35  ANI, 'India sends first "oxygen express" to Bangladesh to help out with Covid-19,' *Hindustan Times*, 25 July 2021, https://www.hindustantimes.com/india-news/india-sends-first-oxygen-express-to-bangladesh-to-help-out-with-covid19-101627177550677.html. Accessed 14 December 2021.

36  https://twitter.com/ArvindKejriwal/status/1394576958973911047?ref_src=twsrc%5Etfw%7Ctwcamp%5Etweetembed%7Ctwterm%5E1394576958973911047%7Ctwgr%5E%7Ctwcon%5Es1_&ref_url=https%3A%2F%2Ftheprint.in%2Fdiplomacy%2Fkejriwal-sparks-singapore-variant-row-singapores-upset-mea-embarrassed-jaishankar-angry%2F660963%2F. Accessed 23 December 2021.

37  'There is no "Singapore variant": Health ministry of Singapore counters Arvind Kejriwal,' DNA, 19 May 2021, https://www.dnaindia.com/india/report-there-is-no-singapore-variant-health-ministry-counters-arvind-kejriwal-2890948. Accessed 23 December 2021.

38  Ibid.

39  https://twitter.com/DrSJaishankar/status/1394885676588421123?ref_src=twsrc%5Etfw%7Ctwcamp%5Etweetembed%7Ctwterm%5E1394885676588421123%7Ctwgr%5E%7Ctwcon%5Es1_&ref_url=https%3A%2F%2Ftheprint.in%2Fdiplomacy%2Fkejriwal-sparks-singapore-variant-row-singapores-upset-mea-embarrassed-jaishankar-angry%2F660963%2F. Accessed 23 December 2021.

40  'Singapore netizens accuse Delhi CM Kejriwal of "spreading misinformation" on Covid, seek apology,' *The Economic Times*, 19 May 2021, https://economictimes.indiatimes.com/news/india/netizens-in-singapore-accuse-delhi-cm-arvind-kejriwal-of-spreading-misinformation-on-covid-19-seek-apology/articleshow/82767063.cms. Accessed 23 December 2021.

41  Scroll Staff, 'Covid-19: Arvind Kejriwal asks Centre to open vaccinations for all above 18,' *Scroll.in*, 18 March 2021, https://scroll.in/latest/989887/covid-19-arvind-kejriwal-asks-centre-to-open-vaccinations-for-all-above-18. Accessed 23 Decemeber 2021.

42. Tabassum Barnagarwala, 'Vaccines falling short, Maharashtra Health Minister's Jalna district got extra doses,' *The Indian Express*, 5 May 2021, https://indianexpress.com/article/india/vaccines-falling-short-maharashtra-health-ministers-jalna-district-got-extra-doses-7302302/. Accessed 14 December 2021.
43. Nikhil Inamdar and Aparna Alluri, 'How India's vaccine drive went horribly wrong,' BBC News, 14 May 2021, https://www.bbc.com/news/world-asia-india-57007004. Accessed 14 December 2021.
44. '"India does not need lectures about vaccine supplies", "European Union is leading the way in vaccine donations": President Macron,' *The Statesman*, 8 May 2021, https://www.thestatesman.com/world/india-not-need-lectures-vaccine-supplies-european-union-leading-way-vaccine-donations-president-macron-1502966756.html. Accessed 14 December 2021.
45. https://twitter.com/ani/status/1354901033332273154. Accessed 14 December 2021.
46. Jacob Koshy, 'Fact check: History shows India did not lack access to vaccines as claimed by PM Modi,' *The Hindu*, 8 June 2021, https://www.thehindu.com/news/national/news-analysis-history-shows-india-did-not-lack-access-to-vaccines-as-claimed-by-pm-modi/article34758021.ece. Accessed 14 December 2021.
47. https://twitter.com/adarpoonawalla/status/1382978713302683653?lang=en. Accessed 14 December 2021.
48. 'US to send raw material "urgently required" to manufacture Covishield in India,' *The Times of India*, 25 April 2021, https://timesofindia.indiatimes.com/india/us-to-provide-vaccine-components-medical-supplies-to-india/articleshow/82245992.cms. Accessed 14 December 2021.
49. 'Prime Minister's comments at the Global COVID-19 Summit: Ending the Pandemic and Building Back Better Health Security to Prepare for the Next,' 22 September 2021, https://pib.gov.in/PressReleasePage.aspx?PRID=1757110. Accessed 14 December 2021.
50. Rahul Srivastava, 'Did ventilators from PM Cares Fund fail or states failed to manage them?' *India Today*, 17 May 2021, https://www.indiatoday.in/india/story/did-ventilators-from-pm-cares-fund-fail-or-states-failed-to-manage-them-1803473-2021-05-17. Accessed 4 January 2021.
51. 'Over 250 new ventilators gather dust at Punjab government's warehouse,' *The Tribune*, 19 March, https://www.tribuneindia.com/news/punjab/over-250-new-ventilators-gather-dust-at-punjab-goverenments-warehouse-227712. Accessed 23 December 2021.
52. Rahul Srivastava, 'Did ventilators from PM Cares Fund fail or states failed to manage them?' *India Today*, 17 May 2021, https://www.indiatoday.in/india/story/did-ventilators-from-pm-cares-fund-fail-or-states-failed-to-manage-them-1803473-2021-05-17. Accessed 23 December 2021.
53. Rohan Dua, 'Re-calibrate, change flow, O2 sensors,' *The Times of India*, 16 May 2022, https://timesofindia.indiatimes.com/india/re-calibrate-change-flow-o2-sensors-centre-chides-states-on-faulty-ventilators/articleshow/82674494.cms. Accessed 23 December 2021.

54. Suchitra Karthikeyan, 'Rajasthan: Govt Hospital In Bharatpur Leases Out 20 PM CARES-funded Ventilators To Pvt Hospital,' Republic World, 10 May 2021, https://www.republicworld.com/india-news/politics/govt-hospital-in-bharatpur-leases-out-20-pm-cares-funded-ventilators-to-pvt-hospital.html. Accessed 23 December 2021.
55. https://www.facebook.com/watch/?v=999558623915046. Accessed 23 December 2021.
56. 'Ashok Gehlot demands probe into "defective ventilators" issued under PM Cares,' *The Indian Express*, 14 May 2021, https://indianexpress.com/article/cities/jaipur/ashok-gehlot-demands-probe-into-defective-ventilators-issued-under-pm-cares-7314665/. Accessed 23 December 2021.
57. Rekha Dixit, 'Has judicial overreach impeded COVID-19 pandemic management?' *The Week*, 23 May 2021, https://www.theweek.in/theweek/specials/2021/05/13/has-judicial-overreach-impeded-covid-19-pandemic-management.html. Accessed 23 December 2021.
58. PTI, 'SC wants national plan on COVID-19 situation, including on oxygen supply,' *The Hindu*, 22 April 2021, https://www.thehindu.com/news/national/sc-wants-national-plan-on-covid-19-situation-including-on-oxygen-supply/article34382911.ece. Accessed 23 December 2021.
59. Rekha Dixit, 'Has judicial overreach impeded COVID-19 pandemic management?' *The Week*, 23 May 2021, https://www.theweek.in/theweek/specials/2021/05/13/has-judicial-overreach-impeded-covid-19-pandemic-management.html. Accessed 23 December 2021.
60. Mason Bissada, 'Supreme Court Rejects Request To Block Covid-19 Vaccine Mandate For Massachusetts Hospital System,' *Forbes*, 29 November 2021, https://www.forbes.com/sites/masonbissada/2021/11/29/supreme-court-rejects-request-to-block-covid-19-vaccine-mandate-for-massachusetts-hospital-system/?sh=f4a0335f2fd2. Accessed 23 December 2021.
61. Lawrence Hurley, 'U.S. Supreme Court rejects religious challenge to Maine vaccine mandate,' *Reuters*, 1 November 2021, https://www.reuters.com/world/us/us-supreme-court-rejects-religious-challenge-maine-vaccine-mandate-2021-10-29/. Accessed 23 December 2021.
62. Russell Williamson and Megan Curzon, 'UK Supreme Court unanimously finds in favour of policyholders in landmark COVID-19 business interruption insurance test case,' Bird & Bird, February 2021, https://www.twobirds.com/en/news/articles/2021/uk/uk-supreme-court-covid19-business-interruption-insurance-test-case. Accessed 23 December 2021.

## CHAPTER 20

1. https://www.france24.com/en/asia-pacific/20210903-japan-pm-suga-to-resign-following-criticism-of-his-covid-19-response. Accessed 14 December 2021.
2. PR Ramesh, 'It is important that every youngster get opportunities, not assistance

that keeps them dependent but the support that makes them self-reliant to fulfil their aspirations with dignity', *Open*, 2 October 2021,307https://openthemagazine.com/cover-stories/important-every-youngster-get-opportunities-not-assistance-keeps-dependent-support-makes-self-reliant-fulfil-aspirations-dignity/. Accessed 14 December 2021.

3. 'At CoWIN Global Conclave, PM Modi urges countries to work together to fight Covid,' *Hindustan Times*, 5 July 2021, https://www.hindustantimes.com/india-news/pm-modi-addresses-cowin-global-conclave-101625474729118.html. Accessed 14 December 2021.

4. 'Proud to say that CoWIN is fastest tech platform in world: RS Sharma,' Telecom.com, 6 July 2021, https://telecom.economictimes.indiatimes.com/news/proud-to-say-that-cowin-is-fastest-tech-platform-in-world-rs-sharma/84161642. Accessed 14 December 2021.

5. 'PM Modi's remarks at Global Covid-19 Summit,' YouTube, 22 September, https://www.youtube.com/watch?v=uEoojgqx09Y. accessed 14 December 2021.

6. Ruchir Sharma, 'The pandemic stimulus has backfired in emerging markets,' *Financial Times*, https://www.ft.com/content/37e8e350-71a7-4c00-a4de-a5a6ba776bfb.

7. R. Jagannathan, 'Modi socio-nomics starts to pay off,' *Business Standard*, 2 November 2021, https://www.business-standard.com/article/opinion/modi-socio-nomics-starts-to-pay-off-121110201928_1.html. Accessed 23 December 2021.

8. Sandeep Phukan and Sobhana K. Nair, 'Coronavirus: Opposition demands a "true stimulus",' *The Hindu*, 22 May 2020, https://www.thehindu.com/news/national/coronavirus-federalism-has-been-forgotten-as-all-power-is-now-concentrated-in-pmo-office-says-sonia-gandhi/article31650613.ece. Accessed 23 December 2021.

9. '100 crore vaccinations a reflection of the strength of the country: PM Modi,' 22 October 2021, https://www.narendramodi.in/2021-oct-text-of-prime-minister-narendra-modi-s-address-to-the-nation-557999. Accessed 23 December 2021.

10. Ibid.

11. Ibid.

12. https://www.narendramodi.in/india-s-100-crore-and-counting-covid-vaccine-doses-show-what-people-s-participation-can-achieve-557997. Accessed 14 December 2021.

13. Ibid.

14. https://twitter.com/drtedros/status/1451078629232979969. Accessed 14 December 2021.

15. Bill Gates, '5 Steps to 1 Billion Doses,' *The Times of India*, 21 October 2021, https://timesofindia.indiatimes.com/india/5-steps-to-1-billion-doses/articleshow/87188969.cms. Accessed 14 December 2021.

16. 'Covid: South Africa new cases surge as Omicron spreads,' BBC News, 2 December 2021, https://www.bbc.com/news/world-africa-59503517. Accessed 13 January 2022.

17. Erika Edwards and Berkeley Lovelace Jr., 'Omicron symptoms: What we know

| | |
|---|---|
| | about illness caused by the new variant,' NBC News, 21 December 2021, https://www.nbcnews.com/health/health-news/omicron-symptoms-covid-what-to-know-rcna9469. Accessed 13 January 2022. |
| 18 | Paul Dennis, 'International update: "Blanket booster programs are likely to prolong the pandemic"– WHO,' Pharmaceutical Technology, https://www.pharmaceutical-technology.com/author/dennis/. Accessed 13 January 2022. |
| 19 | Rakhi Bose, 'Covid-19: "Super Immunity" Might Save India from Omicron but Here's the Catch,' *Outlook*, 22 December 2021, https://www.outlookindia.com/website/story/india-news-covid-19-super-immunity-might-save-india-from-omicron-but-heres-the-catch/406210. Accessed 13 January 2022. |
| 20 | *The Lancet*, https://www.thelancet.com/journals/lancet/article/PIIS0140-6736(21)02754-9/fulltext. Accessed 13 January 2022. |
| 21 | 'Lancet Study Stating Protection Offered by Covishield Declines after 3 Months Is Misquoted: Experts,' India.com, 23 December 2021, https://www.india.com/news/lancet-study-covishield-astrazeneca-oxford-protection-covid-vaccine-three-months-90-days-misquoted-experts-5152759/. Accessed 13 January 2022. |
| 22 | Ibid. |
| 23 | Poulomi Ghosh, 'PM Modi announces vaccine for children, precaution doses for frontline workers, senior citizens,' *Hindustan Times*, 25 December 2021, https://www.hindustantimes.com/india-news/no-need-to-panic-take-precaution-pm-modi-addresses-nation-amid-omicron-101640448442267.html. Accessed 13 January 2022. |
| 24 | https://twitter.com/mansukhmandviya/status/1475699946544570372. Accessed 13 January 2022. |
| 25 | Himani Chandna, 'In the time of Omicron, immunity war and the Endgame: What we may or may not avenge in 2022,' *First Post*, 25 December 2022, https://www.firstpost.com/india/in-the-time-of-omicron-immunity-war-and-the-endgame-what-we-may-or-may-not-avenge-in-2022-10235021.html. Accessed 13 January 2022. |
| 26 | https://secureservercdn.net/50.62.198.70/1mx.c5c.myftpupload.com/wp-content/uploads/2021/12/MEDRXIV-2021-268439v1-Sigal.pdf. Accessed 13 January 2022. |
| 27 | https://twitter.com/ScottGottliebMD/status/1475853849684586497. |

# INDEX

2019-NCoV, 18

Aadhaar, 115, 128, 170, 249
Aarogya Setu, 87, 88, 99
Adityanath, Yogi, 120, 226
aerosol droplets, xiv, 29, 99
Agricultural Produce Market Committees (APMCs), 155, 156, 159
AgVa Healthcare, 105
All India Institute of Medical Sciences (AIIMS), 6, 24, 135, 183, 202, 204, 219
Alternative Energy Promotion Centre, 103
Andhra Pradesh MedTech Zone, 104
AstraZeneca, 133, 167, 250, 258
Atmanirbhar Bharat Package 3.0, 142

B.1.1.7 strain (Alpha), 164
B.1.617.2 variant (Delta), 232
barbell strategy, 107, 139
Bharat Biotech International Limited (BBIL), 124, 144
Bharat Electronics Limited, 104, 240
Bharat Heavy Electricals Limited, 105
Bharat Immunologicals and Biologicals Limited, 150
Bhargava, Balram, Dr, 24
Bhat, S. Ravindra, 242
Biden, Joe, 172
BioNTech, 123
Board of Control for Cricket in India (BCCI), 35
Bobde, S.A., Justice, 86, 242
Bureau of Indian Standards (BIS), 103

carbon molecular sieve (CMS), 207
Center for Disease Dynamics, Economics & Policy, 185

Center for Global Development, 225
Centers for Disease Control and Prevention, 20, 29, 70
Central Drugs Standard Control Organisation (CDSCO), 162, 165
Chidambaram, P., 47, 186
Chief of Defence Staff (CDS), 130
Civil Registration System (CRS), 224
Confederation of Indian Industry, 103
Consumer Pyramids Household Surveys (CPHSs), 225
Coronavirus Aid, Relief, and Economic Security (CARES), 52
corporate social responsibility, 96
countrywide lockdown, 42, 79
COVAX, 132, 173, 238
Covaxin, 133, 148, 165, 166, 167, 168, 169, 173, 183, 234, 250, 259
COVID-19 Economic Response Task Force, 50, 52
COVID saral ICU, 253
Covishield, 134, 165, 166, 169, 173, 238, 249, 250, 258, 259
CoWIN, 136, 146, 147, 170, 172, 184, 233, 248, 249, 250
credit-linked subsidies, 115
cyclone Amphan, 119

Darbuk–Shyok–DBO Road, 126
death rates, 199, 225
Defence Research and Development Organisation (DRDO), 103, 104, 105, 208
digital vaccination certificate, 128
Disaster Management Act, 9, 27, 67, 86
doom loop, 106
Doval, Ajit, 3, 4, 76
Drugs Controller General of India, 102

Dutt, Barkha, 121, 223

Electronic Vaccine Intelligence Network (eVIN), 136, 146, 170
Ella, Krishna, 148, 169
Ella, Suchitra, 148
Empowered Group, 34, 63, 136, 137, 170, 184, 205, 242, 252
Epidemic Diseases Act, 1897, 95
Essential Commodities Act, 115
Essential Commodities (Amendment) Bill, 155

Fadnavis, Devendra, 222
Farmers (Empowerment and Protection) Agreement on Price Assurance and Farm Services Bill, 155
Farmers' Produce Trade and Commerce (Promotion and Facilitation) Bill, 155
Finance Minister Nirmala Sitharaman, 50, 66, 142
Food Corporation of India (FCI), 78, 79, 156
food security, 79, 155
foreign direct investments (FDIs), 131
foreign exchange reserves, 109

Gadkari, Nitin, 230
Galwan River Valley, 125
Gamaleya National Research Institute of Epidemiology and Microbiology, 136
Gandhi, Rahul, 48, 84, 128, 161, 226, 251
Garib Kalyan Rojgar Abhiyaan, 139, 142
Gennova, 135, 146
Ghebreyesus, Tedros, 256
Global COVID-19 Summit, 238, 250, 251
Good Clinical Practice (GCP), 143
Goyal, Piyush, 88, 119, 198, 214
Gujarat Biotechnology Research Centre, 150
Guleria, Randeep, Dr, 24, 219
Guterres, António, 172, 235

Haffkine Bio-Pharmaceutical Corporation Ltd, 150
Hasina, Sheikh, 44
healthcare workers, 26, 42, 50, 67, 94, 147, 169, 170, 183, 223, 243, 253, 256
Hester Biosciences, 150
high-flow nasal oxygen, 197
high positivity rate, 118
Housing Finance Companies, 114
HP Inc, 105

inactivated virus, 124, 133, 134, 148, 166
Indian Council of Medical Research (ICMR), 10, 24, 45, 47, 55, 57, 62, 74, 100, 101, 102, 123, 124, 133, 148, 185
Indian Premier League (IPL), 35
Indian SARS-CoV-2 Consortium on Genomics (INSACOG), 163, 164

Jaishankar, S., 12, 232
*jan bhagidari*, 41, 57, 199, 256
Jinping, Xi, 11, 13, 71
Johnson & Johnson, 124, 134, 137, 144, 145
Joint Monitoring Group, 9
Joshi, Shashank, Dr, 180, 197
Jumbo COVID-19 Centres, 97
junta curfew, xiv, 38, 41, 42, 59, 64, 65

Kant, Amitabh, 102, 137
Kejriwal, Arvind, 32, 75, 85, 251
Kerala, 16, 19, 47, 116, 180, 181, 186, 197, 203, 220
Kisan Credit Cards, 115
Kumbha Mela, 179, 187–192

Lifeline Udan mission, 112
Line of Actual Control, 126, 127
liquid medical oxygen, 202, 215

Mahatma Gandhi National Rural Employment Guarantee (MGNREGA), 67, 138, 142
Mahindra, Anand, 104
Make in India initiative, 102
Maruti Suzuki, 105

messenger ribonucleic acid (mRNA), 123, 134, 135, 144, 234
micro-containment zones, 100
Micro, Small and Medium Enterprises (MSME) sector, 109
Middle East Respiratory Syndrome (MERS), 7, 10, 29, 33
minimum support prices (MSP), 156, 157, 158
Mission COVID Suraksha, 143
Moderna, 123, 124, 136, 144, 234, 247
Modi, Narendra, x, 3, 219, 256
Municipal Corporation of Greater Mumbai (MCGM), 36, 37, 97, 208, 218
Mutual Fund Investments, 114

Namami Gange, 226
Naravane, M.M, Army chief, 130
National Centre for Biological Sciences, 6
National Democratic Alliance (NDA), 121, 158
National Executive Committee, 27
National Expert Group on Vaccine Administration for COVID-19 (NEGVAC), 135, 136, 137, 144, 145, 146, 147, 170, 185, 200, 234, 235, 242, 247, 248
National Food Security Act, 115
National Health Mission, 43
National Institute of Virology (NIV), 10, 16, 18, 35, 123, 124
National Technical Advisory Group on Immunisation, 135
Neighbourhood First Policy, 43
NITI Aayog, 23, 87, 88, 102
Non-banking Financial Institutions (NBFCs), 114, 115

Obama, Barack, 128
Office of the Registrar General & Census Commissioner, 224
Omicron, 257, 259
Omnibrx, 150
Operation PPE Coverall, 103
Operation Warp Speed, 123

Oxygen rationing, 197

Patel, Pankaj, 69, 148
Patel, Sharvil, 148
Paul, V.K., Dr, 5, 23, 24, 123, 233
People's Liberation Army, 125
Personal protective equipment (PPE), 8, 10, 14, 18, 26, 56, 63, 80, 92, 98, 100, 101, 102, 103, 112, 172
Pfizer, 123, 124, 136, 144, 145, 162, 165, 234, 237, 247
PM SVANidhi, 115
Poonawalla, Adar, 150, 173, 237
Poonawalla, Cyrus, 150
Poonawalla, Natasha, 150
Pradhan Mantri Awas Yojana (PMAY), 142
Prasad, Ravi Shankar, 88
President Emmanuel Macron, 235
Prime Minister of Denmark Mette Frederiksen, 125
Prime Minister's Citizen Assistance and Relief in Emergency Situations Fund (PM CARES), 77, 95, 96, 97, 105, 182, 207, 239, 241
Prime Minister's National Relief Fund (PMNRF), 96, 97
Production Linked Incentive Scheme, 142

Radhakrishnan, K.S., 242
Rao, L. Nageswara, 86, 242
rapid antigen testing, 100, 101
Rawat, Bipin, General, 18, 130
Redington 3D, 105
relief measures, xii, 66, 96, 106, 108
remdesivir, 70, 148, 207, 209, 222, 248
repo rate, 109
reverse migration, 84, 114
Right to Information (RTI) Act, 95
Russian Direct Investment Fund, 136

Sample Registration System (SRS), 224, 225
Samyukta Kisan Morcha, 174, 175, 176
Sanyal, Sanjeev, 108

Sardesai, Rajdeep, 91
SARS-CoV-2, ix, 10, 68, 134, 163, 259
SD Biosensor, 102
Sen, Pronob, 201
seroepidemiology studies, 144
sero-surveys, 100, 260
Serum Institute of India (SII), 124, 132, 133, 134, 144, 150, 162, 165, 166, 167, 173, 199, 238, 259
Severe acute respiratory syndrome (SARS), ix, 5, 7, 8, 10, 29, 33, 68, 74, 134, 163, 259
Shah, Amit, 88, 95, 140, 157, 175, 216
Sharma, K.P., 44
Shiv Sena, 97, 118, 122
Singh, Manmohan, 93, 159
Sisodia, Manish, 213
Society for Biomedical Technology, 104
South Asian Association for Regional Cooperation (SAARC), 43, 44, 45
South India Textile Research Association, 103
Sputnik, 124, 136, 144, 145
Standing Committee on Economic Statistics, 201
State Disaster Response Fund, 43
State Disaster Risk Management Fund, 95
Suga, Yoshihide, 246
Sullivan, Jake, 238
Swachh Bharat Abhiyan (Clean India Mission), 30

Tablighi Jamaat, 31, 75, 192
tax collected at source (TCS), 115
tax deducted at source (TDS), 115
Test-Track-Treat protocol, 194
Tharoor, Shashi, 167
Thackeray, Uddhav, 47, 85, 118, 179, 209
Trade-Related Aspects of Intellectual Property Rights (TRIPS), 172
Tshering, Lotay, 44

Udwadia, Zarir, Dr, 35
United Nations Office for Disaster Risk Reduction, 7
United Progressive Alliance (UPA), 47, 96, 159
Universal Immunization Programme, 146
Uri, 43

vaccine nationalism, 132, 172, 236
Vaccine Maitri, 172, 234, 237, 238, 251
Vaccine Task Force, 110
Vardhan, Harsh, Dr, 9, 103, 230
VijayRaghavan, K., Prof., 5, 6, 7, 23, 24, 32, 33, 34, 54, 110, 124

Wenliang, Li, Dr, 8
wet market, 3, 5
Wuhan, 8

Yadav, Akhilesh, 93, 168
Yadav, Mulayam Singh, 93, 168
Yadav, Tejashwi, 140
Yediyurappa, B.S., 228

zeolite molecular sieve (ZMS), 207
Zydus Cadila, 124, 133, 134, 144, 148, 250